Cell Proliferation in the Gastrointestinal Tract

Edited by

D R APPLETON, MA, MSc, PhD
Senior Lecturer in Medical Statistics
University of Newcastle upon Tyne

J P SUNTER, MB, BS, MRCPath
Lecturer in Pathology
University of Newcastle upon Tyne

A J WATSON, MD, FRCPath
Reader in Pathology
University of Newcastle upon Tyne

PITMAN MEDICAL

First Published 1980

Catalogue Number 21 4200 81

Pitman Medical Limited
57 High Street, Tunbridge Wells, Kent

Associated Companies:
Pitman Publishing Pty Ltd, Melbourne
Pitman Publishing New Zealand Ltd, Wellington

British Library Cataloguing in Publication Data

Cell proliferation in the gastrointestinal tract.
  1. Alimentary canal
  2. Cell proliferation
  I. Appleton, D R
  II. Sunter, J P
  III. Watson, A J
  591.8'762   QP145

ISBN 0-272-79597-6

Text set in 11/12 pt VIP Garamond,
printed and bound in
Great Britain at
The Pitman Press, Bath

Introduction

This book contains the definitive versions of the papers given at a conference on Cell Proliferation In The Gastrointestinal Tract held in Newcastle upon Tyne, England in September 1979. It is not a record of the proceedings of that meeting, for it contains no synopsis of the discussions which took place, nor of the poster presentations. Instead, the authors of the twenty-nine articles were able to incorporate important points which arose as a result of discussions after their oral presentations.

Like the conference, the book is divided into six sections. These start with a consideration of the growth and normal proliferative status of the small and large intestine in experimental animals, and move naturally to hypotheses of growth control and studies on the physiological factors influencing proliferative responses. Most of the articles deal primarily with the intestine, but several deal with the stomach as well, and there is a review article concerned with the rumen of the sheep. There is considerable overlap in subject matter between the section dealing with stem cells and that dealing with the responses of the intestine to cytotoxic drugs and other stimuli, since these responses are usually expressed through the stem cells. This is the area where most controversy exists, different workers with different approaches having arrived at quite different estimates of the number of stem cells in the intestinal crypt. The different points of view are clearly illustrated and the assumptions underlying the techniques used are examined. A discussion of carcinogenesis and cancer in animals leads on to the final section which deals with cell proliferation in a variety of disease states affecting human beings.

We believe that the heterogeneity of approach, which is apparent in the papers at several levels, is of value. There are review articles, especially the first papers in each section which are derived from the six 'keynote talks' at the meeting, and there are hitherto unpublished results; there are reports of detailed research programmes, and of interesting new approaches; there are thorough discussions of the problems of experimental techniques, analysis of data and interpretation of results, and there are interesting speculations on the mechanisms underlying the findings.

In two areas, however, we as editors have endeavoured to produce a degree of uniformity: namely in nomenclature and in the presentation of results. Where different authors have used different terms to describe the same thing (eg mitotic flux, mitotic rate, cell birth rate) we have tried to standardise and, where appropriate, to use a single predefined abbreviation. We have tried to make the figures and tables readily understandable, and to present in a standard way the results of similar experiments by different workers. Thus, not all the authors would have chosen, in isolation, to illustrate their results as we have done, and they should not be held responsible for any deficiencies in the figures, which have all been redrawn for this book. Nor should they be blamed for any apparent lack of detail in terms of the number of significant figures used in the tables, or the frequency with which standard errors of estimates are quoted. We are firmly of the opinion that results should not be presented with more precision than the experimental techniques and methods of data analysis will bear. It is true that standard errors, properly used, can be helpful in this context, but often they are only stepping stones to the carrying out of a statistical test and provide little information in themselves. Furthermore, we believe that their erroneous use is very undesirable; in particular there is a tendency to pool the data from many samples taken from few animals, and to calculate standard errors of means as if all the observations were independent. This can yield many seemingly 'significant' differences between treatments, when in fact only normal inter-animal variation has been observed. On the other hand, sub-optimal tests are sometimes performed, for example between small samples at many different time points, when it is quite clear from the overall pattern of results whether a difference exists. Probably no single author would consider himself competent to judge the interpretation of the data in every paper in this book; we certainly do not consider ourselves so qualified. Sometimes, however, we feel that too much is being made of the data; possibly our colleagues will have reservations about our own methods. Having said this, we nevertheless consider that the articles represent a cross-section of the best in the field at the present time.

The experimental techniques used include morphometry on thin sections or crypt microdissections; point-counting; estimation of mitotic indices, and of cell birth rates using metaphase-arresting techniques; autoradiography using tritiated thymidine, and hence the fraction of labelled mitoses experiment; calculation of tritium activity by scintillation counting; DNA and RNA assays; the use of labelled actinomycin; and the split-dose irradiation technique. Results are presented relating to the effects of starvation; the oestrus cycle; operations of jejunal resection or bypass; castration; ovariectomy; thyroidectomy; hypophysectomy; administration of hormones; cyclic nucleotides; carcinogens; chalones; and cytotoxic agents, especially irradiation, cytosine arabinoside, and hydroxyurea. Human diseases investigated include coeliac disease, dermatitis herpetiformis, familial polyposis, and colorectal cancer.

None of these lists are exhaustive. We have provided a comprehensive table of contents, and every article referred to in the text is indexed in the list of references by the numbers of the articles which refer to it. We consider that this provides a suitable index to the subject matter of the papers, and allows readers to decide quickly which of the articles intestest them particularly. There are over 800 references drawn from about 200 different books and journals; we hope that the distillate of these references which this book represents will prove useful to established workers in this field as well as to beginners. More than half of the articles cited have been published in the last six years, which is indicative of the considerable amount of current interest in cell proliferation in the gastrointestinal tract, but the fact that some sixty come from before 1960 could be taken as showing how slow real progress is, and how dependent we still are on the efforts of earlier workers.

There are several people and bodies whom it is a pleasure to thank for their help in preparing this book; firstly those organisations which contributed financially: the University of Newcastle upon Tyne; the North of England Council of the Cancer Research Campaign; the Boots Company Limited; ICI Limited; Janssen Pharmaceuticals Limited; Lilly Industries Limited; Lundbeck Limited; May and Baker Limited; Montedison Pharmaceuticals Limited; and Upjohn Limited. Secondly, we are grateful to Professor L F Lamerton for his preface and for his encouragement in the past, to Mrs P. Thompson for typing the manuscript, to Miss E Wark for typing the references, and to Dr R E Bolton for help with reading the proofs. We thank Mr and Mrs D Dickens and the Staff of Pitman Medical for their work in publishing the finished product.

Newcastle upon Tyne DRA
JPS
AJW

Foreword

For the student of the cell population kinetics of tissues the gastrointestinal tract offers a very happy hunting ground. It has the great advantage of a clearly defined architecture with cells in sequence through the proliferative and functional compartments, which allow the techniques of cell kinetics to be applied more directly, and more precisely, than in many of the other tissues of the body. The tissue has other interesting characteristics, including a high rate of turnover and a considerable capacity for rapid adjustment of cell output to demand. Also susceptibility to malignant change shows a wide variation over its length, with the small intestine having one of the lowest levels of incidence of cancer in the body, in spite of, or perhaps even because of, its very high rate of cell turnover. The various pathological conditions of the gastrointestinal tract in man lend themselves well to cell kinetic studies, which have helped to define the nature of these diseases in cell kinetic terms and give clues about their origins.

When Charles Leblond and his colleagues in Montreal and Henry Quastler in Brookhaven first demonstrated the potential for quantitative dynamic studies in the small intestine, hopes ran high that the homeostatic mechanisms operating would soon be elucidated. Things have not quite turned out that way, and the tissue has so far kept its secrets fairly well. The relative importance of feedback and of local control mechanisms in the homeostasis of the cell populations, and the nature of the messengers through which they operate, cannot yet be defined with any assurance, but there is a very skilled and enthusiastic effort being put into the attack on these problems, as the present volume shows.

The investigations being made are relevant not only to the problems of the gastrointestinal tract. The studies, for instance, of the response of the tissue to perturbations of various sorts and of the number, position and characteristics of the stem cells present have wide implications in general biology, and the gastrointestinal tract is proving to be one of the most useful models for study of the general principles of cell population control.

This volume presents a comprehensive account of work related to the cell population kinetics of the gastrointestinal tract, both by review of past work and discussion of new approaches. It has avoided many of the disadvantages of most Conference reports by virtue of very careful and thorough editing, with the contributors modifying their presentations in the light of the discussions that took place at the Conference—a procedure that could with advantage be followed more often. The editors and the contributors are to be congratulated on this highly informative and very readable account of the subject, which will be of much value both to the worker already in the field and to the student who has not yet entered this area of work and requires an authoritative survey of the subject and its growing points.

Professor L F Lamerton
Institute of Cancer Research
Chester Beatty Research Institute
London

Contributors

F ALLEN	Gastrointestinal Unit, Western General Hospital, Edinburgh, Scotland
A AL-NAFUSSI	Department of Histopathology, John Radcliffe Infirmary, Oxford, England
D M AL-THAMERY	Gastrointestinal Unit, Western General Hospital, Edinburgh, Scotland
D R APPLETON	Department of Medical Statistics, University of Newcastle upon Tyne, England
D H BARKLA	Department of Anatomy, Monash University, Clayton, Australia
M BERGERON	Department of Physiology, University of Montreal, Canada
M BJERKNES	Department of Anatomy, University of Toronto, Canada
R E BOLTON	Institute of Occupational Medicine, Edinburgh, Scotland
N BRITTON	Department of Biomathematics, University of Oxford, England
W W L CHANG	Department of Pathology, West Virginia University, Morgantown, USA
H CHENG	Department of Anatomy, University of Toronto, Canada
D A CROUSE	Department of Anatomy, University of Nebraska, Omaha, USA
G E CULLAN	Department of Anatomy, University of Nebraska, Omaha, USA
E E DESCHNER	Memorial Sloan-Kettering Cancer Center, New York, USA
S H FATEMI	Department of Anatomy, University of Nebraska, Omaha, USA
A FERGUSON	Gastrointestinal Unit, Western General Hospital, Edinburgh, Scotland
R J M FRY	Department of Radiation Biology, Rush-Presbyterian-St Luke's Medical Center, Chicago, USA
R F HAGEMANN	Cancer Research Unit, Allegheny General Hospital, Pittsburgh, USA
E HAMILTON	Department of Oncology, Middlesex Hospital Medical School, London, England

W R HANSON	Department of Radiation Biology, Rush-Presbyterian-St Luke's Medical Center, Chicago, USA
D L HENNINGER	Department of Radiation Biology, Rush-Presbyterian-St Luke's Medical Center, Chicago, USA
H HIKOSAKA	Department of Biology, Tohuku Dental University, Koriyama, Japan
M B HOFF	School of Medicine, University of Buffalo, NY, USA
R M KLEIN	Department of Anatomy, University of Kansas, Kansas City, USA
M LIPKIN	Memorial Sloan-Kettering Cancer Center, New York, USA
H L LIPSCOMB	Department of Anatomy, University of Nebraska, Omaha, USA
D McLAUGHLIN	Department of Anatomy, University of Nebraska, Omaha, USA
R A MALT	Surgical Services, Massachusetts General Hospital, Boston, USA
T A PHELPS	Division of Biophysics, Institute of Cancer Research, Sutton, England
C S POTTEN	Paterson Laboratories, Christie Hospital and Holt Radium Institute, Manchester, England
A M PREUMONT	Department of Moleculat Biology, Free University of Brussels, Belgium
M de REUCK	Department of Gastroenterology, Free University of Brussels, Belgium
R P C RIJKE	Department of Pathology II, Erasmus University, Rotterdam, The Netherlands
M S B de RODRIGUEZ	Department of Pathology, University of Newcastle upon Tyne, England
J ROWINSKI	Department of Histology and Embryology, Medical School, Warsaw, Poland
T SAKATA	Institute for Zoophysiology, University of Hohenheim, Stuttgart, W Germany
A R SALLESE	Department of Radiation Biology, Rush-Presbyterian-St Luke's Medical Center, Chicago, USA
P SASSIER	Department of Physiology, University of Montreal, Canada
W SAWICKI	Department of Histology and Embryology, Medical School, Warsaw, Poland
R SBARBATI	Department of Anatomy and Embryology, University of Leiden, The Netherlands
J G SHARP	Department of Anatomy, University of Nebraska, Omaha, USA

Y SHIOMURA	Laboratory of Animal Morphology, Tohoku University, Sendai, Japan
G L STOFFELS	Department of Pathology, Free University of Brussels, Belgium
J STRACKEE	Laboratory of Medical Physics, University of Amsterdam, The Netherlands
J P SUNTER	Department of Pathology, University of Newcastle upon Tyne, England
H TAMATE	Laboratory of Animal Morphology, Tohoku University, Sendai, Japan
P J M TUTTON	Department of Anatomy, Monash University, Clayton, Australia
A J WATSON	Department of Pathology, University of Newcastle upon Tyne, England
R C N WILLIAMSON	Department of Surgery, University of Bristol, England
N A WRIGHT	Department of Histopathology, Royal Postgraduate Medical School, London, England

CONTENTS

Section 1 Cell Proliferation in Normal Experimental Animals

1.1 N A WRIGHT

Section 2 Growth Control in Normal Experimental Animals

Section 3 Stem cells

3.3 E HAMILTON

Section 4 Responses to cytotoxic agents and other stimuli

Section 5 Experimental Carcinogenesis and Cancer

Section 6 Normal and Disease States in Man

6.3 A J WATSON, N A WRIGHT and D R APPLETON

6.4 G L STOFFELS, A M PREUMONT and M de REUCK

SECTION 1

CELL PROLIFERATION
IN NORMAL EXPERIMENTAL ANIMALS

1.1 Cell Proliferation in the Normal Gastrointestinal Tract. Implications for Proliferative Responses

Nicholas A Wright

1.1.1 INTRODUCTION

The gastrointestinal mucosa, and particularly that of the small intestine, is a pleasing system to study from the viewpoint of cell population kinetics. Proliferative rates are high making it practicable to obtain accurate measurements, and, unlike the haemopoietic system, the tissue architecture allows a detailed analysis of its kinetic organisation. These observations are reflected in the popularity of the intestinal mucosa as a kinetic model. Much of the literature to date has been of a descriptive nature, and a rich field for future study lies in the operational aspects of intestinal cell proliferation. Clarke in 1973 (111) pleaded most convincingly for a wider approach to the epithelium, to include not only the proliferative portion, that lining the crypt, but also the functional compartment, the epithelium clothing the villi. He suggested that more emphasis should be placed on the sizes of component populations; there are few studies on the organisation of the epithelium, and on number as well as flux and time, with respect to the functional compartment.

It is the purpose of this article to redress this imbalance, and at the same time to review all kinetic organisation and kinetic parameters in the intestinal epithelium, with special emphasis on their contribution to induced or physiological proliferative responses. During this it will become apparent that, although we can measure many kinetic parameters with known precision and can appreciate their contribution to hypoproliferative or hyperproliferative mucosal responses, we are largely ignorant of the controlling mechanisms.

1.1.2 ORGANISATION OF CELL PROLIFERATION IN GASTRO-INTESTINAL TISSUES

In the gastrointestinal tract the epithelial renewal systems are usually divided readily into proliferation and function compartments, cells being born in the proliferation compartment and migrating into the function compartment. Between these compartments a transitional zone can be identified where cells are losing their proliferative capacities and acquiring the characteristics of mature, functional cells; this is usually termed the maturation compartment. Such compartments are not structurally discrete and usually need some kinetic technique for their delineation. Thus in the small intestine, while the villus epithelium is the function compartment, both proliferation and maturation compartments are found in the crypt (Figure 1.1.1); in the colon, proliferating

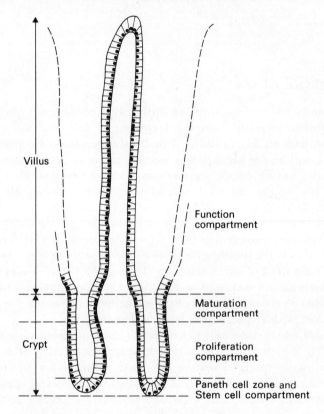

Figure 1.1.1 A schematic diagram of the small bowel crypt and villus, showing the several kinetic compartments

and maturing cells are also found in the crypt, with functional cells both within the crypt and on the surface. A similar though more complex arrangement is found in the gastric gland.

Within crypts, the spatial distinction between proliferating and maturing cells is shown by the distribution of mitotic and tritiated-thymidine (^{3}HTdR)-labelled cells. Figure 1.1.2 shows such data derived from large numbers of

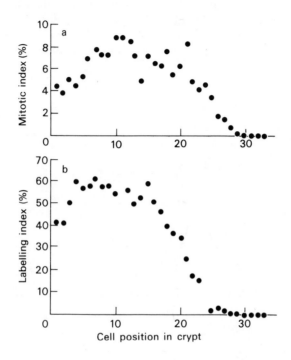

Figure 1.1.2 (a) Mitotic and (b) labelling index distributions in the rat jejunal crypt

perfect longitudinal sections of crypts one hour after injection of ^{3}HTdR. There are three components to these distributions; in basal cell positions proliferative indices are low, but from cell positions 4 to 15 labelling indices are uniformly high. After cell position 15 proliferative indices decline, and from cells 30 to 33 in the crypt column neither labelled cells nor mitoses are apparent. The labelling index (I_s) declines before the mitotic index (I_m). To explain the distributions in dynamic terms it is best to consider each segment in turn.

1.1.2.1 BASAL CELLS

The labelling and mitotic indices in the first few cell positions are smaller than those in immediately higher positions, probably because of the presence of cells with long cell cycle times (T_c). Detailed measurements of T_c at individual cell positions using the fraction of labelled mitoses (FLM), stathmokinetic and continuous labelling methods have shown prolonged cycle times in basal crypt cells (5, 6, 83, 813). In the mouse jejunum, for example, a mean value of 16.7 h was obtained with the FLM method for cell positions 1 and 2, compared with a value of 10.9 h for cell positions 11 and 12. More informative are the distributions of cell cycle times for the various cell positions (Figure 1.1.3); 60

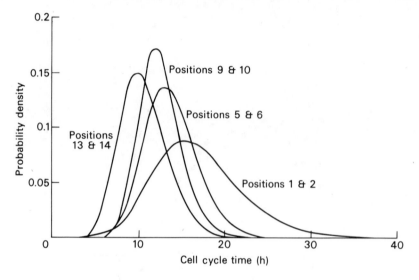

Figure 1.1.3 The distribution of cell cycle times for various cell positions in the mouse jejunal crypt, assuming a gamma distribution for transit times through the cell cycle

percent of cells in positions 1 and 2 have T_c greater than 15 h, compared with only 6 percent in positions 13 and 14.

The importance of the basal crypt cells is their probable role as functional stem cells for the crypt (403, 813) which, in normal conditions, give rise to all the cell types comprising the small-bowel epithelium. In the mouse there are about 20 to 30 cells in this part of the crypt out of a total crypt complement of 250 cells (534). The concept of slowly cycling functional stem cells is certainly attractive; because of their longer T_c such cells would be less sensitive to phase specific insult such as irradiation, and would then be available for crypt repopulation (385); indeed, basal crypt cells are the first to respond after death of proliferating cells induced by hydroxyurea, by a decrease in T_c (10). More contentiously, the basal cells have also been regarded as forming the whole or part of the potential stem cell pool (see Section 3.1 et seq).

1.1.2.2 MID-CRYPT CELLS

In cell positions 4 to 15, in the rat, I_s approaches 60 percent; this is the proliferation compartment proper, the zone of greatest cell production. It is probable that all cells here are cycling, since the theoretical labelling index, calculated from the duration of DNA synthesis, t_s, and T_c, also equals 60 percent.

1.1.2.3 UPPER-CRYPT CELLS

After cell position 15 proliferative indices decline, and early views were that the reason lay in a gradual prolongation of T_c as cells progress up the crypt; however, calculation of T_c by cell position within the crypt indicates that the cell cycle actually shortens somewhat as cells migrate (5, 6, 83). Therefore the fall in proliferative indices must be explained by cells leaving the cell cycle as they migrate; the fall in I_m, which occurs later than the fall in I_s, reflects the completion of mitosis after the final S-phase in the proliferation compartment.

1.1.2.4 THE SLOW CUT-OFF MODEL

This concept was formalised by Cairnie, Lamerton and Steel (84) in their *slow cut-off model*, which proposed an increasing probability of a decycling division occurring over a particular portion of the crypt; with this model they were able to predict reasonable labelling and mitotic indices from a consideration of the changing age distribution at each cell position. It will readily be appreciated that, with a T_c that is not lengthening with increasing position in the crypt, the fall in I_s with cell position, on the basis of the slow cut-off model, will reflect the declining growth fraction, I_p. Given that T_c must have a certain minimum duration, and that in the small bowel the actual T_c probably approaches this, the main factor controlling the size of the proliferation compartment is the site of the zone within which decycling occurs; this effectively decides the position of the trailing edge on the labelling and mitotic index distributions. Movement of this position will reflect changes in the size of the proliferation compartment. Such changes rarely occur in isolation, but an increase in crypt cell production mediated solely by an increase in the size of the proliferation compartment and reflected by an upward movement of the trailing edge of the proliferative index distribution with respect to the top of the crypt has been described (819). A method for determining, from proliferative index distributions, the site in the crypt where cells decycle is given in Section 1.4.5.4.

The slow cut-off model has proved successful in predicting proliferative index distributions, and also in explaining the age distributions of cells in the crypt. Fluxes into and out of S are equal for the whole crypt, and thus a rectangular age distribution is appropriate (635); in the crypt base, where the slow cut-off model predicts an exponential age distribution, the flux into S exceeds the flux out of S which would be expected on the basis of an exponential age distribution (74).

At the top of the crypt are some cell positions where neither labelled cells nor mitoses are present (Figure 1.1.2); these cell positions are therefore occupied exclusively by non-proliferating cells, and are part of the maturation compartment. An increasing number of non-proliferating cells is also present in lower cell positions where cells are decycling, and this makes the lower limit of the maturation compartment difficult to identify. However, methods do exist for the measurement of its size and transit time (see Table 1.1.2).

The jejunal crypt has therefore a distinct kinetic architecture with recognisable component compartments. The colonic crypt is organised in a similar manner (Figure 1.1.4), although there are large quantitative differences. There are also important variations from site to site within the large bowel (689). Moreover, even in as different a mucosa as that of the glandular stomach, the kinetic organisation, and indeed evidence supporting a slow cut-off model, can be deduced from proliferative index distribution curves (Figure 1.1.4).

1.1.3 THE CRYPT CELL PRODUCTION RATE

Perhaps the most important parameter in crypt cell proliferation is the crypt cell production rate (CCPR). Changes in CCPR may result from a change in T_c, in I_p, in the crypt population size, or from combinations of such changes, and it determines the efflux into the functional compartment. Clarke (111) has argued strongly for its accurate measurement as the sole estimator of proliferative activity in the crypt. If the detection of an induced change in proliferative activity is the only objective of a particular investigation then measurement of CCPR is more informative than measurement of any of the parameters which influence it. However, once a change in CCPR is detected, to understand the kinetic mechanism of the change it is necessary to measure each one of the component parameters.

Perhaps the most convenient method of measuring the CCPR is by the stathmokinetic or metaphase arrest method, employing a microdissection technique; this takes advantage of the fact that the crypt is a closed system, and the presence of an arrested metaphase indicates a net output of one cell. This method has been used to obtain a value of 35 cells per crypt per h in the rat upper jejunum and throughout the rat small bowel (109). We have used three further independent methods to estimate the CCPR in the rat jejunum: firstly, the birth rate was calculated from a stathmokinetic experiment and multiplied by the number of proliferating cells per crypt; secondly, the birth rate was

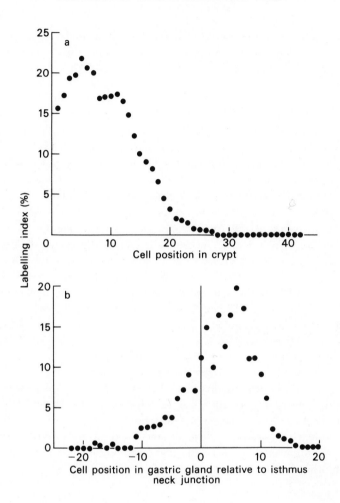

Figure 1.1.4 The labelling index distributions in (a) the crypt of the descending colon of the rat and (b) the gland of the proximal fundal mucosa of the stomach of the rat

calculated from T_c derived from an FLM experiment, and multiplied by the number of proliferating cells; and thirdly, the cell production rate for each column in the crypt was found from a cumulative birth rate curve, and multiplied by the number of columns in the crypt. Values of 32, 36 and 40 cells per crypt per h were obtained.

Our studies using the stathmokinetic technique with microdissection in the small bowel of the mouse yielded values of 16 cells per crypt per h in the jejunum but a lower value towards the terminal ileum (Table 1.1.3). This method has also been used to monitor changes in crypt efflux after proliferative cell death produced by cytosine arabinoside (Section 2.5).

1.1.3.1 THE CELL CYCLE TIME

In the small intestine of both rats and mice T_c, as determined by the FLM method, is about 11 to 12 h in most of the proliferation zone (5, 6). Therefore, in states of increased cell demand, the size of the increase in CCPR effected by a shortening of T_c is limited, although cell cycle times as short as 7 h have been recorded during recovery from irradiation (413). However, in basal cell positions, where many cells have longer cell cycle times, there is more opportunity for a reduction in T_c to produce an increase in CCPR. After treatment with hydroxyurea, I_s in basal cells increased greatly, an effect which was ascribed to a marked decrease in T_c. In the human jejunum however, cell cycle times of 48 h have been described (821), and in hyperproliferative mucosal states CCPR can be doubled by halving of T_c even in the absence of any other adaptive responses (817, 821) (see Section 6.3).

On the other hand, an increase in T_c can effect a reduction in CCPR; for example several groups (281, 333, 334, 785) have ascribed the decrease in CCPR which follows starvation (110) to a longer T_c. Our own results based on stathmokinetic studies in the rat indicated an increase in T_c after 4 days starvation, but FLM experiments have failed to confirm this. After 4 days starvation the mean cell cycle time was 12.3 h compared with a control value of 11.3 h; the coefficient of variation of T_c increased from 21 percent to 56 percent and it is evident that, although the variance of the cell cycle time increased, there was no significant increase in the mean value. We now believe that changes in other factors, such as the growth fraction, may be more important.

1.1.3.2 THE GROWTH FRACTION

The growth fraction in the crypt is defined as the proportion of cells which are engaged in the cell cycle, and, if all cells in the proliferation compartment are cycling, is equal to the relative size of the proliferation compartment. The non-proliferating cells have either left the proliferation compartment to mature and differentiate at the top of the crypt, or could possibly be in a resting phase (G_0). Some authors have assumed that G_0 cells are present in the small-intestinal crypts, but precisely where remains an enigma. In the zone of maximum labelling indices (see Figure 1.1.2) the theoretical labelling index is the same as the experimental labelling index, and it may be deduced that all cells there are cycling. It could be postulated that the lower labelling indices in basal positions are due to G_0 cells, but these lower indices are adequately accounted for by the presence of slowly cycling cells, and non-proliferating, terminally differentiated Paneth cells (818). We therefore agree with Cairnie et al (81) that there are no G_0 cells in the normal small-bowel crypt. That is not to say that in induced hypoproliferative states previously proliferating cells cannot enter a G_0 phase from which they can return when conditions are appropriate.

Of the factors concerned in the control of the size of the proliferating population, the position of the cut-off zone, where cells begin to decycle, is critical; movement of this position will lead to changes in CCPR. The mechanism through which this operates is by controlling the numbers of *transit divisions* possible in the crypt. In the normal mouse there are thought to be about two (120) and in the rat about four (814).

An upward movement of the cut-off zone thus delays the onset of terminal differentiation by increasing the number of transit divisions. In most hyper-proliferative states this change is accompanied by a decrease in T_c with or without an increase in crypt size, and is just one of the possible adaptive responses eg, in the rat after continuous irradiation (7) or administration of hydroxyurea (10), in coeliac disease and in human convoluted mucosae (817, 822). However, treatment of castrated mice with testosterone leads to an increase in I_s from 23 percent in castrate controls to 37 percent in treated animals (819). There was no change in T_c or in the crypt size, but calculations of I_p from the FLM curve indicated an increase from 40 percent in controls to 70 percent in treated animals. The labelling index distributions from the two groups (Figure 1.1.5) show that the main reason for this increase lies in an upward movement of the half-maximum position (HMP) (see Section 1.4.5). These studies show that movement of the cut-off position can occur in isolation, with consequent effect upon the CCPR.

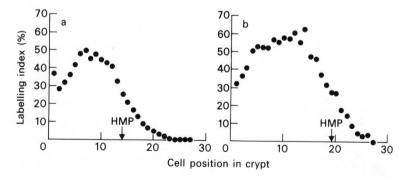

Figure 1.1.5 The labelling index distributions in the jejunal crypt of (a) castrated control mice and (b) castrated mice treated for 3 days with testosterone. The half-maximum positions are indicated

It was suggested previously that cells in the proliferation compartment could decycle in hypoproliferative states; there is some evidence that this occurs during starvation. Figure 1.1.6 shows the labelling index distribution for the rat jejunal crypts in controls and after 96 h starvation (8); the number of cell positions occupied by the proliferation compartment, as indicated by the HMP, is unchanged. However, I_s is reduced in the proliferation compartment. Table

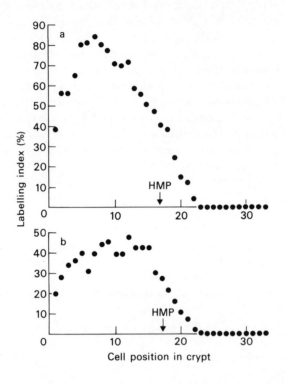

Figure 1.1.6 The labelling index distributions in the jejunal crypt of rats starved for (a) 4 h and (b) 96 h. The half-maximum positions are indicated

Table 1.1.1 Crypt population, mitotic and labelling indices, duration of cell cycle and S-phase, growth fraction, birth rate and crypt cell production rate in jejunal crypts of control rats and rats starved for 96 h

	Crypt population	I_m (%)	I_s (%)	T_c (h)	t_s (h)	I_p (%)	k_B (cells/1000 cells/h)	CCPR (cells/crypt/h)
Control rats	670	6.2	36	11.3	6.5	61	112	39
Starved rats	580	4.5	22	12.3	6.3	45	57	19

1.1.1 shows the duration of the cell cycle parameters in controls and in starved animals, and although they are virtually unchanged there is a reduction in the growth fraction from 61 percent to 45 percent, and the non-cycling cells must be distributed throughout the proliferation compartment. On refeeding there is an immediate increase in I_s, and consequently it is more likely that cells are blocked in G_1 or at the G_1 to S boundary (249), rather than in a true G_0 phase.

Change in the relative size of the proliferation compartment as an adaptive mechanism influencing cell production rate has been referred to as the feedback control mechanism of crypt cell production (579), and considered to be a local control mechanism brought about by a reduction in the size of the function compartment, such as is produced by irradiation (585), or villus damage induced by ischaemia (583). This concept is considered further in Section 2.1.

However, these changes are manifest very rapidly after death of proliferating cells in the crypt (10), possibly before the villus population has decreased; only detailed studies of temporal changes in villus and crypt populations, and their relationship with the various proliferative responses, can establish the physiological mechanisms involved.

1.1.3.3 CHANGES IN CRYPT POPULATION

An increase in the size of the crypt will increase the number of proliferating cells even though I_p remains constant, as occurs in lactation (300) and after ileo-jejunal transposition or intestinal bypass (579).

An isolated change in the crypt size in the absence of any alteration in I_p has been envisaged (579), but as a result of studies on human mucosae showing different degrees of villus cell depletion, we believe that the increase in crypt size may have a place in a defined sequence of events which also includes a decrease in T_c and an increase in I_p (Figure 1.1.7).

The mechanism by which an enlargement or reduction in crypt size is achieved is unknown. An increase could be due to a shortening of T_c, but it is difficult to see how this would work unless some other mechanism caused the cells to remain in the crypt, rather than migrate at a faster rate. Studies on recovery from injury induced by hydroxyurea (10) and by starvation (8) indicate that the number of cells in the crypt circumference (the column count) increases before the number of cells along its length (the crypt column). The kinetic mechanism is likely to be complex and involve changes in the planes of cell division (187).

1.1.3.4 INTERDEPENDENCE OF FACTORS CONTROLLING THE CELL PRODUCTION RATE

The hypothesis set out in Figure 1.1.7 postulates a sequence of events which

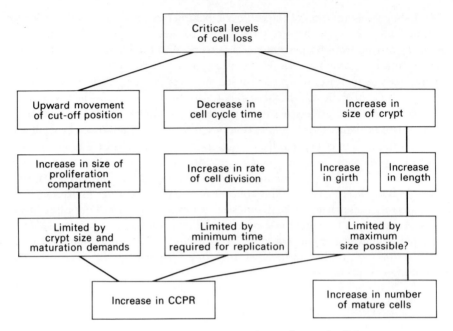

Figure 1.1.7 Compensatory crypt reactions to increased cell loss

follows an increased demand for cells, possibly induced by a depletion in villus cell number. It is based upon studies of the convoluted and flat mucosae of human beings suffering from a variety of diseases, especially coeliac disease (768). The connecting thread is that the three mechanisms are brought into play probably as a result of different levels of cell demand. The observations behind this hypothesis are also discussed in Section 6.3.

1.1.3.5 OTHER KINETIC PARAMETERS

There are several other parameters which go to make up a kinetic definition of the crypt; for example the number of transit divisions, and various transit times. They are themselves largely determined by T_c, I_p and crypt size, and are detailed in Table 1.1.2 for the rat and mouse jejunal crypt.

1.1.3.6 CIRCADIAN VARIATION

In any study of cell proliferation it would be unwise to ignore the changes due to circadian variation (652), and Figure 1.1.8 shows the changes in I_s and I_m in rat jejunum (9). The timing of the variation appears to be different from species to species and from study to study; at the moment the mechanisms involved are

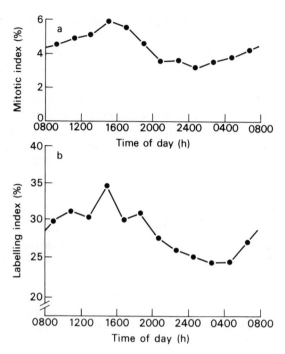

Figure 1.1.8 (a) Mitotic and (b) labelling indices at different times of day in
the rat jejunal crypt; each point is the mean of three animals

not understood. Any system with coincident peaks in I_s and I_m, such as that
illustrated, probably has control points in both G_1 and G_2. Whatever the
mechanism, such physiological changes will complicate the interpretation of
cell kinetic experiments.

Table 1.1.2 A summary of kinetic parameters in the jejunal
crypts of rats and mice. Estimates vary according to the
experimental method and the assumptions made in their
calculation (7, 773)

	Rat	Mouse
Crypt length (cells)	32.9	25.1
Column count	22.3	14.6
Total population	650; 735	280; 365
Growth fraction	61; 62	61; 65
Proliferating population	395; 455	170; 235
Number of mitoses/crypt	22.5	20.4
Migration rate (cells/h)	1.43; 1.78	1.48; 1.85
CCPR (cells/crypt/h)	32.4; 39.7	13.6; 21.5
Crypt transit time (h)	34	25

1.1.4 VILLUS CELL POPULATION KINETICS

The preceding sections have dealt almost exclusively with quantitative description of the crypt and factors within it which influence the CCPR. However, from a functional viewpoint, the most important part of the mucosa is the villus epithelium, which is concerned with the secretory and absorptive functions. Where cell proliferation in the gut is concerned, any control process, local or systemic, effects a change in the CCPR whatever its kinetic mechanism. Furthermore, arguing teleologically, what is essential to the villus cell population is not even the CCPR, but the net influx into the villus population, which is the product of the CCPR and the number of crypts serving each villus, ie, the crypt-villus ratio (109). Most current ideas of growth control stem from the Weiss and Kavanau (779) model of negative feedback, and for such concepts to be studied in the gut the only measurement of cell production needed is an accurate estimate of the *net villus influx*. Accurate estimates of the villus cell population and of the crypt cell population are also needed; but it is the present author's opinion that we must move away from the kinetic factors which determine the magnitude of any response, and take a more comprehensive view of the epithelium, and especially of the villus cell population, concentrating less on time than on population size and flux (111).

1.1.4.1 THE STEADY STATE REQUIREMENT

There is a tacit assumption that the intestinal mucosa is in a steady state, that is to say that cell production and cell loss are balanced so that the cell population remains (generally) constant; the caveat is necessary because of diurnal variation. For a villus cell population of n_v with net influx k_{cv} and transit time t_v:

$$t_v = \frac{n_v}{k_{cv}}$$

Consequently, to test such a hypothesis it is necessary to measure the villus cell population, the influx into it, and the transit time on the villus. Moreover, it is the measurement of these parameters which is so important in the elucidation of feedback mechanisms (see Section 2.5).

Clarke (111) pointed out large inconsistencies in the transit time as calculated from the above equation and as measured. For example in rat ileum, with a villus size of 3000 cells (334) and a villus influx of 360 cells per villus per hour, the equation gives a transit time of 9 h, obviously at variance with the published value of 40 h (83). For this reason we have measured the above three parameters.

1.1.4.2 VILLUS CELL POPULATION SIZE

Despite warnings (82, 111) some workers have relied on simple length measurements as estimators of villus cell population size in both animal and human villi. It is often forgotten that villi are three-dimensional structures, they contain smooth muscle fully capable of contracting; and, possibly most importantly, in abnormal states they vary a good deal in shape. Thus we obtained good correlations between villus cell population and morphometric parameters such as villus length in normal mouse intestine, but in villi regenerating after cytosine arabinoside, and in the abnormal villi found in patients with treated coeliac disease after gluten challenge (837), there were poor correlations. For these reasons an accurate estimate of villus cell population entails actually counting it.

Using standard microdissection methods, ten villi were dissected from each of five defined sites in 6 Balb/c mice; they were stained in bulk by the Feulgen reaction, then squashed, and the epithelial nuclei counted. Results are shown in Table 1.1.3; counting variation in these analyses was between 2 and 3 percent;

Table 1.1.3 Size and flux parameters for the villus, measured as described in the text, for sites in the small bowel (i) 0 (ii) 25 % (iii) 50 % (iv) 75 % and (v) 100 % of the distance from the pylorus to the ileocaecal junction

Bowel position	i	ii	iii	iv	v
Villus population (cells)	7650	6150	4840	3400	2160
CCPR (cells/crypt/h)	12.4	16.4	11.6	10.6	13.0
Crypt-villus ratio	13.7	11.4	10.7	9.1	6.2
Net villus influx (cells/villus/h)	170	187	125	97	81
Calculated villus transit time (h)	46	33	43	35	27
Observed villus transit time (h)	38	37	45	36	33

the relative standard error of the observations was less than 10 percent in each case. In the duodenum, values of about 8000 cells were obtained, whereas in the terminal ileum the villus population was much smaller at around 2000 cells. Incidentally, the best morphometric estimator of the villus cell population for this sample of normal villi was found to be the linear height multiplied by the basal width, both measured in longitudinal section of villi.

From this study it may be concluded that the villus cell population can be measured accurately and precisely. There is a diminution in the size of the population from proximal to distal small bowel.

1.1.4.3 INFLUX ONTO THE VILLUS

This is the rate at which cells enter the functional villus compartment, and is evaluated as the product of the CCPR and the crypt-villus ratio. Methods for estimating these are given in Section 2.5.2.

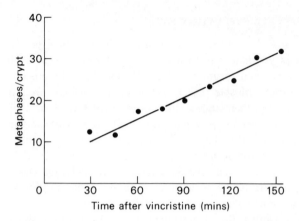

Figure 1.1.9 Stathmokinetic data for a position in the mouse small bowel, 75 percent of the distance from the pylorus to the ileocæcal junction, fitted by linear regression

Figure 1.1.9 shows the results of a typical stathmokinetic experiment for a position 75 percent of the distance along the small bowel from the pylorus; the CCPR was 10.6 ± 0.8 cells per crypt per h. The results for different positions are shown in Table 1.1.3.

Table 1.1.3 also gives the values of crypt-villus ratios in the several bowel positions; there was a steady decrease in the ratio from 13.7 ± 0.7 crypts per villus in the proximal duodenum, to 6.2 ± 0.2 in the terminal ileum.

Values for the net villus influx calculated from these figures vary from 187 ± 16 cells per villus per h in the jejunum to 81 ± 5 cells per villus per h in the terminal ileum. We may conclude from Table 1.1.3 that the large villi in proximal positions have the largest influx.

1.1.4.4 THE VILLUS TRANSIT TIME

When measuring this it has been usual in the past to measure the shortest time taken for a cell labelled with ³HTdR to reach the villus tip. This will give something approaching a minimum villus transit time. However if it is intended to compare a calculated transit time as computed from the population size and influx, with the measured transit time, estimation of an average transit time is necessary.

The villus transit time is the time taken for cells to pass from the foot of the villus to the villus tip. After labelling with ³HTdR, labelled cells are found only in the lower two-thirds or so of the crypt. Therefore, to exclude the time required to traverse the upper third, both the average transit time to the crypt-villus junction, and the average transit time to the villus tip should be measured.

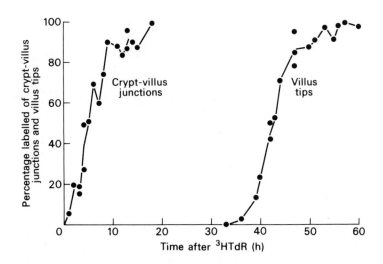

Figure 1.1.10 The percentage of crypt-villus junctions and villus tips labelled at various times after injection of ^{3}HTdR

Mice were injected with ^{3}HTdR and killed serially over 60 h. Autoradiographs were prepared and, in each animal, the proportion of crypt-villus junctions labelled and the proportion of villus tips labelled were counted. Figure 1.1.10 illustrates the results for the upper duodenum; both curves are sigmoid in shape and they show for example that the minimum time for a labelled cell to reach the crypt-villus junction is very short, while by 15 h virtually all crypt-villus junctions are labelled. Similarly the shortest transit time to the villus tip is 35 h with virtually all villus tips labelled by 55 h. The best estimate of the villus transit time can be found from the difference in the times of 50 percent labelling. This is given for the different bowel positions in Table 1.1.3 and values vary from 33 to 45 h.

Table 1.1.3 compares the villus transit times calculated from villus size and influx with the measured transit times. The result is not inconsistent with the steady state model.

There are two further considerations which may affect this conclusion. Firstly as is demonstrated in Figure 1.1.8 there is circadian variation in proliferative indices, and therefore probably in the CCPR. The measurements of villus cell population size were carried out on animals killed at 0900 h, and the metaphase arrest data were obtained from animals injected with vincristine at 0900 h and followed over the next 2.5 h. In contrast, the transit time experiments lasted for at least 42 h. The agreement between transit times may indicate that circadian variations are not large, but for definitive analysis changes in villus influx and population should be investigated throughout the day.

Secondly, there is the anatomical site of cell loss to be considered; this is generally thought to be at the villus tip (134), but studies using scanning electron microscopy have produced morphological evidence for cell death and cell loss on the sides of the villus (539). The measured transit time referred to above assumes that cell loss is confined to the villus tip and would be affected by loss of cells before this site, resulting in overestimation of the life span on the villus.

1.1.5 THE EQUIVALENCE OF VILLUS AND CRYPT CELL POPULATIONS

At first sight, the relatively small crypt cell population would appear to be dwarfed by the larger villus cell population. However, the set of crypt cells supplying one villus is the crypt cell population multiplied by the crypt-villus ratio, the *crypt cell population per villus*. If this is compared with the villus population in the small intestine of the mouse (Table 1.1.4) it is evident that at

Table 1.1.4 Relationship between the sizes of crypt and villus populations. Bowel positions are as in Table 1.1.3

Bowel position	i	ii	iii	iv	v
Crypt population (cells)	530	510	470	380	360
Crypt-villus ratio	13.7	11.4	10.7	9.1	6.2
Total crypt cells/villus	7250	5790	5090	3500	2250
Villus population (cells)	7650	6150	4850	3400	2060
Ratio of villus cells to crypt cells/villus	1.06	1.06	0.95	0.97	0.96

each site the crypt cell population per villus is almost equal to the villus cell population. This important relationship, together with the response of the two populations after pertubation (Section 2.5), suggests that control processes are directed to maintaining the equivalence of the two populations sizes, by a series of regenerative compensatory mechanisms in which changes occur in both the CCPR and the crypt–villus ratio.

Zajicek (832) has suggested that an intestinal 'proliferon' or proliferative unit exists. Our results indicate that this may consist of the villus and the whole of its attendant crypt population.

1.1.6 CONCLUSIONS

This short survey has shown that it is now possible, in the normal animal, to define the crypt and villus cell populations in terms of size, flux and time. Much attention has been paid to the measurement of kinetic parameters in the crypt, but when analysing adaptive responses which are often short-lived these may not be the appropriate measurements to make. In the analysis of growth control in the small bowel, and in particular with respect to feedback studies, it is necessary to pay attention to changes in population size. Methods are available by which the numbers of crypt and villus cells and their rates of flux, can be measured with precision, and only such studies can be relied on in the analysis of feedback control of cell proliferation.

ACKNOWLEDGEMENTS

These studies were carried out with the assistance of Dr D R Appleton, Dr A J Watson and Dr A R Morley of the University of Newcastle upon Tyne, Dr H S Al-Dewachi of the University of Mosul, Iraq and also Dr A Al-Nafussi, Dr N Britton, Dr M Irvin and Mrs J Carter, all of the University of Oxford.

I thank the Cancer Research Campaign for generous financial support.

1.2 Aspects of the Growth of Epithelium and Mesenchyme in the Intestine of Mouse Embryos

Rosella Sbarbati and Jan Strackee

1.2.1 INTRODUCTION

A recent work (625) has presented data relating to the growth in volume of the intestine in mouse embryos from 12 days after fertilisation until birth, and has demonstrated that it follows an exponential pattern. However the intestinal wall is formed by two layers, the epithelium and the mesenchyme, which grow one inside the other and differentiate during the last week of gestation. As we could find no published data about the separate growth in volume during embryonic life of these two components of the intestine we conducted the investigation described here. Our results throw some light on the roles of, and the interactions between, epithelial and mesenchymal tissues during the morphogenesis of the previllous ridges and the villi.

1.2.2 MATERIALS AND METHODS

In the present study we have defined the *mesenchyme* as the sheath of loose connective tissue surrounding the *epithelium* in the intestine of the youngest embryos, and as the sheath of lamina propria, muscularis mucosae, submucosa and muscularis externa which are differentiated and recognisable as such in the intestine of the older embryos. The small and large intestines have been considered together. The investigation was carried out on a series of 28 mouse embryos of the CPB-S strain aged between 11.9 days after fertilisation and birth (255).

The material was divided into two groups: 9 embryos younger than 14.8 days, and 19 older. In the younger group the intestinal cross-sections show a rather immature pattern, with the previllous ridges either not yet present, or just beginning to form.

The same morphometric technique used to estimate the volume of the whole intestine (V_I) (625) was adopted to estimate the volumes of the intestinal epithelium (V_E) and mesenchyme (V_M) in these embryos; the volumes were estimated by means of a point-counting method (775) in 20 systematically sampled sections of intestine.

With increasing age, more profiles of newly formed villi appear in the cross-sections of the small bowel, with a considerable increase of epithelial and mesenchymal surfaces. Furthermore, the spatial texture of the sectioned villi becomes so fine as to require high magnification (eg ×400) for the tissue components to be distinguishable. We therefore decided to infer the volume for the older group of embryos using samples of the intestinal tissue.

1.2.2.1 SAMPLE SIZE

A square grid of 25 points (Zeiss Integrationsplatte I) was inserted into the eye-piece of the microscope. If λ is the distance between adjacent lattice points, the projected portion of intestinal cross-section (the *field*) has an area of $25\lambda^2$. Since the total area of the intestinal cross-sections is known for each embryo (625) the total number of fields containing samples of intestinal cross-sections, ie, of epithelium or mesenchyme or both, can be estimated. The number of grid points (η) hitting epithelium or mesenchyme in each of the fields is a random variable; we can reasonably assume that it has a unimodal distribution in the population of possible fields, so that adequate population parameters are the mean μ and the variance σ^2. We chose the sample size such that the sampling distribution of the means of all the possible samples of that size was approximately normal and had a 95 percent confidence interval of length 0.05 μm. By randomly sampling about 100 fields in each of two embryos of different ages (15 and 17.8 days) and counting η for both epithelium and mesenchyme we concluded that a sample size of about 25 fields satisfied both these conditions. The number of fields actually sampled in each of the 20 sections was proportional to the cross-sectional area of the intestine. The fields were selected with the help of a cross-stage and a table of random numbers. Overlapping of the fields was avoided.

If η_E and η_M are the total number of points hitting epithelium and mesenchyme respectively, then V_E and V_M at age t were estimated from:

$$V_E(t) = \eta_E V_I(t)/(\eta_E + \eta_M) \quad \text{and} \quad V_M(t) = \eta_M V_I(t)/(\eta_E + \eta_M)$$

1.2.2.2 STATISTICAL ANALYSIS

The study of the specific growth rates of the two tissues, ie the relative increase of the volume per unit time, was performed by applying polynomial regression analysis to the logarithmically transformed data (625). If the log volume can be described by a polynomial, the volume itself has a basically exponential form. However exponential functions are not 'summable', ie, the sum of two exponentials is not an exponential, and this is true for most of the functions commonly used to describe growth. Therefore it would be convenient to have three functions of the same form such that:

$$V_E(t) + V_M(t) = V_I(t)$$

The exponential description represents adequately each growth process but does not reflect this basic property of the additivity of volumes. We believe this to be a major issue in this context but we shall treat it elsewhere.

1.2.3 RESULTS

Figure 1.2.1 shows the growth curves, on a logarithmic scale, for epithelium

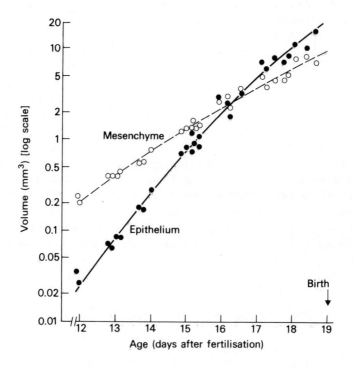

Figure 1.2.1 Growth curves for epithelium and mesenchyme; volume is plotted logarithmically against age

and mesenchyme separately; the data are satisfactorily represented ($r^2 = 0.99$) by the equations:

$$\log_e V_E(t) = -24.76 + 2.275 \, t - 0.04283 \, t^2$$

$$\log_e V_M(t) = -11.64 + 1.033 \, t - 0.01592 \, t^2$$

At the beginning of the observations, epithelial volume doubles every 14 h and mesenchymal volume every 26 h; at birth these volume doubling times have lengthened to 23 h and 36 h respectively. Neither the epithelial data nor the mesenchymal data would be satisfactorily fitted without the quadratic term which provides for the slowing down of the specific growth rates. The volumes of epithelium and mesenchyme are equal about 2.5 days before birth. Over the period of 7 days from 11.9 days after fertilisation to 18.7 days after fertilisation epithelial volume increases over 700-fold and mesenchymal volume only about 40-fold.

1.2.4 DISCUSSION

The present results show that the epithelium and the mesenchyme in the intestine of mouse embryos have different patterns of growth. During the period under study the epithelium is growing in volume almost twice as fast as the mesenchyme. The rate at which the specific growth rate slows down, given by twice the coefficient of the quadratic term, is less marked in the mesenchyme than in the epithelium. The volume of the epithelium at 11.9 days is almost 9 times less than the volume of the mesenchyme, while just before birth it is twice as big. Therefore the growth curve of the intestine as a whole (625) reflects more the growth of the mesenchyme, until the volume of the epithelium becomes comparable.

During the last seven days of embryonic life the intestine not only grows considerably in volume but also differentiates from an immature into an adult-like organ. The epithelium in particular increases strikingly in volume and changes its spatial pattern from a simple stratified tube, which lines the tiny intestinal lumen, into one layer of specialised cells which cover a complex pattern of villi and crypts. Little is known about the normal morphogenesis of the villi in the intestine of mouse embryos, though more is known about rats and chicks. It has been suggested that the formation of the previllous ridges in the duodenum of chick embryos is caused by the contraction of the newly formed muscularis mucosae and muscularis externa (128); but contradictory evidence has also been presented (73, 326). It has been found that although smooth muscle does not seem to influence the formation of the previllous ridges, the mesenchyme as a whole does; intact epithelial tubes isolated from the mesenchyme do not fold (73). The interaction between epithelium and mesenchyme seems to be of fundamental importance in the morphogenesis of the intestine, even if there is controversy about its nature.

The present results seem to substantiate indirectly the idea that the mesenchyme exerts a passive role of support and delimitation of the rapidly expanding epithelium, and aids its folding. The epithelium and mesenchyme can be thought of as two elastic tubes which grow one inside the other while the inner tube grows twice as fast in volume as the outer one. We can assume that the physical properties of the two tissues prior to differentiation are similar. It also seems reasonable to assume that the outer layer exerts a passive resistance to the expansion of the inner layer and forces it to fold into the large previllous ridges. The bulging of the epithelium does not occur at the same time along the intestinal tube, but can be considered entirely completed at about the 16th day. The rates of increase in length and cross-sectional area of the intestine are quite constant before the 16th day, during which time the suggested under-estimation of the length and over-estimation of the cross-sectional area are less perceptible than in older embryos (625). The folding of the epithelium does not seem to produce significant changes in the proportional increase of the cross-sectional area of the tube.

Recently it has been shown that cell degeneration contributes to the formation of the villi in the foetal rat duodenum (462). We too have observed a considerable number of degenerated cells in the epithelium of the intestine during growth. Villus and crypt formation (196) and cell degeneration do not have the same spatial and temporal characteristics along the intestinal tube. That the degenerated cells observed first in the epithelium and later in the lumen are the product of a morphogenetic process and not of cellular turnover has been indirectly confirmed (503), since cell turnover in the epithelium covering the villi of the mouse duodenum does not occur during embryonic life, as the extrusion zones at the top of the villi form only after birth. Further investigation is needed on the characteristics of the morphogenesis of the villus and crypt and on the role of cell degeneration in the mouse intestine. Whether a different balance between the incremental and the decremental components during the two growth processes contributes to the different rates of slowing down of the two growth curves is also a matter of interest.

1.3 Spatial Distribution of Proliferating and Specialised Cells and Cell Cycle Analysis of the Guinea Pig Colonic Crypts

W Sawicki and J Rowinski

1.3.1 DISTRIBUTION OF PROLIFERATING AND SPECIALISED CELLS IN THE CRYPT

The intestinal crypt represents a specific geometrical model: it is a cylinder open at the mouth and closed at the bottom. The epithelium of the crypt is of simple columnar type consisting of tightly packed polygonal, mostly octahedral, cells which are attached to the basement membrane. The colon of the guinea pig is a particularly good model for the study of cell proliferation and differentiation since there are groups of crypts differing in length according to their localisation in the colonic wall (Figure 1.3.1). Although many ultra-structural and histochemical features of epithelial cells change along the length of the crypt, the height of cells and their light-microscopic appearance vary only slightly at different positions in the crypt (512).

1.3.1.1 DISTRIBUTION OF PROLIFERATING CELLS ALONG THE CRYPT

Knowledge of the distribution of both the proliferating and the specialised cells in the crypt epithelium is important in respect of any assessment of the kinetics of cellular proliferation, migration and differentiation in normal and patho-logical conditions, as well as in respect of studying the mechanisms controlling these processes. The distribution of proliferating cells was found to be non-random along the crypts of the small and large bowel of rodents (83, 624, 819). The pattern of this non-randomness is such that the proliferating cells occur most frequently between 0.2 and 0.4 of the distance from the bottom to the top of the crypt. The interrelationship between cellular proliferation and differentiation has been well documented (603). Since in the epithelium of intestinal crypts both the mitotic and DNA-synthesising cells represent the proliferation compartment, whereas goblet cells together with other differenti-

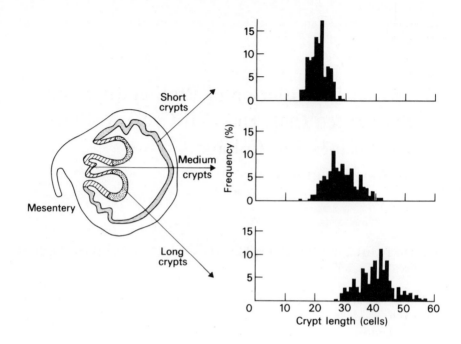

Figure 1.3.1 Schematic representation of a transverse section of the guinea pig ascending colon, showing longitudinal folds; and the distribution of crypt length for the crypts at various regions of the colonic wall

ated columnar cells represent the function compartment of differentiated cells, the proliferation and differentiation as well as the relationship between both processes can be simply analysed using this model.

Guinea pigs were pulse-labelled with tritiated-thymidine (^{3}HTdR) to mark the nuclei of DNA-synthesising cells. Transverse, paraffin sections of the ascending colon were cut and autoradiographed (595). The DNA-synthesising cells were recognised by the appearance of at least 3 emulsion grains over the nucleus, and mature goblet cells by staining with the PAS method (622), in longitudinally sectioned crypts. The analysis involved data from more than 500 crypts grouped into four classes differing in length and position in the colonic wall: short (20 to 29 cells) and medium crypts (30 to 39 cells) situated either at the base of a colonic fold or out of the fold, and medium (30 to 39 cells) and long crypts (40 to 49 cells) situated at the top of a colonic fold (Figure 1.3.1). The mitotic (I_m) labelling (I_s) and mature goblet cell (I_g) indices were computed for each cell position.

In order to obtain a consistent description of the distribution of mitotic and labelled cells along the crypt, a truncated normal distribution curve was fitted to the experimental data by the method of least squares and tested for goodness of fit. Since the fit was found to be reasonable, the mode and standard deviation were taken to describe the chief characteristics of the experimental distributions of either I_m or I_s. Statistical errors of the parameters of the distributions were found automatically by the fitting algorithm, taking into account statistical errors of the experimental data.

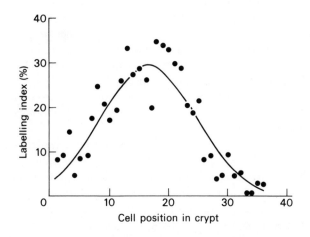

Figure 1.3.2 The labelling index distribution in medium length crypts, and the fitted truncated normal distribution curve

An example of the relationship between experimental I_s values and the fitted curve is presented in Figure 1.3.2. It was found that the distributions of I_m and I_s along the crypt of the guinea pig colon could be described, in each of the four crypt classes, by truncated normal curves. The modes, standard deviations and areas delimited by such curves for the four crypt classes were calculated. Estimated modes of I_m distributions differed significantly between crypt classes, being higher in long than in short crypts. When the modes of these distributions were normalised and expressed in fractions of crypt length the differences disappeared. The mode of the I_m distribution was 0.442 ± 0.019 of the crypt length.

At that fraction of the crypt length I_m was between 5 and 8 percent, independent of the crypt class. Similarly, the estimated modes of I_s distribution along the crypt were proportional to the crypt length. When the modes of these distributions were normalised the difference disappeared. The mean value of the mode of the I_s distribution was 0.375 ± 0.004 of the crypt length. At that fraction of crypt length I_s was between 30 and 35 percent, independent of the crypt class. It is noteworthy that the areas delimited by the I_s distribution curves for medium crypts situated at the tops of colonic folds were significantly higher than those for medium crypts situated at the base of the fold.

All these results as well as those obtained by others for intestinal crypts of the small and large bowel of mouse and rat (82, 83, 553, 574, 819) seem to indicate that the distribution of proliferating cells along the crypt is a stable and characteristic spatial feature. At least some factors, like the length of crypts and their position in the intestinal wall, as well as variation of some physiological conditions, such as lactation (82), did not modify this feature. Furthermore, the stability of the distribution pattern of proliferating cells along the crypt, ie, the occurrence of the highest frequency of mitotic and DNA-synthesising cells between 0.2 and 0.4 of the distance from the bottom, was also pointed out in a number of experimentally induced conditions. However variations in the length of the proliferation zone along the crypt, and in I_m and I_s values, were noted. Thus, neither maintaining the animals in germ-free conditions (247), nor castration and testosterone treatment (819), X-irradiation followed by cutting off the villi (247), partial resection of the small bowel (296) or early changes brought about by a carcinogen (574), caused the distribution of proliferation in the crypt to change, although I_m and I_s and the length of the proliferation zone varied. Similar modifications of I_m, I_s and the length of the proliferation zone were observed between crypts of the same length but situated at different sites in the colonic wall. It may be therefore inferred that extrinsic factors affect groups of crypts rather than individual crypts, modifying the intensity of proliferation by increasing or decreasing the proliferative indices and broadening or narrowing the proliferation zone along the crypt, without changing the distribution pattern of proliferating cells.

On the other hand, the stability of the distribution of proliferating cells along crypts of various lengths strongly supports the hypothesis that this pattern depends upon intrinsic factors connected equally to the bottom and the mouth of the crypt. An alternative though speculative explanation of the pattern is the occurrence of some regulatory factors along and out of the crypt. One candidate for such a factor is the distribution of capillary vessels along the crypt, and the relationship between the frequency of mitoses and the distance from blood vessels has been pointed out by Tannock (703) for tumours. Their frequency distribution along the crypt was found to be non-random and the pattern of such non-randomness coincided with the distribution pattern of the proliferating cells along the crypt (593). However, there is no evidence whether the variations in blood vessel arrangement remain in a *propter hoc* or a *post hoc* relationship to the distribution of proliferating cells along the crypt.

1.3.1.2 DISTRIBUTION OF GOBLET CELLS ALONG THE CRYPTS

The mature goblet cell index (I_g) calculated for each position along the colonic crypts of the guinea pig was obtained. The experimental distribution of I_g can be approximated by curves of exponential decrease given by:

$$I_g(j) = a \exp\left\{-\ln2 \frac{j-1}{k-1}\right\}$$

with two parameters: a is I_g at position 1 (the crypt bottom) and k is the cell position where I_g falls to half its maximum; j is cell position in the crypt column. The parameters a and k giving the best least squares fit to the exponential function were found. At position 1, I_g differs significantly between various crypt classes, being proportionately higher for longer crypts. Parameter k showed no significant differences among crypts of various classes: its mean value was calculated as cell position 6.7 ±0.3 for all crypt classes of the colon.

The distribution of goblet cells in the crypt of the small bowel, with most frequent accumulation close to but not at the bottom, (which in the small bowel is occupied by Paneth cells) and gradual decrease of their number toward the crypt mouth has been previously demonstrated (476). The distribution of goblet cells along the crypt of the large bowel is different in that the highest frequency of these cells is at the crypt bottom. The simple mathematical formula describes this distribution. It should be emphasised that I_g at the crypt bottom is strictly related to the crypt length: in long crypts it was 30 percent, whereas in the short crypts 15 percent. On the other hand, the rate of decrease of I_g along the crypt does not depend upon the crypt length since for all three groups of crypts I_g was half of its maximum value at cell position 6 or 7.

It can therefore be concluded that the goblet cell index at the crypt bottom, and therefore the rate of cell differentiation and cell proliferation in that region of the crypt, are regulated by factors connected to the crypt length.

1.3.2 THE CELL CYCLE TIME IN THE COLONIC CRYPT

The study of cell proliferation, including analysis of the cell cycle, in intestinal epithelium has been extensive (6, 83, 98, 427, 553, 595, 819). Cell proliferation is normally restricted to the crypts and it appears neither in the epithelium covering the villi of small bowel nor in that lining the lumen of large bowel (83, 427). It recently became evident that the rate of proliferation in the epithelium of the large bowel is generally lower than that in the small bowel. This is revealed by appropriate differences in the cell cycle time and particularly by the variation in the duration of the G_1 phase, as well as by the variations of other proliferative parameters.

Two features make the analysis of cell proliferation in the large bowel interesting: a small number of recognisable cell types in crypt epithelium (principal-columnar, goblet and enteroendocrine cells) and the high frequency of human cancer of the large intestine. The former facilitates the analysis of cell proliferation and the interrelationship between cell proliferation and differentiation, whereas the latter allows for step-by-step study of the transition from normal to cancerous cell proliferation and differentiation.

The advantage of the histological appearance of the crypts of the guinea pig colon has been briefly discussed in the introduction to this paper. Here, another advantage of the ascending colon of the guinea pig should be emphasised, the lack of circadian rhythm of mitoses (594) which would complicate any analysis of cell proliferation.

1.3.2.1 THE CELL CYCLE TIME IN THE GUINEA PIG ASCENDING COLON

Three groups of crypts differing by their length and localisation in the colonic wall were separately analysed: short (20 to 29), medium (30 to 39) and long (40 to 49 cells) (Figure 1.3.1). In order to analyse the cell cycle at various positions in the crypt, each of them was divided into three segments. The division was based on the normal distribution of DNA-synthesising cells along the crypt (Figure 1.3.2), which revealed the maximum at 0.38 of the distance from the bottom and a standard deviation of 0.16. Accordingly, the middle segment of crypt was taken to extend from 0.30 to 0.46 of the crypt length (mode $. + \frac{1}{2}$ standard deviation), the lower segment from the bottom to 0.30 of the length and the upper segment from 0.46 of the length to the crypt mouth. As a result of such division, roughly equal samples of mitoses in calculating fractions of labelled mitoses (FLM) at different times after ^{3}HTdR injection could be obtained.

1.3.2.2 CHARACTERISTICS OF FLM CURVES

The calculation of the cell cycle time (T_c) and its phases may be obtained from FLM curves (557). The mitotic duration was determined with the use of a stathmokinetic method using colchicine (401). Duration of mitosis was estimated as ranging from 1.1 h to 3.2 h with a tendency to longer duration in the lower crypt segments (595). The FLM curves were calculated separately for all three segments of short, medium and long crypts.

The FLM curves for the cells of the guinea pig colonic crypt have first waves which reach approximately 100 percent and flattened second waves (Figure 1.3.3). The latter may be either unimodal or bimodal, depending upon crypt length and crypt segment. The interpretation of such FLM curves, which differ in shape from that predicted for the simple model of cell cycle (557), represents a problem of general importance since this type of curve has been obtained also

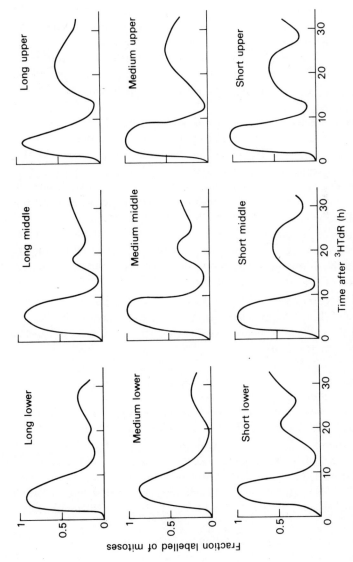

Figure 1.3.3 FLM curves for short, medium and long crypts in lower, middle and upper crypt segments

for a variety of human and animal tumours (647, 669). It should be emphasised that the interpretation of FLM curves with damped second waves may be as arbitrary as it is erroneous. Therefore, the interpretation should be as careful as possible and, besides the measurement of interpoint distance on the FLM curve, it ought to involve the analysis of grain counts per mitosis and the measurement of the areas delimited by the curve under the first and the second waves.

In the case of the guinea pig colon the FLM curves were similar for all three segments of short crypts and for the upper segments of medium and long crypts (Figure 1.3.3). The cell cycle time for these crypt segments was estimated as between 13 and 19 h.

In the middle segments of medium and long crypts the second wave of the FLM curve was found to be bimodal. The question arose, therefore, whether both modes represented the same (ie, the second) wave of the FLM curve, or belonged to two separate waves. To answer this question the grain count of labelled mitoses at 6, 20 and 32 h after ^{3}HTdR injection was calculated (595). Since no difference was found in mean grain count per mitosis 20 h and 32 h after labelling it was concluded that both modes represented the second wave of labelled mitoses. Accordingly, two estimations of T_c, 13 h to 16 h and 22 h to 26 h, were made. It was concluded that proliferating cells in the middle segment of medium and long crypts consisted of two subpopulations differing in duration of G_1 phase by about 9 h.

The FLM curves for the lower segments (including the crypt bottom) of medium and long crypts have unimodal second waves with their maxima shifted to the right as compared with the respective maxima of FLM curves for the upper crypt segments. The cell cycle time was estimated as between 22 and 26 h.

The measurements of the area under the second wave of the FLM curves indicate that about 50 percent of cells located in the middle and especially in the lower segments of the crypts had a cell cycle longer than 26 h. The G_1 phase of these cells was 16 h and could be considered as a G_0 phase.

The estimates of T_c for short crypts were the same for all segments of crypts and contrasted with the variations along medium and long crypts. However, when additional data are taken into consideration, it seems that short crypts also contain some cells of long cell cycle in their lower segments, and therefore they are not an exception to the rule that T_c is longer in lower than in upper crypt segments.

These additional data are as follows: the area under the second wave of the labelled mitoses curve is only 0.75 of that under the first wave, and the ratio of the mean grain counts per labelled mitosis for 20 h and 32 h after labelling is 1.45 instead of the expected value of 2.

1.3.2.3 PITFALLS OF INTERPRETATION

The general feature of the FLM curve for the crypt cells of the large bowel is that the second wave does not reach 100 percent (98, 427, 553, 574, 595, 623). The second wave for three classes of crypts of the guinea pig ascending colon attains a level of between 0.25 and 0.6 varying with the crypt segment and the crypt-length class. This may be a source of erroneous calculations of the cell cycle duration. Usually, for calculation of the overall cell cycle time, the following inter-point measurements of FLM curve can be carried out:

(a) between the ascending limb of the first wave and that of the second, at the level of 50 percent;

(b) between the ascending limb of the first wave and that of the second, at the level of 25 percent;

(c) between the maximum of the first wave or the middle of the plateau and the maximum of the second wave or the middle of the plateau.

The first measurement could not be used for FLM curves of the guinea pig colon, since the maximum values of the second wave, at least of some curves, were lower than 50 percent. Therefore only the two latter measurements were applied. An alternative method which could be used is the fitting of a computer-simulated FLM curve to the experimental data (670); but this was not applied here. The damping of the second FLM wave could be interpreted in various ways. One possibility is that it is an effect of the considerable spread of G_1-phase times of individual cells. The other explanation includes the concept of the G_0-phase, which is characterised by a fixed rate of cell release into a G_1-phase and not by a definite duration (75). Damping of the second wave of labelled mitoses is expected when the FLM curve relates to a cell population composed of two or more sub-populations differing in G_1-phase duration, and it can be supposed that this occurs in the middle segments of long and medium crypts of the guinea pig colon. Nevertheless, the rate of damping, and the rather poor resolution of the two peaks of the second wave of FLM curves, calls for additional explanations, eg, a spread of G_1-phase duration or the occurrence of a G_0-phase. The experimental data available at present cannot distinguish between these interpretations.

Yet another model for the interpretation of the diversity in shape of the second FLM wave has been proposed (268). The model assumes a branching of the G_1-phase, which is composed of a number of sub-phases. The cells have the option of proceeding from mitosis to DNA synthesis through different sequences of the G_1 sub-phases. Therefore, the various shapes of the second waves of FLM curves could be explained as resulting from variation of the proportion of cells which pass through different sequences of G_1 sub-phases. In terms of a branching structure of G_1-phase, the majority of proliferating cells in the upper segment of the colonic crypt of the guinea pig would pass through the shortest possible sequence, while a substantial fraction of cells in the lower segments would spend some additional time when passing through side branches of the G_1-phase. Although speculative, the hypothesis of a branching structure of G_1-phase can explain the variation of G_1-phase time.

With all these reservations on the interpretation of FLM curves, it can be concluded that proliferating crypt cells in the ascending colon of the guinea pig consist of at least two subpopulations of cells in respect of cell cycle time. One subpopulation is characterised by a T_c of between 13 h and 16 h and occurs along the entire length of short crypts and in the upper and middle segments of medium and long crypts. The second subpopulation is characterised by a T_c of between 22 h and 26 h and the cells which comprise this subpopulation are located in the middle and lower segments of medium and long crypts. The difference in the duration of cell cycle of these two subpopulations is chiefly caused by a change in G_1-phase, which is about 9 hours longer in the latter than in the former subpopulation. Besides the changes in G_1-phase duration, a pronounced modulation of duration of mitosis was also evident along the crypt. In the region close to the bottom mitosis lasted 3 h, while in the region close to the mouth it was only 1 h.

Furthermore, it may be assumed that a third separate cell sub-population occurs in lower segments of medium and long crypts, with T_c longer than 26 h, and including a G_0 phase.

A number of studies indicate that epithelial crypt cells of the intestine of adult mammals are heterogeneous in respect of their cell cycle duration (6, 83, 553, 595, 623). Thus the cells situated in the crypt region close to the bottom were found to have longer T_c than those situated close to the mouth. The differences found along the crypt were chiefly due to changeable G_1-phase duration, which is in accordance with the results of cell cycle analysis of the guinea pig colon (595). The difference between cells located at various heights of the crypt was more pronounced in the large than in the small bowel, as the direct comparative studies of small and large bowel of the rat indicated (553). The only studies which show no changes in cell cycle time along the crypt are those done on mouse descending colon (98) (see Section 1.4).

1.3.3 CELL GENERATIONS IN THE COLONIC CRYPT

The labelling indices, I_s, calculated for each cell position in the crypt, and the cell cycle phases in various segments of crypts, provide sufficient information to design a model of successive generations of cells along the crypt. For this, a method described earlier (98) can be applied. The calculation of the number of cell divisions, d, in each cell position along the crypt, accounting for the difference between the efflux, k_{out}, and influx, k_{in}, of cells for this cell position is given by

$$k_{out} = k_{in}2^d,$$

where k_{in} for a given cell position, n, is assumed to be the cumulative birth rate, I_s/t_s, for cell positions 1 . . . n − 1, and k_{out} is calculated as the sum of k_{in} and the birth rate for cell position n.

The medium-sized crypts were selected to design the model of successive generations of crypt cells. The I_s for each cell position has been calculated previously (624); t_s was taken to be 7.5 h (595).

The numbers of successive divisions along the crypt were deduced according to the values of the cumulative number of divisions for each cell position (98).

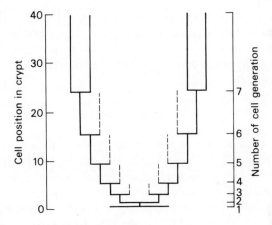

Figure 1.3.4 Cell generations along the length of the colonic crypt

The results of calculation show that there are on average seven successive divisions, beginning with the stem cells at the crypt bottom, through the proliferating but 'committed' cells, to the non-proliferating cells in the upper segment of colonic crypt. The first five divisions occur in the lower segment of the crypt, the sixth division appears in the middle segment, whereas the seventh division is in the upper segment of the crypt (Figure 1.3.4).

The comparison between the distribution of the seven cell generations along the crypt and that of proliferating cells of long (23 to 26 h) and short (13 to 16 h) cell cycle seems to indicate that the first six cell generations of the crypt have a relatively long cell cycle, whereas the seventh cell generation has a short cell cycle. The bimodal character of the second wave of the FLM curve for the middle segment of medium crypts could be interpreted as resulting from partial mixing of the sixth and seventh cell generations in this segment.

The model of cell generations along the crypt does not account for the existence of various cell types (columnar, goblet and enteroendocrine) present in the colonic epithelium. Since the crypt columnar cells are most numerous, the model reflects preferentially the proliferative behaviour of this cell type.

Similar models were proposed previously for the descending colon of the mouse (98) indicating about 3 cell generations, and for jejunum of the mouse and rat (403, 552), suggesting 4 and 14 cell generations respectively.

Six cell generations were deduced for the crypts of the ascending colon of the rat (552); this figure agrees satisfactorily with that of the guinea pig colon.

1.3.3.1 STEM CELLS OF THE COLONIC CRYPT

The model of cell generations for the colonic crypt (Figure 1.3.4) showed that the first division of epithelial cells along the crypt appears in the bottom two cell positions. The assumption can be made that such division is of stem cells (403). If this assumption is correct, the number of stem cells, N_S, can roughly be estimated from the formula:

$$\frac{N_s}{N} = \frac{I_s}{t_s/T_C}$$

where N is the total number of cells in the region of stem cell occurrence, I_s is the labelling index, T_C is the cell cycle time and t_S is the duration of the S phase. This formula is usually applied for the calculation of cell number within the cell cycle and here it is assumed that all proliferating cells situated at cell positions 1 and 2 of the colonic crypt are stem cells. Therefore, for the lower segments of colonic crypts of the guinea pig the experimental data obtained previously (595, 621) were taken and used in the calculation: $I_s = 2.5$ percent,

Table 1.3.1 A dynamic model of the guinea pig colonic crypt

Crypt length (cells)	35
Column count	15
Total crypt population (cells)	520
Number of stem cells	1 to 3
Number of proliferating cells	170
Number of cell generations	7
Cell cycle time (h): first 6 generations	25
7th generation	15
Migration rate at top of crypt (cell positions/h)	0.75
Crypt cell production rate (cells/crypt/h)	10 to 12
Transit time to cell position 10 (h)	236
Transit time between positions 10 and 39 (h)	53

$T_c = 26$ h, $t_s = 7.5$ h, and N is between 15 and 30 cells in cell positions 1 and 2. Then N_s is between 1 and 3 stem cells per crypt.

1.3.4 DYNAMIC MODEL OF THE COLONIC CRYPT

The results obtained from the study of cell proliferation and differentiation (594, 621, 623, 624) in the ascending colon of the guinea pig have been summarised in Table 1.3.1.

ACKNOWLEDGEMENTS

The original research was supported in part by the grants II 1 and PR 6.

1.4 Cell Proliferation in the Mouse Large Bowel, with Details of the Analysis of the Experimental Data

D R Appleton, J P Sunter, M S B de Rodriguez, and A J Watson

1.4.1 INTRODUCTION

The morphometric and cytokinetic characteristics of the colonic mucosa of normal mice have been described in a number of reports, but there are apparent discrepancies between the findings of different groups of workers. For example, the mean crypt height has been reported as 20 cells (427) and 29 cells (95); the tritiated thymidine (^{3}HTdR) labelling activity has been found to be highest in the middle portion of the crypt (427, 472), but has also been described as highest at the bottom and falling steadily with rising cell position (95, 574); estimates of cell cycle time (T_c) have varied between about 16 and 27 h (98, 244, 427, 542).

We have previously described the differences in cytokinetic organisation of the crypts at different sites in the rat colon (689), and this report extends our description of similar variation in the colon of the mouse (589, 685), which may be sufficient to account for some of the inconsistencies in the literature. We have used simple morphometry, the stathmokinetic technique, and autoradiographic methods including the fraction of labelled mitoses (FLM) experiment, at four representative sites in the mouse colon, namely (i) the descending colon (30 percent of the distance from the anus to the ileocaecal valve), (ii) the transverse colon (60 percent of the distance from the anus), (iii) the ascending colon (90 percent of the distance from the anus), and (iv) the caecum (at the junction of the distal and middle thirds of the caecoappendix).

1.4.2 MATERIALS AND METHODS

Male A2G mice 12 weeks old, weighing between 20 and 25 g and convention-ally managed were used throughout. They were fed on 14 percent rat cake (dried milk) and had unlimited access to tap water. In order to minimise the effect on proliferative indices of circadian variation (93, 287, 652) all experiments were begun at 0900 h.

1.4.2.1 MITOTIC AND LABELLING INDICES

Four animals were given ^{3}HTdR of specific activity 5 Ci per mMole by intraperitoneal injection at a dosage of 1 μCi per g body weight. After one hour they were killed by cervical dislocation and their colons removed in continuity with the caecoappendix. The colon was opened along its length, cleaned, and pinned mucosal surface uppermost to a cork board. After fixation for 6 h in Carnoy's solution, transected segments of bowel were taken from the four sites described, and processed through to paraffin wax in the usual way. Autoradiographs were prepared on 3 μm serial sections using a dipping technique, and were exposed for two weeks.

One hundred perfect axially sectioned crypts were located in each sample and the left-hand crypt columns as they presented were analysed. The total number of cells in the column was counted and the positions of mitoses and labelled cells were noted. For each of the selected sites within the bowel, overall mitotic (I_m) and labelling (I_s) index distribution curves were produced by combining the data from the 4 animals and expressing them in terms of a crypt column whose length was the mean of all crypt columns counted at each site (82, 818).

1.4.2.2 STATHMOKINETIC EXPERIMENT

Eleven animals were given an intraperitoneal injection of 1 mg per kg body weight of vincristine sulphate and killed at 15 minute intervals thereafter. The colons were fixed in Carnoy's solution and samples taken from the same 4 sites as before. Serial 3 μm sections were prepared and stained with Harris's haemotoxylin. Again the left sides of 100 axially sectioned crypts were studied, the number of cells per column and the positions of arrested metaphases being recorded. That the stathmokinetic agent was effective in material taken 30 min and longer after administration was confirmed by the absence of any post-metaphase mitotic figures.

In 4 animals from this group the numbers of cells appearing in transverse sections of crypts (the column count) were calculated from 50 such sections at each site in each animal. From the same sections estimates were also made of the correction factors (Tannock's factor) which must be applied to mitotic indices observed in axial sections to compensate for the displacement of mitotic figures towards the lumen of the crypt (702).

1.4.2.3 FLM EXPERIMENT

Thirty-six mice were given ^{3}HTdR by intraperitoneal injection at a dosage of 1 μCi per g body weight, and one animal was killed at hourly intervals for 24 h and thereafter at two-hourly intervals until 48 h. Autoradiographs were prepared as before for each of the four sites in the bowel. The cells in the crypts were divided into groups of 4 cell positions starting at the base of the crypt, and in each group at least 20 mitoses were examined for the presence of label. Thus an FLM curve was constructed for each of the cell position groups, and the phase durations and their variability were estimated (251). An FLM curve for the crypt as a whole was derived by calculating the mean proportion of mitoses labelled, weighted according to the distribution of mitoses within the crypt.

Table 1.4.1 Morphometric and mitotic index data for the whole crypt

	Descending colon	Transverse colon	Ascending colon	Caecum
Crypt column length (cells)	31.1	34.7	19.3	25.3
Number of columns per crypt	22.5	19.6	16.2	25.0
Total number of cells per crypt	700	680	310	630
Observed mitotic index (%)	2.15	1.58	2.04	1.79
Tannock's factor	0.62	0.53	0.57	0.61
Corrected mitotic index (%)	1.33	0.84	1.16	1.09
Birth rate (cells/1000 cells/h)	26	13	16	18
Mitotic duration t_m(h)	0.5	0.7	0.7	0.6

1.4.3 RESULTS

The mean crypt length and the mean column count for each of the 4 sites in the bowel are shown in Table 1.4.1. In the descending and transverse colon, crypts are of a similar length, but in the ascending colon they are much shorter; in the caecum they are of intermediate length, though of a greater circumference. An approximate estimate of the total number of cells per crypt has been found from the product of these two measurements; in the ascending colon there are about half as many cells per crypt as in the other sites.

The data from the stathmokinetic experiment treating the crypt as a whole are presented in Figure 1.4.1; the solid lines have been fitted by least squares to the points from 30 min onward when we are sure that vincristine is fully effective. If the age distribution is known the slopes of these lines can be used to give estimates of k_B, the cell birth rate (see Section 1.4.5.1). The mitotic duration, t_m, can be found, albeit imprecisely, from the ratio of the mitotic index at time zero, I_m, to k_B, and is given in Table 1.4.1 along with the values

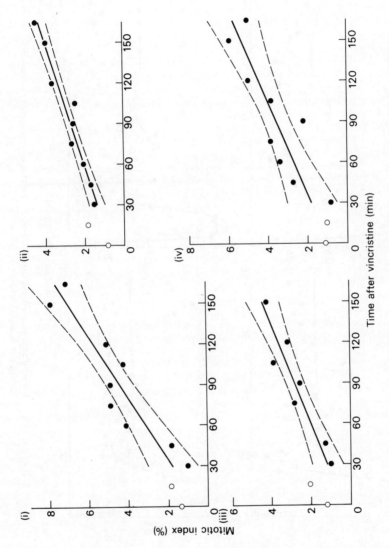

Figure 1.4.1 Mitotic accumulation data for the whole crypt after administration of vincristine, showing fitted lines and 95% confidence limits. Figures (i)–(iv) correspond to the sites in the bowel described in Section 1.4.1

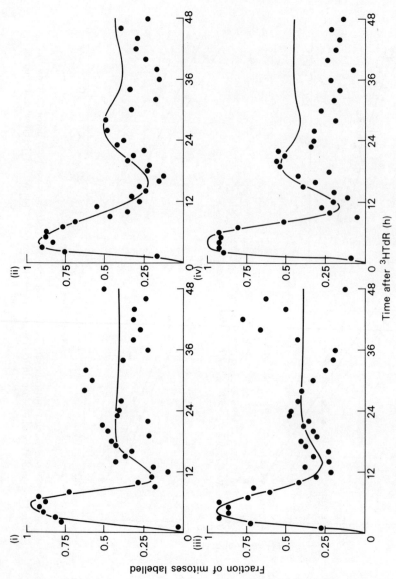

Figure 1.4.2 FLM data for the whole crypt, showing fitted curves. Figures (i)–(iv) correspond to the sites in the bowel described in Section 1.4.1

of these other variables. I_m is presented as it was observed and as it has been corrected by Tannock's factor; the indices in Figure 1.4.1 have all been corrected.

The results of the FLM experiment for the crypts as a whole, and the curves fitted (see Section 1.4.5.2) are shown in Figure 1.4.2. The estimates of the phase durations and the coefficient of variation of T_c are detailed in Table 1.4.2.

Table 1.4.2 Autoradiographic data for the whole crypt

	Descending colon	Transverse colon	Ascending colon	Caecum
t_{G_1} (h)	7.0	10.3	9.4	6.7
t_s (h)	6.2	8.8	7.4	6.8
t_{G_2} (h)	1.8	1.4	1.4	1.2
Cell cycle time T_c (h)	15.5	21.2	18.9	15.3
Coefficient of variation of T_c (%)	43	27	45	30
Theoretical labelling index (%)	43	45	44	48
Observed labelling index (%)	11.7	12.1	12.3	13.5
Growth fraction (%)	27	27	28	28
Total number of proliferating cells per crypt	190	180	90	180
Birth rate (cells/1000 cells/h)	21	14	19	20

The quality of fit is poor for later times, but estimates are probably reasonably accurate since the fit over the first 24 h is adequate. Cell cycle times vary from 15.5 h in the descending colon to 21.2 h in the transverse colon. From the age distribution and the cell cycle parameters a theoretical value for the labelling index if all cells were proliferating may be found, and the proportion of this which is actually observed is an estimate of the growth fraction (see Section 1.4.5.3). Taking this in conjunction with the total number of cells per crypt we can estimate the number of proliferating cells, and from the growth fraction and the cell cycle time we can obtain an estimate of the birth rate independent of that given in Table 1.4.1 (see Section 1.4.5.1). Values for all these variables are given in Table 1.4.2.

By treating each cell position in the crypt separately and performing a total of 110 regression analyses we may calculate the birth rate at each cell position in

Table 1.4.3 Data from mitotic indices at each cell position

	Descending colon	Transverse colon	Ascending colon	Caecum
Cumulative mitotic index (cells/column)	0.36	0.28	0.25	0.28
Cumulative birth rate (cells/column/h)	0.93	0.44	0.36	0.43
Mitotic duration t_m (h)	0.39	0.64	0.69	0.65
Crypt cell production rate (cells/h)	20.9	8.6	5.8	10.8
Cut-off position (cells from crypt base)	8.9	16.7	7.2	8.4

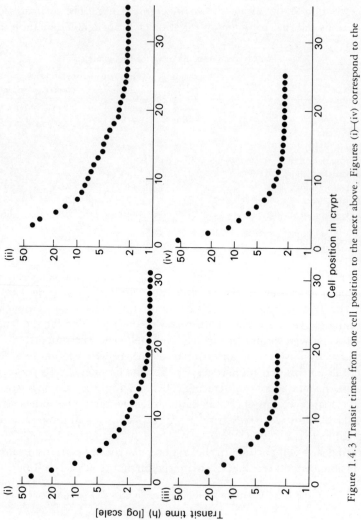

Figure 1.4.3 Transit times from one cell position to the next above. Figures (i)–(iv) correspond to the sites in the bowel described in Section 1.4.1

the four sites. Table 1.4.3 shows the resulting cumulative birth rate or migration rate at the top of the crypt. By dividing this into the cumulative mitotic index an estimate of the mitotic duration may be obtained, which is probably better than the one previously found (589). We may also calculate, from the cumulative birth rate and the column count, the rate of cell production by the crypt; the crypts of the descending colon are producing about 21 cells per hour, some 3 or 4 times more than the short crypts of the ascending colon.

Estimates of the average cell position at which a cell last undergoes a mitosis which gives rise to two proliferating daughter cells (the cut-off position (84)) may also be calculated from the birth rates at each cell position. This involves the derivation of the transit time from a particular cell position to the one above (see Section 1.4.5.4) and these times are shown in Figure 1.4.3. The estimates of the cut-off positions given in Table 1.4.3 suggest that the growth control mechanisms in the transverse colon are rather different from those in the other sites.

Figure 1.4.4 shows the labelling index distribution diagrams for each of the four sites. In the descending colon highest values are found at the bottom of the crypt and there is a steady fall towards the top. In the ascending colon, however, maximum I_s occurs in the middle of the crypt; the transverse colon shows an intermediate pattern, and in the caecum highest values, which are greater than at other sites, are again near the bottom of the crypt.

The cell cycle times derived from the 18 FLM curves resulting from treating each group of 4 proliferative cells separately are given in Table 1.4.4. There are

Table 1.4.4 Cell cycle times (h) for different parts of the crypt

Cell position	Descending colon	Transverse colon	Ascending colon	Caecum
1–4	15.3	22.0	20.6	15.3
5–8	14.9	21.7	18.2	15.5
9–12	15.8	22.0	20.4	16.0
13–16	16.3	20.9	20.0	12.9
17–20	15.4	20.1		

no obvious differences in T_c between different cell position groups within the crypt at any site. From the observed labelling indices of Figure 1.4.4 and the cell cycle phase durations at any cell position we can calculate how the growth fraction (I_p) varies in the crypt (see Section 1.4.5.3), and this is shown in Table 1.4.5. Even in the areas of maximum proliferative activity the growth fraction is well below unity.

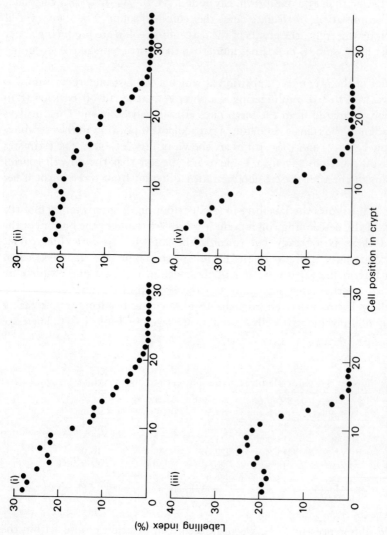

Figure 1.4.4 Labelling index distribution within the crypt. Figures (i)–(iv) correspond to the sites in the bowel described in Section 1.4.1

Table 1.4.5 Growth fraction (%) in different parts of the crypt

Cell Position	Descending colon	Transverse colon	Ascending colon	Caecum
1–4	53	48	44	76
5–8	49	50	54	74
9–12	41	49	53	42
13–16	24	43	10	10
17–20	9	39		

1.4.4 DISCUSSION

We have calculated for the descending colon a mean crypt length of 31 cells, which agrees closely with previous estimates of 29 cells (95) and 28 to 32 cells (574) in two communications where the site in the descending colon from which the material was taken was described in precise anatomical terms. In the transverse colon we have found that the mean crypt length is slightly greater, whereas in the ascending colon it is only 19 cells, close to the value of 20 cells obtained in material from both ascending and sigmoid colon (427), though it is not known whether these two sites were morphologically similar. Our approximate estimates of the total number of cells per crypt show that the ascending colon with 310 cells has less than half the population of the other sites investigated. This number is close to the 358 cells calculated from whole crypt squashes (378) in material whose precise site of origin was not given, but which has the type of distribution of labelled cells which we and others (427, 472) have observed in ascending colon. The distribution of labelled nuclei in the crypts of the descending colon is quite different, with labelling most intense at the bottom of the crypt and falling steadily with rising cell position. This is the sort of pattern previously described in studies on the descending colon (95, 574). In the transverse colon there is an intermediate pattern of distribution of labelled cells.

From the analysis of FLM data we have derived estimates of T_c for the whole crypt at each of the sites in the bowel: the mean values of 15.5 h in descending colon, 21.2 h in transverse colon, 18.9 h in ascending colon and 15.3 h in caecum lead to estimates of cell birth rate similar to those obtained from analysis of the stathmokinetic experiment, after taking the growth fraction and the age distribution into account. Other cell cycle time estimates based on FLM data are to be found in the literature: 19 h (707) and 23 h (98) in descending colon, 16 h in ascending colon (427). We have analysed FLM curves for separate cell position groups within the crypts, and in none of the sites have we demonstrated any differences in T_c within the crypt, though cell migration during the experiment could be masking these.

It has been calculated that between 35 percent and 52 percent of colonic crypt cells are in the 'proliferative zone' (378) while the 'proliferative compartment size' has been estimated as 37 percent of the total crypt cell population (281). We have estimated I_p for the whole crypt from labelling index data and the cell cycle parameters. The values are virtually the same at all sites, just under 30 percent, though lower than those cited because within that zone of the crypt broadly termed the proliferative compartment I_p is, as we have demonstrated, by no means 100 percent. In absolute terms the crypts of the ascending colon contain about 100 proliferating cells, whereas in the other sites the figure is about 200. However, it is the transverse colon which stands out as being different in terms of the average position at which cells begin their final cycle, where it is twice as far up the crypt as at the other sites.

There are therefore many differences in the kinetic organisation of the crypts at different sites in the mouse colon. Similar differences occur in the large bowel of the rat (688), and, while the two species do not exhibit quite the same pattern of variability, it should be remembered that we have chosen to sample our tissues from anatomically well defined regions rather than from morphologically or functionally equivalent sites.

1.4.5 METHODS OF ANALYSING CELL KINETIC DATA FROM THE INTESTINAL CRYPT

Many of the variables whose values have been derived in this description of cell proliferation in the mouse large bowel are merely the product or the ratio of other variables which have been observed directly; these present no problem, save that it is worth remembering that errors present in the original data are magnified in quantities derived from them, even if the relationship used to calculate them is exact. Usually this effect is compounded by the necessity to make assumptions about the system under consideration before being able to calculate what we may regard as its most useful descriptors. We may be tacitly ignoring known complications such as circadian rhythm, variability in cell cycle phases, or experimental artifacts, or we may be making certain assumptions with regard to the age distribution of cells or their mode of migration. Some of the methods we have used are worthy of further explanation.

1.4.5.1 STATHMOKINETIC EXPERIMENTS

The stathmokinetic experiment has frequently been employed rather uncritically, but carefully used it can give good estimates of the cell birth rate (815). It generally provides only poor estimates of the mitotic duration, and unless the age distribution of cells is known, good estimates of the turnover time cannot be obtained.

For the crypt as a whole we have assumed a rectangular age distribution for proliferating cells, and the values we give for the birth rate are the slopes of the lines relating mitotic index to time after administration of vincristine. For the individual cell positions we have assumed exponential age distributions; this is a good approximation over the most highly proliferative part of the crypt, and the fact that it is far from true near the top of the crypt does not greatly affect the estimate of cumulative birth rate.

We have estimated so many values for this report that to give standard errors of all the estimates would be cumbersome, but it is important to have some idea of the precision of the principal analytical methods. Assuming that the mitotic indices on which we base our calculations are correct, which implies among other things that Tannock's factor exactly compensates for the preferential counting of mitoses, we may expect the standard error of the birth rate to be about 15 percent of the estimate itself; the standard error of the cumulative birth rate is about half this. In fact, as we have indicated, such correction factors as Tannock's and the one for birth rate given below are also subject to uncertainty. By using them we increase the imprecision of our calculated values, but we gain greatly in accuracy.

We have estimated birth rates from autoradiographic data which compare well with those estimated from the stathmokinetic experiment. We shall discuss later the FLM method of obtaining an estimate of the cell cycle time (Section 1.4.5.2) and how the growth fraction should be calculated (Section 1.4.5.3), but even if these quantities are known it is not as straightforward as it seems to estimate the birth rate. For a rectangular age distribution, for instance, the relationship $k_B = I_p/T_c$ has been used (120), but it can be shown (29) that this leads to an underestimate of k_B and that a better estimate is found by dividing this estimate by $1 - CV^2$ where CV is the coefficient of variation of the cell cycle time expressed as a proportion. This correction factor must also be borne in mind when estimates of turnover time or cell cycle time are made from stathmokinetic data.

1.4.5.2 FLM EXPERIMENTS

Most of the methods of analysing FLM experiments in current use make broadly similar assumptions and give comparable estimates of the cell cycle phase durations (301). We have shown in the previous section how important it is to obtain and use estimates of the coefficient of variation of the cell cycle time. It is also important to have some idea of the standard errors of the estimates of phase times. The method we use (251) gives standard errors, and those for the cell cycle time in the 22 FLM curves we analysed averaged one hour. We have already stated (6) that we regard these standard errors as being too low by a factor of between 2 and 3 in the small bowel, and can only emphasise this opinion in the light of the poorer fits we obtain in the colon.

Another point which is sometimes overlooked by using the simplistic terminology 'the cell cycle time at cell position x' is that by the end of an FLM experiment lasting 48 h, a cell which began as low as position 8 could have migrated right out of the crypt. Thus it is not clear what precisely it is that such an FLM is estimating, and it may be largely because of migration that no differences in cell cycle times at different positions were apparent. A comprehensive model of the crypt is required so that estimates of 'the cell cycle time of a cell born at position x' may be found.

1.4.5.3 ESTIMATING THE GROWTH FRACTION

Estimates of the growth fraction may be made by calculating what proportion the observed labelling index is of a theoretical index which would occur if all cells were cycling. To calculate this latter quantity it is necessary to know the durations of the phases of the cell cycle and the age distribution of cycling cells. However, the usual formulae (120):

$$I_s^{theoret} = t_s/T_c$$

for a rectangular age distribution and

$$I_s^{theoret} = \{1 - \exp(-0.693 \, t_s/T_c)\} \exp\{0.693 \, (1 - t_{G_1}/T_c)\}$$

for an exponential age distribution do not take into account variability in phase durations, and can lead to quite erroneous estimates (27). Figure 1.4.5

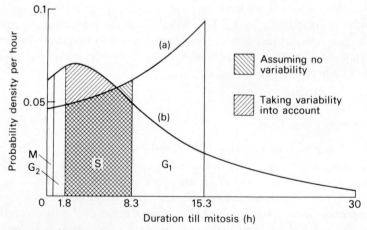

Figure 1.4.5 Distribution of times remaining till the end of mitosis for an exponential age distribution with $t_{G_1} = 7.0$ h, $t_s = 6.5$ h, $t_{G_2} = 1.2$ h and $t_m = 0.6$ h assuming (a) a constant cell cycle time and (b) a CV of T_c of 51%

illustrates the case of the bottom 4 cell positions of the caecum. Straightforward application of the formula for an exponential age distribution yields a value for $I_s^{theoret}$ of 0.37, and since the labelling index is 0.34 (see Figure 1.4.4) a growth fraction of 92 percent would be obtained, implying that virtually all cells in this region were proliferating. However, the coefficient of variation of the cell cycle time is 51 percent, and calculation of the area corresponding to labelled cells, which lies under the correct distribution of times remaining until the end of mitosis, gives $I_s^{theoret}$ as 0.45, and hence a considerably lower growth fraction of 76 percent, as shown in Table 1.4.5. When there is little variability in cell cycle time the usual formulae are adequate, but when the coefficient of variation is greater than about 25 percent it is advisable to take it into account. Either overestimates or underestimates of growth fraction may result from ignoring the variability, depending on the relative position in the cycle of the S-phase.

1.4.5.4 ESTIMATING THE CUT-OFF POSITION

Different measurements have been employed to quantify the size of the 'proliferative compartment' (120) in the crypt. In our previous reports on the cell kinetics of the small bowel (814) and the large bowel (689) we have calculated the cell position at which the labelling index falls to half of its maximum value; this was done by projecting individual crypts onto one of average length (82, 818). Another possible method is to calculate the mean position over a number of crypts of the highest labelled cell (287). Both these methods are less than completely satisfactory because the cell position they define will be moved up the crypt not only by a real increase in the extent of the proliferation zone caused by more transit divisions, but also by a decrease in cell cycle time or an increase in growth fraction within the proliferation compartment (28). It is possible to calculate the number of transit divisions from stathmokinetic and FLM data (814), but we believe that the best single descriptive measurement is the cut-off position (84): the average position at which a cell enters its final cycle. We have described a simple calculation (28) based on working out from transit times where a cell at the position of half maximum mitotic index near the end of a stathmokinetic experiment would have been a certain time previously. This calculation does not take into account all of the aspects of the 'slow cut-off model' (84) but we feel that it is adequate to draw clear distinctions between crypts with different characteristics.

ACKNOWLEDGEMENTS

This work was supported by a grant from the North of England Council of the Cancer Research Campaign. We would like to thank Mrs E Wallace and Mrs M Hughes for preparing the histological sections.

SECTION 2

GROWTH CONTROL IN NORMAL EXPERIMENTAL ANIMALS

2.1 Some Speculations on Control Mechanisms of Cell Proliferation in Intestinal Epithelium

R P C Rijke

2.1.1 INTRODUCTION

When in 1972, I started to work in the field of cell proliferation of the small intestinal epithelium, one of the most basic questions for me was why the prevalence of malignant tumours was so low in the small intestine, particularly in comparison with the colon. I was impressed by the very orderly appearance of the small-intestinal epithelium. Also, it was difficult to imagine the very fast turnover of the epithelium when looking at microscope slides. My preliminary idea was that very efficient regulating mechanisms must be operating in the small-intestinal epithelium, and so I set out to investigate them, and here I present my findings.

Epithelial cell proliferation of the small intestine and the colon differ in some respects and are similar in others (194, 422, 587). Both epithelia are cell renewing systems which have been found to adapt to altered circumstances and to respond to damage. In this paper we shall speculate on the control mechanisms underlying the changes in epithelial cell proliferation which occur under various circumstances. This will be done largely in relation to the small-intestinal epithelium, since relatively little is known about cell proliferation in the colon, but some comments on the differences in epithelial cell proliferation between large and small bowel will be included, and the implications for carcinogenesis discussed.

2.1.2 SMALL-INTESTINAL EPITHELIUM

The epithelial lining of the small intestine is a cell renewing system in which cells are continuously lost from the villi and replaced by newly formed cells from the crypts (43, 47, 406, 407). The size of the functional villus cell population is dependent on the balance between cell production and cell loss, while flexibility would make it possible to meet with perturbations of the system and with new functional situations. The regulatory mechanisms which are responsible for maintaining the balance between cell production and cell loss in this epithelium are still largely unknown, although much knowledge has been gathered on the many factors which may influence the intestinal epithelium.

2.1.2.1 EPITHELIAL CELL PROLIFERATION IN THE SMALL INTESTINE

The functional capacity of the small-intestinal epithelium depends primarily on the number of villus cells in the small intestine (see Figure 2.1.1), since adaptive changes in enzyme activities do not occur (56, 181, 254, 319, 470, 578, 586, 783). Marked changes in enzyme activities have only been found when an increase in crypt cell production was brought about by an enlargement of the proliferation compartment in the crypt: then enzyme activities were reduced (54, 56, 176, 246, 578, 583).

Since the number of villi in the small intestine seems to be constant (85, 110, 235), the size of the functional villus cell population in the small intestine depends on the size of the individual villi. Although available techniques for the determination of the number of cells per villus are not completely satisfactory, changes in the number of villus cells may be found by counting them in two-dimensional tissue sections; the three-dimensional structure of the villi, however, should always be borne in mind (20, 113). Our experience is that the changes in the three-dimensional structure are even more pronounced than the changes in the number of cells per villus column (299, 586).

The number of cells per villus is determined by the rate of cell supply from the crypts and by the time that an epithelial cell is present on the villus (transit time on the villus) which may be determined by calculating the migration rate of the cells along the villus column. In several studies it has been found that no large variations in the transit time on the villus occur under a variety of circumstances including recovery after irradiation (584) and adaptive changes in which the villus cell population is either enlarged or reduced (300, 582, 586). Exact knowledge of the lifespan of epithelial villus cells under various conditions is, however, still lacking.

The *crypt-villus ratio*, the number of crypts per villus, has been shown to increase with age (110, 116), and from the ileocaecal valve to the pylorus (110, 243). Although new crypts may be formed by fission following high doses of X-irradiation (85), and occasionally in normal animals (110, 297), the crypt–villus ratio has been found not to change under a number of circumstances such as fasting, lactation, and experimental bypass, transposition or resection of

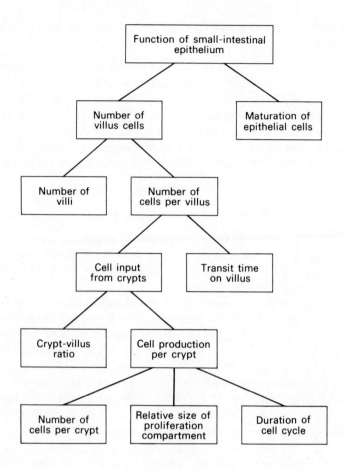

Figure 2.1.1 Schematic representation of the interrelationships of cytokinetic parameters in small-intestinal epithelium

intestinal segments (110, 112, 114, 197, 300, 586). Hence the cell production
rate per crypt determines the number of cells per villus, and hence the number
of functional villus cells in the small intestine.

The cell production rate per crypt is determined by the number of cells per
crypt, the relative size of the proliferation compartment in the crypt (the
'growth fraction'), and the duration of the cell cycle of the proliferating crypt
cells. These three parameters of crypt cell proliferation have all been shown to
change in various circumstances.

2.1.2.2 CONTROL MECHANISMS OF CELL PRODUCTION IN SMALL-INTESTINAL CRYPTS

It appears that cell production in small-intestinal crypts may change in two ways. In recent years we have put forward the hypothesis that these reflect two separate control mechanisms regulating crypt cell production (578, 579). The first, which would regulate the relative size of the proliferation compartment in the crypt, has tentatively been termed the *feedback control mechanism of crypt cell production*. The second mechanism, which would regulate the total size of the crypt, has been termed the *adaptive control mechanism of crypt cell production*.

2.1.2.3 FEEDBACK CONTROL MECHANISM OF CRYPT CELL PRODUCTION

A reduction of the functional villus cell population leads to a rapid rise in crypt cell production. This is brought about by an increase in the relative size of the proliferation compartment in the crypt, which decreases again after recovery of the villus cell population.

This hypothesis is derived from studies on coeliac disease (724, 823), on the influence of X-irradiation on the intestinal epithelium (247, 584, 585, 620), and on the effect of villus cell loss which was induced by temporary ischaemia (583). It was also found that this feedback control is a local mechanism in the small intestine (583), and that experimental bypass has no influence on it (578).

It seems that some shortening of the cell cycle time of the proliferating crypt cells occurs during recovery of the villus cell population (78, 411, 415). However, since the cell cycle time is normally so short in the small-intestinal crypt, this probably contributes little to the observed increase in cell production.

A similar increase in the relative size of the proliferation compartment was also observed in several studies in which surgical procedures were carried out on the small intestine. In these experiments a small increase occurred throughout the small intestine 2 to 4 days after surgery (586, 587). This may reflect a perturbation of the feedback control mechanism by the surgical procedures or a nonspecific effect of temporary changes in blood flow or innervation. Although the changes which were observed after surgery were small, this may present an argument against a feedback control mechanism of crypt cell production by the villus cell population, and in favour of a nonspecific 'wound response'.

2.1.2.4 ADAPTIVE CONTROL MECHANISM OF CRYPT CELL PRODUCTION

The adaptive control mechanism would regulate the total size of the crypt without changing the relative size of the proliferation compartment in the crypt, and hence regulate the size of the villus cell compartment by changing crypt cell production. When the relative size of the proliferation compartment in the crypt remains constant, the cell production rate per crypt is determined by the total number of cells per crypt, provided large variations in other parameters (eg the cell cycle time) do not occur. A shortening of the cell cycle time was found during lactation (300) and after partial resection of the small intestine (296, 466), but the differences were too small to explain the large increases in crypt cell production. Consequently, the size of the functional villus cell compartment is determined by the rate of cell production in the crypt, since the life span of the epithelial cells does not change under the circumstances in which the epithelium shows an adaptive response (300, 582, 586).

Such an adaptive response of crypt cell production to altered circumstances has been found after partial resection of the small intestine (296–299, 466), after ileojejunal transposition (582), after bypass of an intestinal segment (299, 586), and during lactation (300). The adaptive response starts between two and four days after the change in circumstances and stops after approximately 14 days when a new equilibrium has been reached (298, 582, 586). A similar response has also been observed after prolonged administration of the carcinogen dimethylhydrazine (686).

The mechanism by which the crypt is enlarged or reduced in the adaptive response is still unknown. The enlargement of the crypt which has been found after partial resection of the small intestine and during lactation is accompanied by some shortening of the cell cycle time in the crypt (296, 300, 466). It is possible that this is due to a shortening of the cell cycle time in all proliferating crypt cells, which could lead to an increase in crypt size. Theoretically, it seems more likely that a decrease in the cell cycle time of the functional stem cells in the bottom of the crypt (403, 534) would cause this increase. The cell cycle time of these cells in the bottom of the crypt is longer than that of the cells higher in the crypt (6, 83, 818), and a considerable decrease in the cell cycle time specifically in this stem cell compartment would only lead to relatively little shortening of the overall cell cycle time in the crypt. A small shortening of the cell cycle time specific to the bottom of the crypt has been found in enlarged crypts after prolonged administration of dimethylhydrazine (686).

The adaptive control mechanism of crypt cell production may act locally (112, 582, 586), or, after partial resection of the small intestine, systemically (299). Studies on the systemic response of the small-intestinal epithelium to resection have shown that the response is not mediated by a humoral factor (365) (but see Section 4.4).

Many factors have been proposed to account for the great potential of the small-intestinal epithelium to adapt to various circumstances in which the demands on the intestinal epithelium change, such as during lactation or after surgical procedures leading to an altered luminal environment (17, 181, 220, 299, 300, 577, 734). However, all these influences, like blood flow, innervation, local hormones and luminal factors, affect each other and are intimately interwoven in the micro-environment of the epithelial cells. They probably act in combination to induce an adaptive response of the intestinal epithelium, as has been shown for the response to lactation (300). However, the underlying mechanism leading to an increase or a decrease in the number of cells per crypt is still unknown.

In conclusion, it seems that the number of cells per villus, and hence the number of functional villus cells in the small intestine, is determined by the rate of cell production per crypt. This may be indicated by a change either in the total number of cells per crypt, or in the relative size of the proliferation compartment. We suggest that two separate control mechanisms of crypt cell production underlie these two patterns of change in crypt cell production. Obviously, more data are needed to test this hypothesis, especially on the cell cycle time, the life span of the epithelial cells, and the constancy or inconstancy of the number of crypts.

2.1.3 COLONIC EPITHELIUM

Epithelial cell proliferation in the colon has been studied much less than that of the small intestine (194). Especially, disturbances of cell proliferation in the colon have scarcely been investigated. It is therefore purely speculative to talk about control mechanisms of epithelial cell proliferation in the colon. However, some observations are worth mentioning here.

In a number of respects the crypts of the colon resemble those of the small intestine. The size of the crypts is approximately the same, although of course no villi are present in the colon. Also the distribution of proliferating cells in the lower half of the crypt shows a striking resemblance (587, 689), and in some colonic epithelia, at least in the descending colon of the rat, the growth fraction in the lower half of the crypt, the proliferation compartment, approaches unity (but see Section 1.4). The cell cycle time and the life span of the epithelial cells after thay have left the proliferation compartment are much longer in the colon than in the small intestine. The cell cycle time in rat descending colon is between 50 and 60 h compared with approximately 12 h in the small intestine (6, 83, 587, 689).

In the colonic epithelium two important determinants for the rate of cell production in the proliferation compartment seem to be the size of the compartment and the cell cycle time within it (see Figure 2.1.2). Both these variables have been found to change to a considerable extent under different conditions.

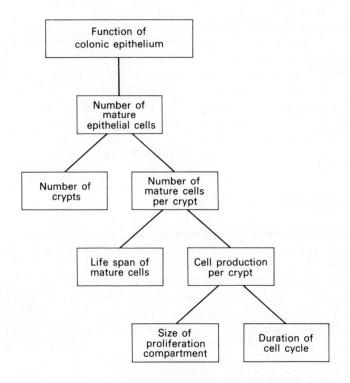

Figure 2.1.2 Schematic representation of the interrelationships of cyto-kinetic parameters in colonic epithelium

Under experimental conditions, like starvation and ischaemia-induced epithelial cell loss, temporary changes in crypt cell production were brought about by changes in the cell cycle time (281, 580, 581), contrary to the situation in the small intestine in which changes in the cell cycle time probably play a minor role in changing cell production rates. From the labelling indices for each cell position in the crypt it was calculated that the cell cycle time may decrease from 50 h to approximately 20 h (580). Also, in the colonic epithelium after experimental bypass an adaptive response was found which consisted of a decrease in the crypt size, whereas the relative size of the proliferation compartment remained the same (581).

The size of the proliferation compartment in the colonic crypts has been found to change in association with premalignant and malignant lesions of the colonic mucosa (155, 424, 456, 736). Recently, a transient increase in the size of the proliferation compartment has also been described as taking place during a hyperplastic disease of the colon in mice (35).

From the data which are now available it seems that there is in the colonic epithelium a difference in cell proliferation of, on the one hand, malignant and premalignant lesions and, on the other, the responses to tissue damage and changes in the luminal environment. Our findings support the hypothesis that an expansion of the proliferation compartment in the colonic crypt indicates malignant or premalignant changes, as has been put forward by Lipkin and his co-workers (423). Whether such a change is reversible, as in a hyperplastic disease of the colon in mice (35), is an important and as yet unanswered question.

2.1.4 CONCLUDING REMARKS

Have we come any closer to answering the basic question: why is cancer so rare in the small intestine in comparison to the colon? Are we now able to formulate better, more precise questions than seven years ago?

From the data that are presently available it is clear that the development and course of cancers is not a simple case of one cause, one effect; factors at all levels from DNA-repair mechanisms to losing a life-partner have been suggested as having associations. On this occasion we shall confine ourselves to the level of epithelial cell proliferation, leaving out even the subepithelial fibroblast layer which is so intimately connected with the epithelium.

Looking at the data on the small-intestinal and colonic epithelia, several differences apart from that in architecture have been observed.

Firstly, the cell cycle time is much longer in the colon than in the small intestine: approximately 50 h versus 10 to 12 h; secondly, the life span of the epithelial cells after their last cell division is approximately 72 h in the colonic epithelium and 40 h in the epithelium of the small intestine; thirdly, an expansion of the proliferation compartment in the crypt is associated with damage to the epithelial cell layer in the small intestine and with premalignant changes in the colon; and fourthly, damage of the non-proliferating cell compartment is associated with an expansion of the proliferation compartment in the crypt in the small intestine, and with a shortening of the cell cycle time in the colon.

In conclusion, let us add one speculation. The proliferation of epithelial cells in the upper half of the crypt is a phenomenon which does not occur under normal circumstances, nor in response to epithelial damage or changing environment. The possibility of colonic epithelial cells departing from the normal, regulated pattern may be a contributory factor to the high incidence of carcinomas in the colon. In the small intestine, cell proliferation in the upper half of the crypt is part of a normal, regulated pattern which would make it less likely for carcinomas to develop in the small intestine.

ACKNOWLEDGEMENTS

I am very grateful to Professor Marco de Vries for his criticism and advice during the preparation of this paper, and to Alie van der Panne for typing it.

2.2 Preliminary Studies of the Effects of Hormones on Cell Proliferation in the Gastrointestinal Tract of the Rat

John G Sharp, Helen L Lipscomb, George E Cullan, Sy H Fatemi, Dee McLaughlin, and David A Crouse

2.2.1 INTRODUCTION

Hormones have a significant role in the regulation of growth and have been implicated in the control of cell proliferation in the gastrointestinal tract (65, 88, 136, 200, 270, 300, 352, 353, 402, 417, 730, 733, 819). However, the relative importance and degree of interaction of the various groups of hormones (pituitary, adrenal, gonadal, gastrointestinal, and neurergic agents) remain to be defined, as do the specific actions and interactions of each hormone with regard to gastrointestinal cell production and intestinal growth (194). In order to understand the role of these hormones, more information about their levels and distribution in healthy individuals and in disease states is needed (175, 516, 679, 759, 826). The distinctions made between different groups of hormones on an anatomical and historical basis may be artificial since, for example, hormones originally described in the gastrointestinal tract (491, 515) have also been found in the brain (515, 681, 836). On the other hand, there is evidence for an interaction between pituitary and gastrointestinal hormones since hypophysectomy leads to a decrease both in antral and in serum gastrin levels (205, 705). At the same time, there is a need to assess the effects of these various hormones alone and in combination on potential target tissues throughout the gastrointestinal tract. We have attempted to apply methods which will permit a systematic analysis of such effects. This report presents the results of our initial studies including our evaluation of inherent methodological problems.

The effects of hormones on gastrointestinal tissues have been investigated previously using surgical techniques (135, 136, 193, 270, 511, 733), administration of hormones (88, 352, 353, 402, 447, 514, 815, 819) and pharmacological agents which modulate specific receptors to alter hormone levels (367, 372, 527, 731, 732, 738, 745). The ultimate effective concentration of hormone at the target tissue level is nearly always inferred because of difficulties in the measurement of these values. A variety of techniques have been employed to determine the effects on the target tissue, including the calculation of mitotic index in histological sections (88, 402), and stathmo-kinetic analysis (730, 732, 733, 738, 745). These and many other kinetic techniques are time consuming and of limited scope, and it would be difficult to perform and analyse all the necessary experiments employing them. Some workers (352, 353, 511) have studied the effects of several gastrointestinal hormones employing radio-isotope uptake by mucosal scrapings in vitro. Unfortunately this technique does not permit an adequate definition of the localisation of radioactivity in the crypt-villus unit. A useful compromise appears to be the technique of crypt dissection (279) complemented whenever appropriate by morphometric and autoradiographic analyses. In our experience this has been a powerful tool for the study of the effects of X-irradiation and resection on the gastrointestinal tract (59, 296–298, 365, 508, 545), and these previous studies have conditioned our approach to the present study of the effects of hormones. In order to illustrate our rationale, some of the relevant aspects of these earlier studies are summarised in Table 2.2.1.

Table 2.2.1 Summary of some effects of X-irradiation and resection on cell proliferation in the gastrointestinal tract which are relevant to the rationale of studies of the effects of hormones on the gastrointestinal tract

Effect	Occurrence
1. Effects at a distance within the gastrointestinal tract	Following both X-irradiation and resection. Involves the colon after X-irradiation of the small bowel and after large resections of the small bowel, but no effect can be demonstrated in the stomach after either treatment
2. Changes in crypt number	Only when density of crypts is altered ie, following X-irradiation but not resection
3. Changes in size of crypt proliferation zone	Transiently during recovery from X-irradiation; permanently after resection
4. Involvement of a circulating humoral factor	Not easily demonstrated during the compensatory phase following either X-irradiation or resection

Our findings are generally compatible with those of other workers, and indicate that compensation in the gastrointestinal tract following a reduction in the density of crypts is by production of new crypts from surviving cryptogenic stem cells (85). In contrast, compensation following a reduction in the total number of crypts, but with no change in crypt density, is by an increase in the size of the crypt proliferation zone and entire crypt-villus unit (297, 298).

There is an effect at a distance in the gastrointestinal tract following both X-irradiation and resection of the small intestine. This effect extends to the remaining uninvolved small bowel and after treatments involving a large amount of small bowel, affects the colon (501), but unlike others (637) we have been unable to demonstrate effects in the stomach.

There is no easily demonstrable circulating factor present, except perhaps very early during the compensatory phase following X-irradiation or resection (112, 365, 508, 800), which argues against the obvious involvement of circulating hormones in the permanent adaptation of the intestine to resection, but does not exclude a role for locally acting factors and luminal contents. Studies of isolated loops of bowel under various experimental circumstances strongly support a role for some type of humoral mechanism in the control of intestinal epithelial cell production (192, 299, 586). Gastrin has been put forward as a primary candidate for a humoral factor involved in the compensatory response to resection (34) but the experimental evidence to date does not fully support this hypothesis (292, 485, 511). Perhaps, as an alternative, a glucagon-like factor is involved (34, 200, 501). Luminal factors also influence intestinal cell proliferation and morphology (17, 19, 21, 114, 117, 796). The factors which might be elicited by a meal and which might contribute to stimulation of the gastrointestinal mucosa have been summarised (353).

If the compensatory mechanisms described above are representative of mechanisms of normal intestinal growth, this suggests that growth can occur by an increase in the number of crypts (81, 110), or by an increase in the size of the crypt-villus unit with a corresponding increase in the size of the crypt proliferation zone, or by a combination of both of these processes. Both can be detected using crypt dissection combined with morphometric analysis. We have not yet attempted as detailed an analysis of epithelial cell cycle parameters as has been undertaken, for example, following testosterone administration (819) and in young hypophysectomised animals (828). Since in the adult the cell cycle time of the majority of proliferating cells is short, a further reduction would not be expected to make a very large contribution to the overall rate of cell production. This is less true of newborn and suckling rats in which the cell cycle times of intestinal epithelial cells are longer than in the adult (367, 828). Consequently, this remains an important area of future investigation in those instances where hormones appear to alter the rate of epithelial cell production.

Since our studies are currently in progress, we report here only on some aspects of the effects of hypophysectomy, prolactin-producing ectopic pituitary transplants, castration and the administration of testosterone, pentagastrin, gastrin and isoprenaline to adult rats. Because of the suggestion of a difference in the response of the stomach and that of the remainder of the gastrointestinal tract, we have attempted whenever possible to obtain data for stomach glands although the dissection of these glands is difficult. We have found that there are problems in providing adequate and appropriate controls in these experiments and because of this we have had to re-evaluate the adequacy of our methods. It is becoming increasingly evident that significant events affecting intestinal maturation occur in the rat during the third week of life, around the period of closure of the intestine; these involve hormones, particularly thyroid hormone and glucocorticoids (315, 830, 831). Consequently, we shall present preliminary data on some indices of intestinal cell proliferation in adult rats which have been subject to thyroidectomy, castration or thymectomy at about this time.

2.2.2 MATERIALS AND METHODS

2.2.2.1 ANIMALS AND EXPERIMENTAL CONDITIONS

These studies have involved inbred rats of three strains: Fischer 344, Lewis, and Wistar. Originally, our intent was to use Fischer 344 rats throughout these studies; however, a supply problem necessitated the use of Lewis rats in some experiments. Subsequently, we discovered that under certain circumstances Lewis rats may be susceptible to autoimmune endocrine disease (430) and thus may not be entirely suited for some experiments employing endocrinological manipulations. This has prompted us recently to use Wistar strain rats.

All rats purchased from outside suppliers were allowed a minimum of two weeks to acclimatise to their new environment. They were housed under conventional conditions. Rats, with the exception of mothers with pups, were caged alone or in pairs in wire bottom cages. Mothers with pups were housed singly in plastic shoe-box cages. All rats were allowed standard lab chow and water ad lib. Initially, we attempted to maintain pair-fed controls in the longer term experiments, but food loss and the evident alteration in the feeding pattern made this a difficult and unsatisfactory control which was therefore discontinued. However, the food consumption of the various groups was estimated throughout and all rats were weighed weekly. In those instances where experimental protocols altered food intake and caused changes in body growth the measured weight of the intestine was compared to a weight predicted on the basis of body weight (661). Because of the existence of a diurnal rhythm in proliferative indices in normal rats (9, 93, 537, 629) all animals were maintained on a strict 0600 h to 1800 h light, 1800 h to 0600 h dark, cycle. They were handled, weighed and cleaned in the mornings at the same time as subsequent surgical procedures and autopsy. Injections during the dark period were carried out under a red light.

2.2.2.2 AUTOPSY PROCEDURES

All rats were autopsied during the period 0800 h to 1100 h and when, for example, 5 rats at 5 doses of hormone were involved, the autopsies were spread over a 5 day period, with one rat at each dose autopsied in a different order each day. Each intestinal segment (stomach, duodenum, etc) was removed in a different order on different days. These precautions were designed to minimise systematic errors. One hour prior to autopsy each rat was injected intraperitoneally, unless specified otherwise, with 1 μCi per g body weight (0.33 μCi in studies of the effects of hypophysectomy) of tritiated thymidine (^{3}HTdR) of specific activity 2 Ci per mM.

Rats were killed by decapitation, trunk-blood collected and the serum removed and stored frozen at $-90\,°C$. Complete intestinal segments were removed, their length measured and any attached mesentery dissected away. The cardiac portion of the stomach was discarded. The small intestine was sectioned midway between the ligament of Treitz and the ileo-caecal junction. For convenience, the proximal half will be referred to as jejunum and the distal half as ileum. Each segment was slit along its mesenteric border, washed clean in ice-cold saline, carefully blotted dry and weighed. Multiple samples were removed from the stomach, the mid-duodenum, mid-jejunum, mid-ileum and around the mid-point of the descending colon. In most experiments the samples of stomach and colon were not processed further.

Samples were employed in triplicate to determine the percentage water content, the tritium activity per mg of wet weight or dry weight, and the tritium activity per crypt (or, in the case of the stomach, per gland). Some samples were fixed, either in formol saline or 2 percent glutaraldehyde, for subsequent light and electron microscopic examination. The number of crypts per mg intestinal dry weight or crypts per intestinal segment were calculated (279). Tritium content reflecting the incorporation of ^{3}HTdR into DNA was determined using a Searle liquid scintillation counter. At autopsy tissues were examined macroscopically for completeness of surgical procedures and appropriate samples removed for histological examination. Rats with unsatisfactory surgical procedures were excluded from the study. Selected tissues whose size and morphological appearance provided information on the effectiveness of procedures designed to alter hormone levels were also removed, weighed and fixed in formol saline for histological examination. In hypophysectomised rats paraffin sections 5 μm thick were prepared and stained with haematoxylin and eosin.

The height of the villi, depth of the crypts and thickness of the muscle layers were measured using a calibrated micrometer on 10 complete crypts and villi per section. The number of cells per crypt and villus section was counted. A minimum of three sections was used for each tissue.

2.2.2.3 EXPERIMENTAL PROTOCOLS

Hypophysectomy. Fischer 344 female litter-mates were hypophysectomised or sham-hypophysectomised by the parapharyngeal approach at 6 to 8 weeks of age. Completeness of the hypophysectomy was judged initially by noting their lack of weight gain and confirmed at autopsy by histological examination of the contents of the pituitary fossa. One hour prior to autopsy at 7 months of age each rat was injected with 0.33 μCi ^{3}HTdR per g body weight. At autopsy small-intestinal weight and crypt values were obtained together with morphometric data on the intestine of the hypophysectomised and sham-operated animals.

Administration of prolactin. Daily vaginal smears were performed on a group of 3-month old female Fischer 344 rats to identify those which were ovulatory. These animals then received ectopic pituitary grafts from syngeneic donors in order to produce elevated prolactin levels (498). One pituitary was transplanted by trocar to a site beneath the left renal capsule through an incision in the left lateral body wall. If the first insertion of the trocar beneath the kidney capsule failed to deliver all the donor tissue, the remainder was inserted by trocar beneath the capsule of the spleen. At 6 months of age the ovulatory status of these rats was determined by vaginal smears and only anovulatory rats with their ovulating sham-operated littermate controls were retained for study. One hour before autopsy at 7 months of age each rat was injected with 1 μCi ^{3}HTdR per g body weight. At autopsy small-intestinal weight and crypt values were obtained.

Administration of pentagastrin and gastrin. Pentagastrin was administered intraperitoneally at doses of 0 (diluent only), 100, 250, 500 and 1000 μg per kg body weight to adult male Lewis rats weighing 250 g (352). Each received one injection every 8 h over a fasting period of 40 h for a total of 6 injections. Eight hours after the last injection and 1 h prior to autopsy each rat was injected with 1 μCi ^{3}HTdR per g body weight. At autopsy intestinal crypt values were determined.

Gastrin was administered subcutaneously at doses of 0 (vehicle only), 10, 20 or 40 μg per kg body weight to adult male Wistar rats weighing 250 g. Each rat received a single injection after 24 h of a 48 h fasting period prior to autopsy. One hour prior to autopsy each rat was injected with 1 μCi ^{3}HTdR per g body weight. At autopsy the tritium content, reflecting the incorporation of tritiated thymidine into DNA, was determined. Because there are conflicting reports regarding the tropic effects of gastrin and pentagastrin on the gastrointestinal tract the data for gastrin has been compared to similar data obtained using pentagastrin.

Administration of isoprenaline. Isoprenaline was administered intraperitoneally to adult male Lewis rats weighing 250 g at doses of 0 (diluent only) 0.001, 0.01

and 0.1 μg per kg body weight. Each rat received six injections every 4 h over a fasting period of 24 h. Three hours after the last injection and 1 h prior to autopsy each rat was injected intravenously with 1 μCi ^{3}HTdR per g body weight. At autopsy intestinal crypt values were determined.

Administration of testosterone. Testosterone was administered by gradual release (482) to castrated and sham-castrated 3-month old male Lewis rats. Silastic tubes of a volume calculated to provide an average release of 1 mg per day for a 30 day period were packed with testosterone acetate, or left empty, and implanted subcutaneously in the dorsum of the neck of male Lewis rats which had been castrated or sham-operated two weeks previously. One month later and 1 h before autopsy each rat was injected with 1 μCi ^{3}HTdR per g body weight and at autopsy small-intestinal weight and crypt values were determined.

Thyroidectomy of suckling rats. Male Lewis rat littermates were either thyroidectomised or sham-thyroidectomised at 12 or 17 days of age. Following surgery the pups were returned to their mothers until weaning at about 28 days of age. These rats were maintained until autopsy at 3 months of age. Their drinking water was supplemented with 1 percent calcium lactate. One hour prior to autopsy each rat was injected with 1 μCi ^{3}HTdR per g body weight and intestinal weight and tritium content reflecting the incorporation of ^{3}HTdR into DNA were determined.

Castration of suckling rats. Male Lewis rat littermates were either castrated or sham-castrated and female Lewis rat littermates ovariectomised or sham-ovariectomised at 15 days of age. Following surgery the pups were returned to their mothers until weaning at about 28 days of age. These rats were maintained until autopsy at 3 months of age. One hour prior to autopsy each rat was injected with 1 μCi ^{3}HTdR per g body weight and intestinal weight and tritium content reflecting the incorporation of ^{3}HTdR into DNA was determined.

Control experiments. Our concern over problems of providing appropriate controls for the experiments described above prompted several additional experiments. We wondered if changes in the water content of the intestine might occur after some of the procedures, in particular hypophysectomy, prolactin administration and castration; we therefore monitored the water content in all segments of the intestine in all experiments.

A second concern related to the age at which a rat can be considered as an 'adult'. The number of intestinal crypts increases, albeit at a continuously decreasing rate, until 3 to 4 months of age (81, 110); we therefore examined the number of crypts in various segments of the intestine of untreated female control Fischer 344 rats at several times between 2 and 12 months of age.

For convenience, ^{3}HTdR was administered intraperitoneally in all experiments with the exception of the study of the effects of isoprenaline where it was given intravenously. This exception was prompted by our desire to measure intestinal blood flow at the same time by using radiolabelled microspheres in isoprenaline-treated rats. Our results appeared to show that various hormones had very different effects on different segments of the gastrointestinal tract and we became concerned that this might represent an artifact related to the site of intraperitoneal injection of ^{3}HTdR, so we compared the intestinal crypt values obtained in adult male Lewis rats following intravenous and intraperitoneal administration of ^{3}HTdR.

Finally, because of our dissatisfaction with pair-feeding experiments as an adequate control for the effects on the intestine of reduced food intake and growth, we attempted to approach this problem by an alternative method. Thymectomised rats consistently eat less and grow more slowly than their littermate controls. Since there is no known direct effect of thymectomy on the intestine and since the surgical trauma is not unlike that of some of our other procedures, eg thyroidectomy, we studied the effect on female Lewis rat littermates at 7 months of age of thymectomy using a suction cannula at 5 days of age or sham-thymectomy. One hour prior to autopsy each rat was injected with 1 μCi ^{3}HTdR per g body weight and at autopsy intestinal weight and crypt values were obtained.

2.2.2.4 ANALYSIS OF RESULTS

Because of the preliminary nature of the results obtained in these studies, only a simple analysis of the data has been performed, using Student's t-test to compare experimental and control values.

2.2.3 RESULTS

2.2.3.1 HYPOPHYSECTOMY

The hypophysectomised rats included in the results (Table 2.2.2) were judged to be completely hypophysectomised on the basis that they did not show significant growth following surgery and there was no anterior pituitary tissue evident in the pituitary fossa at autopsy. They weighed significantly less than the sham-operated rats and consumed about half as much food as the controls. We did not quantify the water consumption of these groups of rats. The small intestine of the hypophysectomised rats was considerably smaller than in the controls, and overall was very similar in weight to the value predicted on the basis of body weight (661). This suggests that the intestine fails to continue its normal pattern of growth following hypophysectomy. Its length was reduced to about 86 percent of the control, whereas weight was

Table 2.2.2 Effects on small-intestinal crypts 5 months after hypophys-ectomy, by parapharangeal approach, on Fischer 344 female rats 2 months old. Values significantly different from those of sham-operated controls are indicated by * (p <0.05), ** (p <0.01), or *** (p <0.001)

	Sham-hypophysectomy	Hypophysectomy
Number of rats	9	9
Body weight (g)	231	130
Intestinal wet weight (g)		
Duodenum	0.43	0.28***
Jejunum	1.76	1.23*
Ileum	1.94	1.03*
Total	4.13	2.53**
Intestinal length (cm)		
Duodenum	7.6	5.8***
Jejunum and ileum	89.4	77.6***
Total	97.0	83.4***
Tritium activity (dpm/crypt)		
Duodenum	4.4	3.6
Jejunum	4.5	4.3
Ileum	4.5	3.8
Crypts/intestinal segment ($\times 10^6$)		
Duodenum	0.11	0.08**
Jejunum	0.52	0.39***
Ileum	0.56	0.47*
Total	1.19	0.94***

reduced to about 60 percent of the control. Tritium activity per crypt was also slightly but consistently reduced. The number of crypts per segment and the total number of crypts in the small intestine were significantly reduced to about 80 percent of the control values. Morphometric analysis demonstrated that the values for crypt length and cells per crypt column in the duodenum, jejunum and ileum of the hypophysectomised rats were similar for each segment and were 71 percent of sham-operated control values. Similarly villus length and cells per villus column were 79 percent of control values, the thickness of the circular muscle layer 85 percent and the thickness of the longitudinal muscle layer 81 percent. It appears that hypophysectomy has effects on all the values for all segments of the small intestine.

2.2.3.2 PROLACTIN

The rats with ectopic pituitary grafts included in this experiment were judged to have elevated prolactin levels on the basis that they had entered a persistent anovulatory state. The treated rats were slightly hyperphagic when compared to sham-transplanted controls. However, their body weight and intestinal weight, although greater than control values, were not significantly elevated (Table 2.2.3). Tritium activity per crypt was elevated by about 20 percent in

Table 2.2.3 Effects of prolactin on small-intestinal crypts. Three-month old ovulating Fischer 344 rats were given intrarenal and intrasplenic pituitary transplants from non-lactating syngeneic donors. They were maintained non-pair-fed for 3 months, then checked for anovulatory status and autopsied at 7 months of age. Values significantly different from those of sham-transplanted controls are indicated as in Table 2.3.2

	Sham-transplant	Transplant
Number of rats	6	7
Body weight (g)	206	226
Intestinal wet weight (g)		
Duodenum	0.36	0.36
Jejunum	1.74	1.88
Ileum	1.42	1.73
Total	3.52	3.97
Tritium activity (dpm/crypt)		
Duodenum	12.9	15.8
Jejunum	13.3	16.0
Ileum	19.8	27.5*
Crypts/μg		
Duodenum	1.97	1.98
Jejunum	2.32	2.12
Ileum	2.71	1.87
Crypts/intestinal segment ($\times 10^6$)		
Duodenum	0.23	0.20
Jejunum	1.40	0.98
Ileum	1.04	0.77
Total	2.67	1.95

duodenum and jejunum and about 40 percent in ileum. This increase was statistically significant only in the ileum. The numbers of crypts per mg were unaltered in the duodenum and jejunum but there was a suggestion of a decreased crypt density in the ileum, though there was a large variance in the control value. Similarly there was a suggestion of a decrease in the number of crypts per segment which was more evident distally. We do not yet have any morphometric confirmation of these observations. Overall the data suggest that prolactin might increase tritium activity and intestinal mass, and either has no effect on crypt number or even reduces it. These effects occur with a proximal to distal gradient with no effect in the duodenum, a slight effect in jejunum and the greatest effect in ileum.

2.2.3.3 PENTAGASTRIN AND GASTRIN

In this study the effects of pentagastrin were seen primarily in the stomach and the colon (Table 2.2.4). The data suggested that low doses of pentagastrin (100 to 250 μg per kg) decreased tritium activity per stomach gland, whereas a higher value (500 μg per kg) increased it. Similar changes were noted in

Table 2.2.4 Effects on tritium activity and density of gastric glands or intestinal crypts in different segments of the gastrointestinal tract of fasted adult male Lewis rats injected intraperitoneally with pentagastrin every 8 h for 48 h in the doses shown

Dose of pentagastrin (μg/kg)	0	100	250	500	1000
Number of rats	11	5	5	4	4
Tritium activity (dpm/gland or crypt)					
Stomach	2.0	1.3	0.8	4.7	2.5
Duodenum	12.1	15.7	12.0	18.6	8.6
Jejunum	10.6	11.9	14.0	15.2	8.9
Ileum	11.4	13.2	11.0	9.9	6.3
Colon	1.9	1.8	2.1	4.3	3.3
Glands or crypts/μg					
Stomach	4.79	6.84	8.73	3.10	3.37
Duodenum	2.42	2.21	2.24	1.67	2.30
Jejunum	2.58	2.99	2.72	2.61	2.77
Ileum	2.87	2.07	2.33	2.90	2.55
Colon	3.68	4.20	3.94	2.37	4.12

Table 2.2.5 Effects on tritium activity (dpm/μg dry weight) at different sites in the gastrointestinal tract, of pentagastrin or gastrin. Pentagastrin was injected intraperitoneally into fasted adult male Lewis rats every 8 h for 48 h, and gastrin was injected subcutaneously into adult male Wistar rats once after 24 h of a 48 h fasting period

Dose of pentagastrin (μg/kg)	0	100	250	500	1000
Number of rats	5	5	5	5	5
Stomach	7.1	5.9	6.5	8.8	6.8
Duodenum	26.7	29.1	29.2	38.2	30.2
Jejunum	31.4	26.9	30.7	34.4	33.0
Ileum	30.2	27.2	23.4	30.1	27.5
Colon	7.4	7.7	6.2	8.4	12.3
Dose of gastrin (μg/kg)	0	10	20	40	
Number of rats	5	5	5	5	
Stomach	6.3	6.6	7.6	6.1	
Duodenum	51.5	42.9	47.3	40.8	
Jejunum	57.6	66.0	66.5	66.2	
Ileum	56.9	63.9	60.3	56.3	
Colon	8.1	12.7	10.2	15.0	

tritium activity per mg dry weight (Table 2.2.5). In the colon the higher doses of pentagastrin appeared to increase tritium activity per crypt but the variance of these values was large. There appeared to be sporadic elevations at intermediate doses in the duodenum and jejunum and at the highest dose there was a decrease in the ileum. The decreases in the stomach were associated with increases in the number of glands per mg. In the other segments, with the exception of duodenum at 500 μg per kg, the density of crypts was unaltered. This implies for the colon that tritium activity per mg at higher doses of pentagastrin should be elevated and this was, in fact, observed (Table 2.2.5). No changes in the total number of crypts was noted in any intestinal segment. The changes in tritium activity per gland and glands per mg in the stomach must be interpreted with caution because of problems evident in the evaluation of cell proliferation in the stomach by our techniques (Table 2.2.10).

The effects of pentagastrin and porcine gastrin on the tritium content of the various segments of the gastrointestinal tract are compared in Table 2.2.5. It should be noted that pentagastrin was studied using Lewis strain rats and gastrin using Wistar strain rats. Tritium activity per mg dry weight was reduced in the stomach at 100 μg per kg pentagastrin and elevated in the stomach and duodenum at 500 μg per kg and in the colon at 500 and 1000 μg per kg. No significant changes were observed in the jejunum and ileum. Following gastrin administration no changes were noted in tritium activity per mg dry weight in any segment of the gastrointestinal tract with the exception of the colon where values were higher (with a much increased variance) at all doses of gastrin. The value at a dose of 40 μg per kg gastrin was significantly elevated.

Table 2.2.6 Effects on tritium activity and numbers of gastric glands or intestinal crypts in different segments of the gastrointestinal tract of fasted adult male Lewis rats injected intraperitoneally with isoprenaline every 4 h for 24 h in the doses shown

Dose of isoprenaline (μg/kg)	0	0.001	0.01	0.1
Number of rats	9	5	4	5
Tritium activity (dpm/gland or crypt)				
Stomach	5.9	1.8	1.9	1.9
Duodenum	11.6	13.2	11.4	12.0
Jejunum	11.0	9.4	9.6	12.5
Ileum	13.2	12.2	13.1	13.4
Colon	2.4	1.8	2.5	2.0
Glands or crypts/intestinal segment ($\times 10^6$)				
Stomach	0.62	3.89	3.69	10.10
Duodenum	0.22	0.23	0.24	0.30
Jejunum	1.08	1.43	1.18	1.54
Ileum	1.08	1.15	1.09	1.29
Colon	4.26	2.04	2.47	13.55

2.2.3.4 ISOPRENALINE

The primary effect of isoprenaline appeared to be a reduction in the tritium activity per stomach gland (Table 2.2.6) with a corresponding increase in glands per stomach at all doses. This must be interpreted with caution because of potential problems with our technique of evaluating cell production in glands of the stomach (Table 2.2.10). However, even if the values obtained following intraperitoneal injections of ^{3}HTdR were employed here, a similar effect would still be evident. At the highest dose of isoprenaline used (0.1 μg per kg body weight) the tritium activity per crypt in the colon was decreased and the number of crypts per colon increased. There was also a suggestion of a slight reduction in tritium activity per crypt in the jejunum at lower doses of isoprenaline. Tritium activity per mg dry weight was decreased only in the stomach at all doses of isoprenaline and was not significantly altered in all other segments.

2.2.3.5 TESTOSTERONE

Over the 25-day period immediately prior to autopsy on day 30, the sham-castrated rats with an empty implant each consumed on average 12.8 g food per day; castrated rats with an empty implant 10.7 g; sham-castrated rats with a testosterone containing implant 11.1 g and the castrated rats with a testosterone containing implant 9.6 g. These values appear to be reflected in the average body weight of these rats (Table 2.2.7) but there is no apparent relationship between body weight and intestinal dry weight. It is likely that the dose of testosterone delivered by the implants is too high, since prostatic weights in the testosterone-treated rats were elevated over control levels and there appeared to be atrophy of the testis in the sham-castrated testosterone-treated group. This high dose of testosterone may have affected the animals' behaviour and feeding patterns. While there was no relation between food intake and intestinal dry weight, there might possibly be a relation with tritium activity per crypt in the duodenum. However, our methods are inadequate to discern such a difference at a statistically significant level. Tritium activity per crypt was elevated (but with a great variance) in the ileum of the testosterone-treated rats. It was also elevated in the castrated rats given an empty implant. Crypt density was unaltered in the duodenum and jejunum but might be decreased by testosterone administration in the ileum. There was a suggestion that the number of crypts in the duodenum might be slightly increased by testosterone administration, whereas the number in the ileum might be decreased. Tritium activity per mg in jejunum and ileum appeared to be elevated by castration and decreased by testosterone administration, and this can be compared to the results of castration of suckling rats (Table 2.2.9).

Table 2.2.7 Effects on the testis, prostate and small intestine of adult Lewis rats 1 month after administration of an empty or testosterone-containing silastic tubing implant. Values significantly different from those of the sham-castrated rats with empty implants are indicated as in Table 2.2.2

	Sham-castration + empty implant	Castration + empty implant	Sham-castration + testo-sterone implant	Castration + testo-sterone implant
Number of rats	4	4	5	5
Weight (g)				
Whole body	385	370	372	342
Testis	2.87	—	2.16*	—
Prostate	0.42	0.08***	0.72**	0.74**
Intestine (dry)	1.21	1.25	1.35	1.54*
Tritium activity (dpm/crypt)				
Duodenum	12.1	10.3	9.9	9.2
Jejunum	12.5	12.7	11.8	13.2
Ileum	12.8	17.3	18.3	19.3
Crypts/µg				
Duodenum	2.88	2.38	2.91	2.88
Jejunum	2.81	2.99	2.87	2.37
Ileum	3.46	2.77	2.51	1.91*
Crypts/intestinal segment ($\times 10^6$)				
Duodenum	0.24	0.24	0.30	0.34
Jejunum	1.54	1.47	1.70	1.55
Ileum	1.71	1.82	1.58	1.43

2.2.3.6 THYROIDECTOMY

As judged by body weight and kidney weight (Table 2.2.8) and gross examination of the neck for residual thyroid tissue at autopsy, significant amounts of thyroid tissue were removed from the operated rats at 12 and 17 days of age. However, we have as yet obtained histological confirmation of the completeness of thyroidectomy only for those rats operated on at 17 days of age and the data suggest that the group operated on at 12 days contained rats with a significant thyroid remnant, although examination of individual rats did not identify a particular individual with an incomplete operation. The difference between these groups, however, provides an interesting opportunity to note the disassociation of effects on intestinal weight and tritium incorporation. The overall small-intestinal weight in both groups was similar to that predicted from the body weight (661). However, in neither group was the weight of the

Table 2.2.8 Effects on weights of different organs and tritium activity in the small intestine of 3-month old Lewis rats, having undergone thyroidectomy at 12 or 17 days old. Histological confirmation of completeness of thyroidectomy was not obtained for the day-12 rats. Values significantly different from those for sham-thyroidectomised rats are indicated as in Table 2.2.2

	Sham-thyroidectomy	Thyroidectomy Day 12	Thyroidectomy Day 17
Number of rats	10	4	4
Weight (g)			
Whole body	318	255	206*
Kidney	1.15	0.81**	0.66**
Adrenal	0.037	0.031	0.027
Prostate	0.27	0.23	0.21
Thymus	0.40	0.20***	0.27***
Small-intestinal dry weight (g)			
Duodenum	0.077	0.075	0.077
Jejunum	0.453	0.347	0.259
Ileum	0.483	0.434	0.314
Total	1.013	0.856	0.651***
Tritium activity (dpm/μg intestinal dry weight)			
Duodenum	35.8	22.1**	33.5
Jejunum	47.4	28.2**	44.2
Ileum	48.7	38.4	45.4

duodenum reduced proportionately as much as that of the jejunum and ileum. Tritium activity per mg dry weight was reduced by thyroidectomy at both ages but the reduction observed in 12-day-thyroidectomised rats was much greater than in 17-day-thyroidectomised rats despite the possibility that the former group might have residual thyroid tissue. We do not yet have values of tritium activity per crypt for these rats.

2.2.3.7 CASTRATION

Removal of the gonads of male and female rats at 15 days of age reduced the subsequent body growth of the males but had no effect in females (Table 2.2.9). Small-intestinal weight was reduced in both groups but not to a significant degree. Interestingly, tritium activity per mg dry weight was consistently increased over the values for the sham-operated control in castrated male rats but consistently decreased over the control values in ovariectomised female rats.

2.2.3.8 CONTROL EXPERIMENTS

The dry weight of all segments of the intestine in all groups in these experiments ranged from 20 to 26 percent, with a mean value of 23 percent, of the wet weight.

Table 2.2.9 Effects on weights of different organs and tritium activity in the small intestine of 3-month old Lewis rats having undergone castration at 15 days old. Values significantly different from those for sham-castrated rats of the same sex are indicated as in Table 2.2.2

| | Male | | Female | |
	Sham-castrated	Castrated	Sham-castrated	Castrated
Number of rats	5	5	7	7
Weight (g)				
Whole body	305	244***	196	204
Kidney	1.11	0.81	0.68	0.60
Adrenal	0.036	0.041	0.044	0.041
Thymus	0.45	0.51	0.40	0.47
Prostate	0.25	0.03***	—	—
Uterus	—	—	0.11	0.02***
Small intestine (dry)	1.23	1.06	0.95	0.86
Tritium activity (dpm/μg intestinal dry weight)				
Duodenum	23.2	29.1	34.6	27.2
Jejunum	28.0	37.5	40.1	36.8
Ileum	36.3	44.1	40.3	35.1

Water content was not significantly different between treated and sham-treated controls and is not a complicating factor in the interpretation of any of the results. Intraperitoneal injections are generally more conveniently carried out than intravenous injections and there appears to be no disadvantage to the use of

Table 2.2.10 Comparison of tritium activity and numbers of gastric glands or intestinal crypts in different segments in the gastrointestinal tract of adult male Lewis rats following intravenous or intraperitoneal injection of 1 μCi ^{3}HTdR/g body weight. Values significantly different from those obtained after intravenous injection are indicated as in Table 2.2.2

	Intravenous	Intraperitoneal
Number of rats	9	8
Tritium activity (dpm/gland or crypt)		
Stomach	5.9	2.6***
Duodenum	11.6	11.8
Jejunum	11.0	10.6
Ileum	13.2	12.5
Colon	2.4	2.6
Glands or crypts/intestinal segment ($\times 10^6$)		
Stomach	0.62	2.48***
Duodenum	0.22	0.28
Jejunum	1.08	1.13
Ileum	1.08	1.30
Colon	4.26	3.96

intraperitoneal injections of ^{3}HTdR when studying small-intestinal and colonic cell production (Table 2.2.10). An unexpected difference was obtained for tritium activity per gastric gland following intravenous and intraperitoneal injection of ^{3}HTdR, the value being higher following intravenous than intraperitoneal injections. The calculated number of glands per stomach was correspondingly reduced following intravenous injection. This observation is currently unexplained and must lead to caution in the interpretation of our data concerning stomach glands. Thymectomised rats eat slightly less than sham-thymectomised littermate controls and by seven months of age their body weight was significantly lower (Table 2.2.11). The small -intestinal weight was

Table 2.2.11 Effects on small-intestinal crypts in female Lewis rats 7 months after thymectomy at 5 days old. Values significantly different from those in sham-thymectomised rats are indicated as in Table 2.2.2

	Sham-thymectomised	Thymectomised
Number of rats	6	7
Body weight (g)	270	248
Intestinal wet weight (g)		
Duodenum	0.43	0.42
Jejunum	2.00	2.08
Ileum	1.94	1.79
Total	4.37	4.29
Tritium activity (dpm/crypt)		
Duodenum	14.5	11.9*
Jejunum	16.1	11.0***
Ileum	13.8	12.9
Crypts/µg intestinal dry weight		
Duodenum	2.49	1.98
Jejunum	1.58	1.94
Ileum	2.07	2.10
Crypts/intestinal segment ($\times 10^6$)		
Duodenum	0.20	0.20
Jejunum	0.79	1.00
Ileum	1.03	0.97
Total	2.02	2.17

not significantly reduced nor were crypt density, the number of crypts per segment or the total number of crypts in the small intestine. Only tritium activity per crypt was reduced in the thymectomised rats.

Our studies of the number of crypts per intestinal segment demonstrated that the value was relatively constant from three to seven months of age but decreased significantly to about 50 percent of maximum in all segments between eight and twelve months of age. Consequently, seven months of age was selected as the oldest at which rats could be autopsied as 'adults' without introducing additional variables related to age changes in intestinal crypt values.

2.2.4 DISCUSSION

It is necessary, first of all, to point out a number of reservations in regard to the interpretation of our results. Studies of the effects of hormones on cell production in the gastrointestinal tract are complicated because the manipulations involved alter not only the endocrine status of the animal but also its behaviour and feeding patterns (40). Alteration of feeding patterns itself changes gastrointestinal cell production and hormone levels, and there does not appear to be a satisfactory mechanism by which these multiple interactions can be controlled in in vivo studies. Consequently, evaluation of these studies is heavily dependent upon inference.

Pair-feeding has traditionally been used to control for the different growth rates of experimental and control animals seen when the animals are given unlimited access to food. Our experience with pair-feeding, like that of others (300), suggests that it is not an adequate solution to the problem because the altered feeding pattern of animals on a limited food intake can itself have significant effects on gastrointestinal cell production. Furthermore, pair-feeding experiments do not usually control for the changes in water consumption of the experimental animals (40). This could be important if, for example, the bulk of material present in the antrum of the stomach alters the secretion of gastrin or other gastrointestinal hormones (352, 353).

It may be simpler to infer the effects of a reduced food intake on gastrointestinal cell production, and make allowances for them when interpreting the data. In fact, there is little information on changes in intestinal epithelial cell proliferation in animals on a reduced food intake, since most studies have employed starvation or isolated loops of bowel (8, 110, 114, 281, 299, 586). It is likely that total food deprivation will have much more severe effects on cell production. On the basis of reports on the effects of starvation we would expect that reducing the food intake of rats would cause a decrease in the number of villus and crypt cells, the size of the crypt cell proliferation compartment, and consequently of the tritium activity per crypt. There might be slight changes in crypt density (299, 586) but there should be no significant reduction in the number of crypts per intestine (110). The effects of thymectomy, which we employed as a control, are therefore compatible with these expectations in that tritium activity per crypt is reduced to between 70 and 90 percent of control values but no other differences are noted.

We have taken precautions to avoid our results being affected by diurnal variations in gastrointestinal cell proliferation, but it must be recognised that certain of the endocrinological manipulations we have performed, for example hypophysectomy and thyroidectomy, may well modify the pattern of circadian variation (40), and we cannot exclude the possibility that some of the changes we observe are a consequence of this. As in the case of food intake, such a variation will probably alter tritium activity per crypt but should not change crypt numbers. This point is not only relevant to studies involving the removal of sources of hormones, but applies also to situations of hormone administration. For example, we used a depot method to produce a continuous slow release of testosterone, but physiologically testosterone is released according to a very specific circadian pattern (360) which we have not reproduced, and this may have indirectly modified the pattern of cell production. Several of the hormonal agents that we have administered have a very short biological half-life (511) and it could be argued that a repetitive injection schedule is much less satisfactory than continuous infusion of such agents. However, we have not yet been able to achieve infusion without restricting the animals and this itself has significant effects on DNA and RNA synthesis in the gastrointestinal tract (344). Also a single injection of such agents is often sufficient to bring about an effect (511) (Table 2.2.5).

We have investigated a number of other possible sources of error in our experiments and feel that we can rule out water content and the effects of age of the animals. One major discrepancy we cannot explain is the difference in the tritium activity per gastric gland between the rats receiving intravenous and interperitoneal injections. It is likely that cell proliferation in the stomach varies with location (194) and in order to obtain sufficient samples we had to use the entire stomach; it is possible, therefore, that the discrepancy we have obtained has arisen because of the selection of different sampling areas in the two experimental groups. Because of differences between the stomach and the small intestine, for example following isoprenaline administration, it is possible that there are some peculiarities of the gastrointestinal circulation which lead to a differential response under some experimental circumstances (387). We have not calculated precursor-product relationships in our study and we are therefore assuming that an increased tritium content implies increased DNA synthesis and therefore cell proliferation, We cannot however exclude the possibility that the agents we have employed simply change precursor entry into cells (511).

With the above reservations, the results of the study on the effects of hypophysectomy suggest that removal of the pituitary interrupts the process by which the intestine grows. This observation was not unexpected and it confirms that of others (402). Additionally, the data indicate that the number of crypts throughout the intestine of the hypophysectomised rats is reduced, and this suggests that pituitary hormones are required for the process of crypt fission by which the number of crypts in the intestine is increased during normal growth.

It would be of interest to know if crypt replication is dependent on pituitary hormones during only the period of growth or whether, for example, replication of crypts from surviving cryptogenic stem cells following X-irradiation, is compromised in the absence of the pituitary gland. It would also be of interest to know if the decrease in crypt numbers which occurs with age in the rat, and which may also occur in man (765), is related to changes in the pattern of secretion of pituitary hormones.

The decrease in intestinal cell production in the hypophysectomised rats which is suggested by the decreased tritium activity per crypt can probably best be explained on the basis of reduced food and water intake. All the segments of the intestine in hypophysectomised rats are reduced to around 75 percent of their size in sham-operated controls. Since the small intestine is reduced to 86 percent of its length in the sham-operated controls then the product of these values (65 percent) might reasonably be expected to predict the effect of hypophysectomy on intestinal weight, and this generally appears to be the case (Table 2.2.2). Our study provides no information on the particular hormones which are involved, although an earlier study (402) implicated growth hormone and thyroid hormone. Thyroidectomy at an early age certainly has a very pronounced effect on tritium activity per mg dry weight (Table 2.2.8), but this could involve modulation of adrenoreceptors by thyroid hormone (380, 733) or a number of other types of gut-thyroid interactions (473). It is evident that the role of pituitary hormones in crypt replication and intestinal growth (828, 830, 831) needs further study.

The effects of the administration of prolactin on cell production can be compared to the effects of lactation (200, 300). The rats given prolactin were only slightly hyperphagic and did not exhibit the large increase in food intake shown by suckled lactating animals (300). Even so, there was considerable increase in tritium activity per crypt in the ileum, suggesting an increase in the size of the entire crypt-villus unit such as is observed in suckled lactating mice (300). At the same time there was a hint of a reduction in the density and number of crypts, particularly in the ileum. Because of the large variances in these values this observation needs confirmation, but it could be that another control mechanism, perhaps regulating total intestinal absorptive area, has been triggered. This would contrast with the situation in the suckled lactating animal where no decrease in the number of crypts in the intestine was observed (300). Our data suggest that prolactin alters intestinal cell proliferation and are at variance with those of others (200). However, the effects of prolactin seem to be directed mainly towards the ileum and certainly do not exclude a role for an additional factor, perhaps enteroglucagon (200).

The role of gastrin as a tropic hormone for the gastrointestinal tract and the relative efficacies of gastrin and pentagastrin are currently controversial (292, 352, 353, 485, 511). In our hands pentagastrin at low doses appeared inhibitory and at a higher dose stimulatory to tritium activity per stomach gland. Related to these changes was a considerable increase in the number of glands per mg in the stomach. Since there was no change in the total number of glands this presumably reflects an alteration in the weight of the stomach, probably because of the secretion-promoting effects of pentagastrin. In contrast, gastrin appeared to have no effect on tritium activity per mg dry weight of stomach. Our data suggest that pentagastrin may have tropic effects in the stomach, albeit in fasted rats at doses which may be too high to mimic the physiological situation (511). Since these effects may also be related to the stimulation of secretion by pentagastrin, we are trying to monitor secretion and DNA synthesis simultaneously. We have been unable to show that gastrin has tropic effects in the stomach (352, 353); our data are more akin to those of other workers (292, 485, 511). However, our sources of both these hormones were different and the gastrin used may contain small amounts of other hormones. The only observation common to both pentagastrin and gastrin was that at the higher doses there was an increase in the tritium content of colonic crypts (447). Because of the lack of a significant and consistent response of the small intestine to gastrin administration, it is unlikely that this hormone is responsible for its permanent compensatory response to resection. It is possible, however, that it is involved in the response of the colon to resection of the small bowel (511). It may be that there is cross-reactivity of these agents with a molecule more directly involved in effecting tropic responses. In all these situations crypt numbers are unaltered.

It has been shown that beta-adrenergic stimulation prolonged cell cycle and mitotic times in the jejunum and therefore presumably decreased cell production (745). Using our methods we noted a slight reduction in tritium activity per crypt in the jejunum following the administration of 0.001 and 0.01 μg per kg isoprenaline, but much more pronounced effects in the stomach and colon. In the stomach even a low dose (0.001 μg per kg) decreased tritium activity per gland; there were also increases in crypt numbers. These observations require confirmation using other techniques because we cannot exclude the possibility that isoprenaline alters the blood supply to these tissues and this modifies the availability or the incorporation of ^{3}HTdR, which would suggest differences in the type of innervation of the blood supply to different parts of the intestine (387).

We have provided only limited information on the effects of steroid hormones on cell proliferation in the intestine. It has been reported that testosterone administered to castrated animals increases cell proliferation in the upper jejunum (819) although no effect was reported in an earlier study (88). In adult animals we saw no effect of testosterone on tritium activity per crypt in the jejunum, but there was an apparent increase in the ileum. However a similar increase was seen in the ileum of castrated rats. In studies of suckling rats, whereas ovariectomy led to decreased tritium activity per mg dry weight, castration of males led to an increase. Testosterone administration increased intestinal dry weight. It appears that steroid hormones do not alter the number of crypts in the small intestine but they do modify the metabolic activity of cells and this could include DNA-synthesis. Because of the possibilities of interconversion, alterations due to the changed circadian pattern of testosterone levels, and the feedback interactions involving the pituitary, it is not possible to be more specific.

On the whole it appears that the hormones investigated in this study have little role in the intestinal compensatory responses to X-irradiation and resection. Pituitary hormones are required for the process of crypt replication which leads to intestinal growth, but it is doubtful whether they are necessary for the process of crypt replication which gives rise to intestinal regeneration following X-irradiation. If they are not needed, two mechanisms of stimulating crypt replication may be postulated: one local, and one systemic. The latter, involving pituitary hormones, would only be operative during the growth period. The pituitary hormones involved are not known, but growth hormone and thyroid hormone are currently the most likely, and may operate by interacting with a local control mechanism.

A number of hormones, such as prolactin, thyroid hormone, gastrin, neurergic agents and probably also steroid hormones, alter cell proliferation in the gastrointestinal tract. Prolactin may be important in the compensatory response of the intestine in lactating animals, but may not be solely responsible (200). None of these hormones has effects which adequately reproduce the permanent compensation seen in the intestine following partial resection; this compensation also appears to be effected locally. Since this response involves the entire small bowel, and its magnitude is proportional to the amount of tissue resected, thus compensating for the absorptive defect, it is possible that the area of the basement membrane underlying the epithelium is important.

Thus in the case of the compensatory response of the intestine to both X-irradiation and resection, humoral factors may be involved other than classical hormones. Instead, local growth factors with paracrine effects may be involved, as appears to be the case in the lympho-haemopoietic system (575, 812), which is similar in being carefully controlled. Such factors appear to act only on stem cells whereas other hormones act on the committed progenitor and differentiating cell compartments (575, 812). They differ from the chalones and antichalones that have been described (62) in that they can be obtained from intact cells without the use of extraction procedures. Because of the likely lack of a role for most classical hormones in these responses, it appears justified to examine the effects on intestinal tissues of various growth factors (263), alone and in combination with hormones. Due to the difficulties encountered in the present studies and inherent in this type of investigation pursued in vivo, it is preferable that a validated in vitro system or separated purified single-cell assay (658) be developed for future studies of this nature.

2.2.5 SUMMARY

Preliminary studies have been undertaken on the effect of hypophysectomy, prolactin-producing ectopic pituitary transplants, castration, and the administration of testosterone, pentagastrin, gastrin and isoprenaline on some aspects of cell proliferation in the gastrointestinal tract of adult rats. Additionally, the effects of thyroidectomy and castration of suckling rats on the incorporation of ^{3}HTdR at 3 months of age were determined. A crypt dissection technique was used. An attempt was made to compensate for the differential food intake and growth of the treated rats by employing pair-fed controls. However, our experiments suggested that this was not an adequate solution because the obviously altered feeding pattern of rats on a limited food intake could itself change gastrointestinal cell production. Consequently, as a different approach, thymectomy at an early age was employed as a control. This surgical procedure is not known to have any direct effects on the gastrointestinal tract but it leads to an experimental group of rats with a lower food intake and mean body weight than the sham-operated control group. This demonstrated, as might be expected on the basis of the literature, that the reduced food intake led to a decreased tritium activity per crypt but did not change the number of crypts in the intestine. The water content of the intestine was determined for the various experimental and control groups of rats and no significant differences were noted.

Hypophysectomy reduced tritium activity per crypt and the size of all segments of the intestine. The length and weight of the intestine and the number of the crypts was also significantly reduced. It was concluded that an intact pituitary is required for the process of crypt replication which leads to intestinal growth. Prolactin increased DNA-specific activity per crypt, particularly in the ileum, and may be important in the hypertrophic response of the intestine in lactating animals, but it may not be entirely responsible for the observed changes. Pentagastrin has tropic effects in the stomach and colon, whereas an effect of gastrin could be demonstrated only in the colon. Isoprenaline appeared to inhibit cell proliferation in the stomach, and to a lesser degree in the colon. This may not be a direct effect of this agent on epithelial cells of the gastrointestinal tract but rather a result of altered blood flow. Thyroidectomy decreased the incorporation of ^{3}HTdR by the gastrointestinal tract. Gastrin, pentagastrin, isoprenaline and steroid hormones modify the metabolic activities of cells of the gastrointestinal tract, including DNA synthesis, but do not change the number of crypts.

Pituitary hormones are implicated in the regulation of cell production in the gastrointestinal tract during the growth of the intestine. However, none of the hormones studied appear to play a major role in the compensatory responses of the intestine to X-irradiation and resection in adult rats. Possibly these latter responses are mediated via local growth factors which have paracrine effects.

ACKNOWLEDGEMENTS

These investigations have been supported by a research grant PCM77-14849 from the National Science Foundation. HLL received post-doctoral support from NSF RIAS funds (SER 77-06922) and SHF and GEC were recipients of University of Nebraska Regents' Scholarships. This support is gratefully acknowledged. We wish to thank Mrs Sally Mann, Ms Sandra Grazulewicz and Mr Jeff Breitkreutz for excellent technical assistance and Mrs Sheila Sharp who typed the manuscript.

2.3 Evidence for a Tissue-specific Inhibitor of Intestinal Cell Proliferation in Rabbit Small-Intestinal Mucosa

Michel Bergeron and Pierre Sassier

2.3.1 INTRODUCTION

Cell proliferation in some adult tissues has been found to be controlled by substances known as chalones, which are synthesised by mature cells of a given organ and specifically inhibit cell proliferation in that organ (71). Their action has been defined as being tissue-specific but not species-specific, rapidly reversible, and not cytotoxic (70, 339). Any reduction in numbers of mature cells would result in lowered levels of this messenger, and would elicit a compensatory increase in cell proliferation in the same organ, as has been observed in the liver (655, 752), kidney (169, 604, 717, 718), and small intestine (435).

Recent data about chalone-like inhibition suggest that several chalones may regulate cell proliferation in the same tissue: in epidermis, a reversible chalone inhibition may take place either at the G_1 to.S (198) or at the G_2 to M junction (199). Some data concerning cell proliferation in the small intestine also suggest the existence of a chalone-like control mechanism. In several mucosal disorders, such as those observed in coeliac disease, or after radiation injury or chemical damage, a non-specific pattern of compensatory hyperplasia is seen in the intestine as in several other organs. Cell proliferation is equally increased in parabiotic rats, one of which has undergone a partial intestinal resection, which suggests in resected animals the presence of a stimulatory humoral factor or the absence of an inhibitory one (436). Several studies in embryonic and adult small intestine have detected the presence of substances inhibiting cell proliferation. A decreased mitotic index has been found in colchicine-treated rats after one injection of a crypt-cell extract from small intestine (728); this effect, not recorded when the rats were injected with a villus-cell extract, was tissue-specific. In the adult newt intestine there are two factors which specifically inhibit the intestinal growth of embryos at the end of G_1 and during G_2

respectively (64). However, the irreversible effect of this G_1 inhibitor is inconsistent with a chalone-like regulation of cell proliferation.

In previous studies (616, 617), we have investigated the effects of aqueous extracts from small intestine in vitro and in vivo. Our experimental data suggest the presence in the small intestine of substances inhibiting cell proliferation in the intestinal crypts. These inhibitory compounds, precipitated with ammonium sulphate in the range of saturation 0 to 50 percent (fraction F_1) are directly effective on DNA synthesis in small intestine and colon. Their effect, specific for intestine and rapidly reversible, could represent a regulatory mechanism of cell proliferation in intestine.

2.3.2 METHODS

2.3.2.1 QUANTIFICATION OF CELL PROLIFERATION AND MIGRATION IN INTESTINE

In the present study we have attempted a physiological approach to the chalone hypothesis, taking advantage of three special characteristics of cell proliferation in the small intestine. The cell population of the small intestine is among the most rapidly proliferating and renewing in the organism, with a well-defined area of proliferation in the crypts, resulting in a rapid incorporation of tritiated thymidine (^{3}HTdR) into DNA (616, 617) and a high mitotic accumulation after colchicine blockade (745); epithelial intestinal cells originate in the crypts and migrate from crypts to villi before being ejected into the lumen at the villus tip (406); and the cell cycle in small intestine and colon is one of the shortest in the organism (557).

Several measurements were thus used in order to investigate intestinal cell kinetics: the *specific activity of intestinal DNA* was measured one hour after a single injection of ^{3}HTdR; the *labelling index of the crypt cells* was determined autoradiographically; the *number of grains per crypt cell nucleus*, considered to be a valid index of the average quantity of ^{3}HTdR incorporated, was also recorded; the *mitotic accumulation after colchicine blockade* was measured after a delay of at least 8.5 h after chalone or control treatment, corresponding to the period of time taken for cells in the S-phase at the time of treatment to reach mitosis; and the *cell migration of labelled cells along the crypt-villus column* was investigated autoradiographically.

2.3.2.2 PREPARATION OF TISSUE EXTRACTS

New Zealand albino rabbits, weighing between 3 and 4 kg, were killed by decapitation after a 12-hour fast, and the small intestinal mucosa removed;

aqueous extracts were prepared according to a procedure previously discussed in detail (617, 618). When ready to use, the lyophilised extracts were dissolved in a 0.02 M phosphate buffer at pH 7, the concentration being 130 mg per ml. Protein was precipitated by progressively adding solid ammonium sulphate to the extracts (w/v = 291 g per 1, corresponding to a final saturation of 50 percent). The precipitates were redissolved in a phosphate buffer and dialysed against the same buffer. The non-dialysable fractions (fractions F_1) were diluted in phosphate buffer to obtain a protein concentration of 20 mg per ml.

The F_1 fractions were then filtered through an Amicon XM 100 ultramembrane filter. The non-ultrafiltrable fraction was diluted to the initial volume of F_1 and subjected to Amicon XM 300 filtration. The XM 100 (U_1) and XM 200 (U_2) filtrates were stored at $-20\,°C$. The XM 300 residue (U_3) was diluted to the initial volume of F_1 and stored at $-20\,°C$.

2.3.3 RESULTS AND INTERPRETATION

2.3.3.1 PRESENCE OF FACTORS INHIBITING DNA SYNTHESIS IN INTESTINAL MUCOSAL FRACTIONS FROM ADULT RABBITS

Mice, between 40 and 47 days old, were injected subcutaneously with 500 μl of the small-intestinal fractions U_1, U_2, U_3 (corresponding to the quantities contained in 10 mg of F_1 protein). The incorporation of ^3HTdR into DNA in the jejunum and colon was recorded at various times after the protein injection by measuring the specific activity of DNA in proximal jejunum and colon as previously described (617). As outlined above, preliminary experiments have shown that crude extracts from adult rabbit intestine strongly inhibit DNA synthesis when injected into adult mice; the inhibitory compound was found to be precipitated by ammonium sulphate in the 0 to 50 percent range of saturation (617).

In the present experiments, the fractions U_1 and U_3 were found to inhibit ^3HTdR incorporation into intestinal DNA. As shown in Figure 2.3.1 a single injection of fraction U_1 (0.15 to 0.30 mg of protein) was followed by a decrease of ^3HTdR incorporation into jejunal and colonic DNA, most pronounced between the second and the third hour with progressive recovery thereafter. Figure 2.3.1 shows that a single injection of fraction U_3 (9 mg of protein) decreased the ^3HTdR incorporation into jejunal and colonic DNA as early as the first hour; the inhibition, immediately maximal, was not reversed after seven hours. No inhibitory action of fraction U_2 was found under identical experimental conditions.

In order to study the tissue-specificity of the inhibitory factors, their effect was investigated on regenerating kidney and on testis (Table 2.3.1). Three

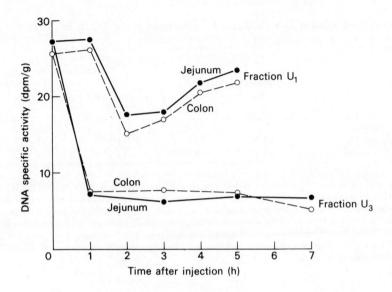

Figure 2.3.1 DNA-specific activity of mouse jejunum and colon at various times after injection of fractions U_1 and U_3

Table 2.3.1 Tissue specificity of inhibitory fractions on thymidine incorporation into DNA

	Jejunum	Colon	Kidney	Testis
Control	27.3	25.7	8.7	9.8
U_1 injected	18.5**	16.9**	13.0	9.9
U_3 injected	9.3***	5.6***	4.3***	3.3***

Mice received, at zero time, a single injection of 500 μl of fraction U_1 (150 μg) or fraction U_3 (9 mg). Three hours later, they were given ^{3}HTdR (34 μCi per mouse) subcutaneously and were killed one hour later. DNA specific activity was measured in jejunum, colon, regenerating kidney (in mice having undergone a mononephrectomy) and testis. Results are mean values of DNA specific activity (dpm/μg) for 6 mice and those significantly different from controls are indicated by * ($p < 0.05$), ** ($p < 0.01$) or *** ($p < 0.001$)

hours after a single injection of fraction U_1, the DNA-specific activities did not differ from control values in either kidney or testis, but after injections of fraction U_3, the DNA-specific activities were significantly decreased in both these organs; the specific activities in jejunum and colon were significantly lowered in mice injected with fractions U_1 or U_3 when compared with phosphate-injected controls.

Since the inhibition exerted by fraction U_1 on intestinal mucosa appeared to

Table 2.3.2 Effect of fractions U_1 and U_3 on incorporation of ^{3}HTdR into DNA and on mitotic accumulation in crypts after colchicine blockade

	Labelling index (%)	Number of grains/nucleus	Mitoses/crypt $3\frac{1}{2}$ h after colchicine Time after buffer or fraction	
			12 h	15 h
Control	35.1	15.8	14.3	14.3
U_1 injected	27.5**	15.6	11.5**	12.3**
U_3 injected	17.9***	8.7***	11.1***	12.0

Six mice per group were given a single injection of phosphate buffer (control), fraction U_1 (0.5 mg protein) or fraction U_3 (9 mg protein) at zero time. Three hours later, they received 30 μCi of ^{3}HTdR, and one hour later jejunal slices were prepared for autoradiography and both the labelling index and the number of grains per nucleus were counted. Different groups of mice also received fractions U_1 and U_3 to study the mitotic index $3\frac{1}{2}$ h after blockade by 60 μg colchicine. The animals were killed at the times shown and their proximal jejunum prepared for histology. The average number of mitoses per crypt was counted in each animal. Values significantly different from controls are indicated as in Table 2.3.1

be tissue-specific and reversible, these results suggest that at least one endogenous inhibitor of DNA synthesis may regulate cell proliferation in the intestine. The effect of U_1 was studied autoradiographically (Table 2.3.2) and found to cause a reversible reduction in the percentage of crypt cells synthesizing DNA in the small intestine without affecting the quantity of ^{3}HTdR incorporated into DNA in each nucleus. This suggests a block exerted by fraction U_1 at the transition from G_1 to S. In contrast, fraction U_3 was found to decrease both the percentage of crypt cells incorporating ^{3}HTdR and the quantity of thymidine incorporated per nucleus, suggesting either a non-specific mechanism inhibiting the uptake of ^{3}HTdR without any change of cell proliferation, or a slowing of DNA synthesis.

2.3.3.2 EFFECTS OF INTESTINAL INHIBITORY FACTORS ON MITOTIC ACCUMULATION

The mitotic accumulation in jejunal crypts after 3.5 h of colchicine blockade was studied in animals which had received the stathmokinetic agent either 8.5 or 11.5 h after fraction U_1 or fraction U_3 was given. Jejunal sections were prepared and stained with haematoxylin-phloxin. The average number of mitoses per crypt was calculated for each animal, and compared with controls given phosphate injections.

Both fractions were found to lower significantly the mitotic accumulation in jejunal crypts over the experimental period from 8.5 to 12 h after the treatment (Table 2.3.2); these data suggest that the block previously induced in DNA synthesis or at the G_1 to S boundary results in a lack of mitotic activity at the time when the blocked cells should have been entering mitosis, In addition, the decrease of mitotic accumulation seems to extend to fifteen hours after the fractions were given, probably due to a progressive desynchronisation of the proliferating crypt cells (7, 83).

2.3.3.3 EFFECTS OF VARIOUS FRACTIONS ON CELL MIGRATION

The migration of epithelial cells in small intestine takes place along the crypt-villus column: a given cell may therefore successively be located in each cell position (83) from the bottom of the crypt to the tip of the villus. The cell position corresponds to the number of cell nuclei separating a given cell from the crypt bottom in either side of the longitudinal axis along the basal membrane of crypts. In order to investigate cell migration in jejunum, sections were prepared for autoradiography from mice which had received twenty hours previously 30 μCi of ^{3}HTdR. In crypt-villus columns cut longitudinally the leading edge of labelled cells was described according to its cell position in three groups of animals: mice injected with phosphate buffer; mice injected with fraction U_1 (100 μg); and mice injected with fraction U_3 (9 mg). Injections were given at three times: 1, 5 and 9 h after ^{3}HTdR administration.

In controls, the leading edge of labelling in jejunal crypts was found to be at cell position 45 twenty hours after thymidine administration. In jejunal crypts of mice given fraction U_1 or fraction U_3, the cell position of the leading edge of labelling was found to be significantly lower: respectively cell positions 33 and 29.

2.3.4 CELL PROLIFERATION IN DAMAGED EPITHELIA

A number of physical and chemical agents have been found to affect cell proliferation in the small intestine, resulting in a general pattern of compensatory hyperplasia, with an increase in the size of the proliferation compartment and shortening of the cell cycle time. In man a massive resection of small intestine has been found to be followed by an anatomical adaptation in the remaining intestine, resulting in an increased absorption capacity per unit length in the small intestine (180).

This phenomenon has been extensively studied in mice and rats. Sixty days after 70 percent resection of jejunum and ileum in rats the total duration of the cell cycle was decreased with a specific reduction of the duration of S; the migration rate from crypts to villi was increased; and the total proliferating population increased in proportion to the increased overall size of crypts, so that labelling index remained unchanged (296). Similar results have been reported in dogs (374).

More complex experimental changes have been reported in the rat small intestine as a result of low doses of X-irradiation: the proliferative activity was temporarily arrested and then, as early as 72 hours after irradiation, substantially increased (245, 416). However, the pattern of compensatory hyperplasia was recorded only in mice and rats subjected to larger cumulative doses. In these experimental conditions a block in G_2 was initially observed, followed after 12 days by a shortening of the cell cycle time principally as a result of a reduction in the S-phase. After a chronic exposure of 35 days in mice and 105 in rats, proliferation returned to normal. This temporary shortening of the cycle duration, already seen in resected animals, appears to be a compensatory reaction (415).

In human pathology, a particular model of compensatory hyperplasia of the small intestine is provided by coeliac disease. Patients with this condition develop malabsorption probably resulting from an enterocyte toxicity induced in some way by gluten. Histological studies have shown a disappearance of villi, a lengthening of crypts, and an increase of mitotic activity related to the mucosal thickness (165). The proliferation compartment has been found to be expanded (776) with a shortened cell cycle time (821, 822) and an accelerated epithelial cell replacement (776) (See section 6.3).

2.3.5 DISCUSSION

In these different experimental and clinical conditions, it is worth noting that the loss of mature cells results in a common pattern of compensatory hyperplasia suggesting that the total number of mature cells is of some importance in proliferation and renewal of cells in the small intestine. As indicated by our data, some compounds of intestinal origin may induce, when injected into mice, a significant decrease of cell proliferation, by blocking specifically the G_1 to S transition, resulting in a decrease of the number of cells synthesising DNA. The effect of fraction U_1, which was diminishing after five hours, was apparent neither in the kidney nor in the testis and was shown to be accompanied by a slowing of cell migration in the small bowel. This suggests that normal intestinal cell proliferation may be regulated by a chalone-like feedback mechanism.

Two hormones extracted from small intestine, secretin (354) and pancreozymin (355), have previously been found to decrease cell proliferation in the small intestine. The effect of both these hormones on DNA synthesis was recorded after a delay of 12 and 8 h respectively. However, as the 2 fractions we have described act much more rapidly than this it is unlikely that the effects observed in our study are due to the presence of these hormones.

The chemical nature of our inhibitors remains to be ascertained, and will require further purification. However, in the area of research into chalones, the lack of a rapid and reliable technology complicates these efforts. In our experiments we used, as the first test, the incorporation of ^{3}HTdR into DNA. However, the pitfalls of this method are well-known and have been discussed elsewhere (617); this test has to be combined with others in order to ascertain that a decrease of ^{3}HTdR incorporation into DNA is linked to a decrease of crypt cell proliferation. Recently, a method has been developed (63) which permits automatic identification and counting of cells in the various phases of the cell cycle; this is less time-consuming than present techniques and may eventually provide a rapid assay to assist in further purification.

In conclusion, an inhibitory effect on cell proliferation in mouse intestine was found in 2 fractions prepared from extracts of rabbit small-intestinal mucosa. The fraction of lower molecular weight, injected into mice, was shown to have some chalone-like properties. The results of this study support the existence of a factor regulating intestinal cell proliferation (619). However, the physiological significance of our data remains to be confirmed by further experiments, including extensive purification with a specific methodological procedure.

2.4 The Role of Underlying Non-Epithelial Elements in the Orientation of Boundaries between Crypt Compartments

M Bjerknes and H Cheng

2.4.1 INTRODUCTION

The intestinal crypt appears to be divided into a number of functionally distinct compartments. From the base of the crypt they comprise firstly the *stem-cell zone*, situated in cell positions 1 to 4, defined as a microenvironment within which stem cells receive no inducement to differentiate (see Section 3.2); secondly the *proliferation zone* in which initiation of stem-cell differentiation begins and where amplification divisions occur in at least two of the four epithelial cell lines, viz. columnar and mucous; and thirdly the *maturation zone* where all proliferative activity ceases and all cells terminally differentiate before moving out of the crypt and into the functional villus compartment.

This compartmentalisation of the crypt is constant, ie, the stem cell zone is always situated at the base of the crypt, the proliferation zone is above this, occupying the middle of the crypt, and the maturation zone occupies the top of the crypt. Here we ask if this apparently constant spatial arrangement has as its basis a one-dimensional coordinate system that provides positional information to the tissue. Perhaps there is a system that stipulates which way is 'up' and which way is 'down'. Apart from accounting for the structural organisation of the tissue, a coordinate system would help to explain the orderly migration, differentiation and ultimate loss of cells. For example, after formation at position 5 or above, ie, at the upper border of the stem-cell zone, most of the columnar, mucous and enteroendocrine cells migrate upwards, traversing the proliferation and maturation zones of the crypt, then the functional compartment of the villus, to be lost from the extrusion zone. We have shown, however, that all Paneth cells, and some columnar, mucous and enteroendocrine cells migrate downwards into the stem-cell zone where they ultimately die (see Section 3.2). In the midst of the downward migration of differentiating cells into the stem-cell zone, there is an upward migration of stem cells from that zone. Such well choreographed movement surely requires the existence of a coordinate system, at least in the vicinity of the crypt base.

The source of such a system would have to bear a special structural relationship to the crypt if it were to provide direction. The elements of the intestinal organ that possess the necessary structural relationships to the crypt are the lumen, the crypt itself and the muscularis mucosae with its associated structures (nerve plexuses, blood vascular system, lymphatics). Each of these structures is so positioned that it could provide the necessary information to the crypt.

We have studied the relationship between the orientation of the crypt axis and the plane of the muscularis mucosae, and the effects of this relationship on the orientation of the borders between the various crypt compartments. These studies provide a means to determine which, if any, of the aforementioned structures have a role in determining the orientation of compartments within the crypt, and specifically to distinguish between co-ordinate systems related to the position of the muscularis mucosae, and those related to the position of the crypt axis.

The orientation of the border between the stem-cell zone and the proliferation zone is reflected in the orientation of the upper border of the Paneth cell

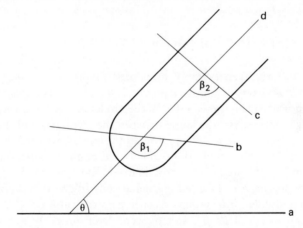

Figure 2.4.1 Schematic diagram of the lines drawn with camera lucida for the measurement of crypt tilt and the orientation of the borders between crypt compartments. Line (a) represents the plane of the muscularis mucosae, (b) represents the line drawn through the highest Paneth cell granule in each crypt column and indicates the orientation of the border between the stem cell zone and the proliferation zone; (c) represents the line drawn through the highest labelled nucleus in each crypt column and indicates the orientation of the border between the proliferation zone and the maturation zone; (d) represents the crypt axis

distribution (see Section 3.2). The orientation of the border between the proliferation and the maturation compartments is reflected in the orientation of the plane of the highest labelled cells within the crypt.

In normal intestine the axes of many crypts are perpendicular to the plane of the muscularis mucosae, and the boundary between the stem-cell zone and the proliferation zone, as demarcated by the upper border of the Paneth cell distribution, is perpendicular to the crypt axis. However in some crypts the axis is not perpendicular to the muscularis mucosae, and may be tilted as much as $40°$ from normal. This offers a tool with which to study the importance of muscle-related factors. If these factors define the coordinate system then tilting of the crypt will result in a change in its position relative to the coordinate system. Furthermore, such a system would imply a change in the orientation of the boundaries between the zones relative to the crypt axis if they were similarly controlled. On the other hand, if the coordinate system was established by crypt-axis-related structures, tilting of the crypts would have no effect on the orientation of the boundaries relative to the crypt axis.

In an attempt to throw some light on this problem we studied the orientation of the boundaries between the crypt compartments in crypts which were perpendicular to the muscularis mucosae and in crypts which were tilted by various degrees relative to it.

2.4.2 MATERIALS AND METHODS

Six hundred and eighteen suitably orientated crypts were studied in serial Epon-embedded sections of mouse jejunum 1 μm thick. For each crypt three angles were measured (Figure 2.4.1): θ, the angle between the crypt axis and the muscularis mucosae; β_1, the angle between the crypt axis and the boundary between the stem-cell zone and the proliferation zone, demarcated by the upper border of the Paneth cell distribution; and β_2, the angle between the crypt axis and the boundary between the proliferation and the maturation zones, demarcated by the highest labelled epithelial cells in the two crypt columns. The crypts were divided into groups according to the values of θ, and for each group the mean values of θ, β_1, and β_2 were determined. In normal animals most of the crypts were found to be nearly perpendicular to the muscularis mucosae. Only a small number of crypts were found with θ less than $50°$. To obtain more data points for the greatly tilted groups an experimental preparation was developed in which the antimesenteric border of a short segment of jejunum was involuted, thus creating a fold of tissue similar in appearance to the plicae circulares of human intestine. The crypts lining the sides and the top of the fold became greatly tilted after two weeks. One hundred and seventy-five crypts from the experimental preparation were used and the mean values of θ, β_1, and β_2 determined for the groups previously defined.

2.4.3 RESULTS AND INTERPRETATION

Results both from intact animals and the experimental preparation showed that as θ decreased β_1 did not change significantly from the values in group 1 ($85° < \theta \leqslant 90°$) until a threshold was reached. In other words as the crypts became tilted, the boundary between the stem-cell zone and the proliferation zone remained more or less perpendicular to the crypt axis until the crypts were tilted by more than $30°$ (ie, $\theta < 60°$). At this point, β_1 became significantly different (p <0.01) from values for group 1. The boundary between the stem-cell and proliferation zones in these rather more tilted crypts was no longer perpendicular to the crypt axis. Furthermore in the greatly tilted crypts of the experimental preparation the boundary was found to be parallel to the muscularis mucosae. On the other hand, β_2 was not significantly different from values for group 1 even in greatly tilted crypts. Therefore, in contrast to the boundary between the stem-cell and proliferation zones, the boundary between proliferation and maturation zones remains perpendicular to the crypt axis no matter how much the crypt is tilted. These results seem to indicate that the orientation of the boundary between the stem-cell and proliferation zones derives positional information from the muscularis mucosae or an associated structure and, beyond a threshold of 30 percent tilt, it tends to become reorientated parallel to the muscularis mucosae. This implies that the boundary between the stem-cell and proliferation zones responds to non-epithelial influences. Presumably, systemic factors related to the muscularis mucosae (neural, vascular or others) play a role in maintaining the coordinate system that governs this boundary. The threshold may exist to permit the slight movements of crypts that surely accompany peristalsis. The boundary between the proliferation and maturation zones, on the other hand, appears to be related to the crypt axis to which it is always orientated perpendicularly. This implies that the boundary between the proliferation and maturation zones responds to crypt-axis-related influences which may be epithelial or luminal. The boundaries between the crypt compartments are orientated relative to their respective coordinate systems. The border between the stem-cell zone and the proliferation compartment is orientated relative to the muscularis mucosae while the border between the proliferation zone and the maturation zone is independent of it, and relates instead to the crypt axis.

ACKNOWLEDGEMENTS

This work was done with the support of grants from the National Foundation—March of Dimes and the Medical Research Council of Canada.

2.5 Growth Control in the Small Intestine after Death of Proliferating Cells Induced by Cytosine Arabinoside

Nicholas A Wright, Awatiff Al-Nafussi and Nicholas Britton

2.5.1 INTRODUCTION

Of the several theories of growth control, the one which has found most favour has been that of negative feedback by the functional cell mass (779). Recently, experimental support for this theory has been obtained in many tissues by the protagonists of the chalone hypothesis (338), and evidence now exists for such a mechanism in the small intestine (see Section 2.3). However, before accepting this proposal as a working hypothesis, the evidence for negative feedback mechanisms operating in the intestine should be considered.

It has been claimed that villus and crypt populations in the mouse intestine show a negative feedback relationship after irradiation (620), but this can be criticised on several grounds: firstly, most workers have used simple linear measurements of villus and crypt length to quantify changes in the size of the crypt population, but it can be shown that, while such simple morphometry is admissible for normally shaped crypts and villi, when abnormal forms are encountered, as after irradiation, then such techniques can be misleading. Secondly, in the assessment of the relationship of the villus population to the crypt population, it is necessary to remember that in all areas of the small bowel numerous crypts supply each villus with cells. A perturbative stimulus such as irradiation could lead to changes in the crypt-villus ratio, and it becomes essential to measure the crypt population as the crypt cell population per villus (Section 1.1). Thirdly, the wrong index of cell proliferation has also been used. So far as the functional villus compartment is concerned, the essential measurement is the net villus influx, which is the crypt cell production rate (CCPR) multiplied by the crypt-villus ratio (109). There is little point in correlating the labelling index or the crypt growth fraction with the villus population, since neither of these parameters need reflect the CCPR; in addition to the growth fraction, the cell cycle time and the crypt population also contribute to the CCPR, so the growth fraction in isolation cannot be used as an estimator.

Consequently, when looking for negative feedback control mechanisms in the small intestine, we must measure three quantities: the villus population, the crypt cell population per villus, and the net cellular influx per villus.

2.5.2 MATERIALS AND METHODS

Female Balb/c mice were given two injections 12 h apart of 400 mg of cytosine arabinoside (ara-C) per kg body weight. All injections were given intraperitoneally and their timing was such as to produce maximum cell kill; labelling index studies had shown that 12 h after the first injection many crypt cells were in the S-phase, and thus susceptible to a further ara-C exposure (11). Animals were killed in groups of three over the next 18 days, and the villus cell population, crypt-villus ratio, crypt cell population, and crypt cell population per villus, were measured in each animal in the upper jejunum (at a site 25 percent of the total length of the small bowel measured from the pylorus).

Samples of intestine were fixed in Carnoy's solution and stored in 75 percent ethanol. After rehydration the tissue was hydrolysed in normal HCl for 6 minutes, and stained in bulk with Feulgen's reagent. Individual villi were microdissected and squashed, and the villus cell population was assessed by counting epithelial cell nuclei in ten villi per mouse. The crypt cell population per villus is the product of the crypt-villus ratio and the crypt population; the crypt-villus ratio was measured as described in Section 1.1, while the crypt population was measured by microdissection of 10 crypts per animal.

On each day after ara-C, nine animals were given 1 mg of vincristine per kg body weight intraperitoneally, and starting 30 minutes after injection, animals were killed every 15 minutes for 2.5 h. Metaphases were counted in 10 microdissected crypts per animal, and plotted against time. The CCPR was measured from the slope of the line, and the net cell influx per villus calculated from the product of the CCPR and the crypt-villus ratio.

2.5.3 RESULTS AND DISCUSSION

Figure 2.5.1 shows the changes in the villus cell population; results are expressed as a fraction of the control value which was 6150 cells. There is only a small decrease in the villus population over the first 2 days after ara-C, but on days 3, 4 and 5 values are about 30 percent of control values. There then follows a rapid increase in villus population size, which reaches a maximum of about 1.4 times the control value on days 9 and 10. The villus population then falls,

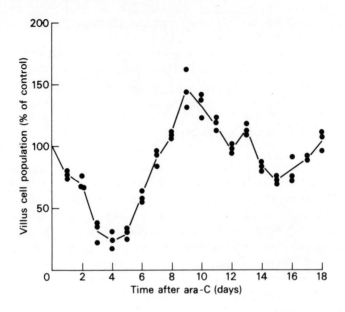

Figure 2.5.1 The villus cell population at different times after ara-C, expressed as a percentage of the normal value

until on days 14 to 16 values are again low, before a further rise occurs to the control level at day 18 after ara-C. The pattern of damped oscillations about the mean is consistent with some form of negative feedback control of the net villus influx by the numbers of functional villus cells.

Figure 2.5.2 shows the changes in crypt population after ara-C; it falls to 20 percent of the control value (510 cells) by 1 day after ara-C, and then recovers quickly with a doubling time of about one day, to reach an initial maximum of about twice the control level on day 5 or 6. By day 12 values are again approaching normal, but there then follows a secondary peak, realising more than twice the control value on day 16; a similarly abrupt fall then follows to the control level at day 18.

Figure 2.5.3 shows the changes in the crypt-villus ratio, and it is evident that the number of crypts per villus has quickly decreased, with a reduction in the crypt-villus ratio from 11 to below 5. This is reflected in the reduction in the number of crypts per circumference of the bowel which occurs at the same time. There follows a slow increase towards normal values.

This change in the crypt-villus ratio has a considerable effect on the crypt cell population per villus, which is plotted against time in Figure 2.5.4. The value is as low as 10 percent of control on day 1, and the subsequent rise is fairly slow,

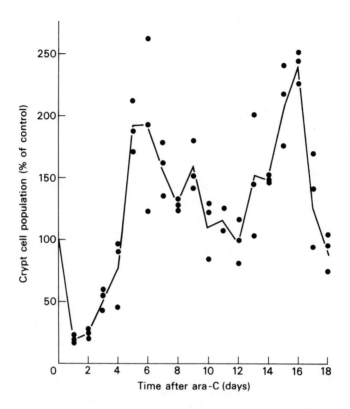

Figure 2.5.2 The crypt cell population at different times after ara-C, expressed as a percentage of the normal value

reaching just about normal on day 6. The timing of the secondary peak on day 16 remains the same although its relative magnitude is decreased.

The finding of the secondary rise is interesting. The initial increase in crypt population is due to crypt repopulation, and the initial peak is presumably due to overcompensation. Although there were always occasional crypts which showed evidence of budding, after day 11 there was a large increase in the number of crypts with buds, and many had more than one bud, as was shown after recovery from irradiation (85). The secondary rise in crypt population is thus due to a large increase in cell population as a result of bud formation in preparation for crypt reproduction by fission.

Figure 2.5.5 combines the curves of Figures 2.5.1 and 2.5.4 and shows the crypt cell population per villus compared with the villus cell population. After the rapid crypt depopulation, caused both by the destruction of crypts and by the large cell kill in surviving crypts, there is a delay of 3 or 4 days before a

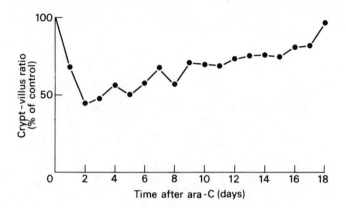

Figure 2.5.3 The crypt-villus ratio at different times after ara-C, expressed as a percentage of the normal value

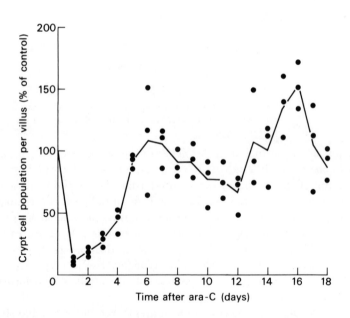

Figure 2.5.4 The crypt population per villus at different times after ara-C, expressed as a percentage of the normal value

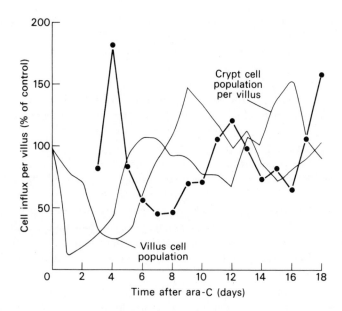

Figure 2.5.5 The cell influx per villus at different times after ara-C, expressed as a percentage of the normal value. Also shown are the villus population and the crypt cell population per villus, as percentages of their normal values

corresponding fall in villus population, no doubt due to the transit time of cells on the villus. There is a tendency for the delay between crypt and villus population changes to lengthen as the response proceeds. Nevertheless, there is a distinct reduction in the villus population at the time of the initial increase in crypt population and, moreover, during the phase of overcompensation of the villus population the crypt population is depressed below normal. Again the results are consistent with a negative feedback hypothesis.

Figure 2.5.5 also shows the villus influx in relation to the crypt cell population per villus and the villus population. Readings on days 1 and 2 proved impossible to obtain, due to difficulties with the microdissection of the small, badly damaged crypts. Nevertheless, by three days after ara-C the villus influx has recovered almost to the control level, even while the crypt cell population is still small; and there is a peak of almost twice the control value on day 4. Then there is a rapid fall, and the initial trough lasts for 3 or 4 days from day 6, at the time of the first peak of crypt cell population and when villus cell population is reaching control levels. A secondary peak ensues at 11 to 12 days, followed by a second decrease below the control value, and on day 18 levels are again well above normal.

The delay between the initial increase in villus influx (and therefore in CCPR since the crypt villus-ratio remains relatively constant at this time) and the rise in crypt cell population is about 2 days, and, moreover, the second increase at 11 to 12 days is about 4 days before the second increase in crypt population, caused by budding in preparation for fission. However, the large initial increase in villus influx occurs at a time when the villus population is declining, but has not reached its lowest levels; the villus influx is increasing at a time when the villus population is also increasing at days 7 to 10, at which time the crypt cell population is in its second trough.

A defect of the present study is the assumption that the crypt-villus ratio times the CCPR is equivalent to the cell influx per villus, which is only true when crypts remain constant in size. After crypt depopulation a certain amount of cell production goes towards crypt repopulation before cells are contributed to the villi, and this may be a cause of delay in the mechanism controlling crypt size. However, we cannot ignore the fact that there may be a feedback from crypt-cell number to proliferating crypt cells, possibly mediated by decycled cells still in the crypt.

Although our experimental findings are consistent with a negative feedback model of control, it must be conceded that we do not yet know whether such control operates from changes in villus-cell number, crypt-cell number, or both.

ACKNOWLEDGEMENT

This work was supported by the Cancer Research Campaign.

2.6 Influence of Guanethidine-Induced Sympathectomy on Crypt Cell Proliferation in the Pre- and Post-closure Ileum of the Neonatal Rat

Robert M Klein

2.6.1 INTRODUCTION

The neonatal development of the ileal epithelium of the rat may be divided into pre- and post-closure phases. During the pre-closure phase villus cells are specialised for macromolecular absorption and are permeable to large macromolecules such as IgG and polyvinylpyrrolidone (118, 119, 282). Between 18 and 21 days after birth permeability of villus cells to macromolecular substances ceases (closure) and permeable vacuolated cells disappear (119). The post-closure period begins after the replacement of the permeable, vacuolated, 'juvenile' cells by 'adult-like', non-permeable villus cells (119).

Several investigators have found that the closure of the ileum in the rat is associated with an increase in turnover of the ileal crypt cells. The progressive removal of vacuolated cells from the ileal villi of the rat during the period from 18 to 21 days after birth has been demonstrated, and it has been proposed that there is an acceleration in crypt cell turnover which accounts for the alteration in villus cells (119). Several laboratories have demonstrated an increase in cell division during the second to third week after birth. Cellular migration in the rat has been estimated to increase by a factor of 4 or 5 in the period between 11 and 28 days of age (376); other workers have found a threefold increase in the rate of extrusion (503) and a decrease of approximately 60 percent in turnover time (602) in the mouse intestinal epithelium between 15 and 21 days after birth. An increase in cellular migration in the duodenum of 18-day-old rats, 48 hours after administration of tritiated thymidine (^{3}HTdR) at day 16, apparently reflects a burst of crypt cell proliferation during this period (828). There are also large increases in the relative weight of the intestine, the depth of intestinal crypts, crypt cell mitotic (I_m) and ^{3}HTdR labelling (I_s) indices, and a decrease in the ratio of height of villi to depth of crypts in rats older than 21 days when compared to those less than 15 days of age (316).

Cell cycle analysis of pre- and post-closure ileal epithelium by the fraction of labelled mitoses (FLM) technique has shown that the cell cycle time, T_c, is longer in 8-day-old rats than in 28-day-old rats (367). The lengthening of T_c is primarily attributed to an elongation of t_{G_1} and is accompanied by a lower I_m, I_s, and growth fraction (367). The present study was undertaken in order to analyse the period of ileal development between the 15th and 23rd days since birth and to quantify specific alterations in crypt cell proliferation. Labelling index, mitotic index, birth rate, (k_B, measured by a stathmokinetic technique with colchicine), the depth of the crypts and the height of the villi were determined. Additionally, the effects of neonatal chemical sympathectomy (with guanethidine sulphate) on crypt cell proliferation associated with closure were studied using these techniques from 15 to 23 days of age, and the FLM method was used on control and guanethidine-treated 15-day-old rats.

2.6.2 MATERIALS AND METHODS

Time-pregnant Sprague-Dawley rats were received in the animal quarters at least 10 days prior to parturition. They were given Purina rat chow and water ad lib and were maintained on a 12-hour light-dark cycle; lights on 0600 h to 1800 h. Rat pups were maintained until being killed by ether overdose.

2.6.2.1 GUANETHIDINE TREATMENT

Beginning on the day of birth and continuing every 48 h for 14 days, rats were injected subcutaneously with 20 μg per g body weight guanethidine sulphate in phosphate-buffered saline (PBS), pH 7.4. Only male rats were used to avoid possible variation due to sex differences. Each rat was given 8 injections. This technique has been shown to produce a 75 to 81 percent reduction in the number of perikarya in the superior cervical and coeliac ganglia of 15-day-old rats (368, 373). Effectiveness of the treatment in these experiments was verified by light-microscopic examination of ganglia from guanethidine-treated rats. Control rats were littermates of guanethidine-treated rats and the same procedure was followed except that guanethidine was omitted from the PBS solution.

2.6.2.2 FLM STUDIES

One hundred and fifty-six 15-day-old rats, 78 controls and 78 guanethine-treated, were injected with ^{3}HTDR of specific activity 6.7 Ci per mmole diluted in saline, by an intraperitoneal injection of 0.5 μCi per g body weight at 1000 h. Groups of 3 control and 3 guanethidine-treated rats were killed hourly for 26 h. A 1 cm section of ileum, 2 to 3 cm proximal to the ileocecal junction, was removed, fixed in neutral buffered formalin for 72 h, washed in running tap water, dehydrated in alcohols, and embedded in paraffin. Sections 4 μm thick were mounted on glass slides and autoradiographs were prepared using a dipping technique, the exposure period being 4 weeks. The slides were stained lightly with Harris's haematoxylin and eosin.

The fraction of labelled mitoses was determined for each hourly interval in the ileum of control and guanethidine-treated rats. At least 500 mitoses were counted per point with a minimum of 150 per rat. All counts were performed on crypts which were cut through their main axis so that the column of cells in the crypt from the base to the junction of the villus could be seen in one section. All mitoses in the crypts were counted. Each mitosis with 4 or more grains above it was considered labelled (674).

The duration of the cell cycle, DNA-synthetic phase (S), $G_2 + \frac{1}{2}M$, and $G_1 + \frac{1}{2}M$ in the ileal crypt were calculated from the FLM curve (120, 557). The duration of mitosis, t_m, was calculated from the product of the cycle time and the mitotic index for each of the groups (557). Labelling and mitotic indices were also determined within the ileal crypt for control and guanethidine-treated rats. A total of at least 3000 cells was counted for each hourly reading to determine these indices.

2.6.2.3 MORPHOMETRY AND PROLIFERATIVE INDICES

Four control and 4 guanethidine-treated rats were killed each day from 15 to 23 days after birth for I_m and I_s estimation. All rats were injected at 0900 h with ^{3}HTdR in the same dosage as in the FLM studies and killed 1 h later; ileal specimens were processed in the same manner as described for FLM analysis. Cells in all stages of mitotis (406) were included in the I_m counts. Changes in the height of the crypts and villi were determined by counting the number of nuclei in areas with a continuous epithelial layer from the tip of the villus to the base of the crypt. Twenty-five villi and crypts were counted per individual rat, ie, 100 for each treatment group per day.

2.6.2.4 BIRTH RATE ESTIMATION

Sixteen rats of each age group from 15 to 23 days after birth were injected with 1 μg/g body weight of colchicine, and 4 control and 4 guanethidine-treated rats were killed hourly for 4 hours. Ileal tissue was removed and processed as described previously. Metaphase cells were scored on sections where the crypt lumen could be seen throughout its length (745). The mean number of metaphases per hour was plotted for each hourly interval, with a minimum of

2000 cells counted per rat. The slope of the line provides an estimated birth rate.

2.6.3 RESULTS

Guanethidine treatment produced no statistically significant alteration in body weight, but at least a 70 percent reduction in sympathetic perikarya of the superior cervical and coeliac ganglia.

2.6.3.1 FLM STUDIES

FLM data for control and guanethidine-treated 15-day-old rats are shown in Figure 2.6.1 and the duration of the cell cycle phases derived from the curves

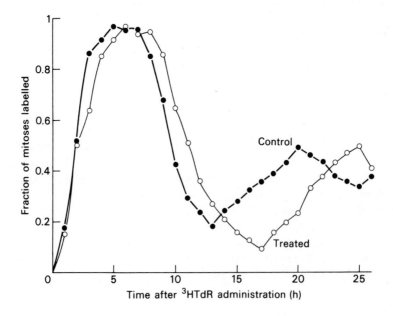

Figure 2.6.1 FLM data for the ileal crypts of control and guanethidine-treated 15-day-old rats. Each point represents the mean of three rats

are listed in Table 2.6.1. The plot of I_s versus time after ^{3}HTdR injection is shown in Figure 2.6.2. There is a rise in the percentage of labelled ileal crypt

Table 2.6.1 Summary of ileal crypt cell cycle parameters for 8, 15, 28 and 45-day-old control rats, and for 15 and 45-day-old guanethidine-treated rats (367, 369)

Age (days)	Treatment	T_c(h)	t_{G_1}(h)	t_s(h)	t_{G_2}(h)	t_m(h)
8	None	16.8	6.8	7.7	2.0	0.3
15	None	18.1	8.3	7.7	1.7	0.4
15	Guanethidine	23.0	11.8	9.0	1.8	0.4
28	None	9.3	0.9	6.6	1.2	0.6
45	None	9.6	1.8	6.6	0.8	0.4
45	Guanethidine	15.0	5.7	7.8	1.1	0.4

cells with time after injection in both groups, as has been demonstrated previously in both neonatal and adult intestinal epithelium (367, 435).

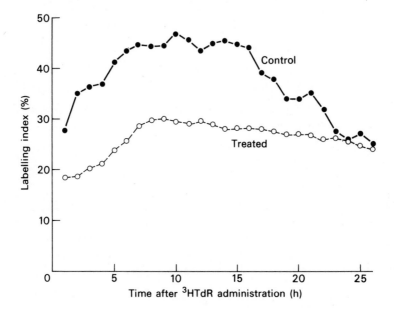

Figure 2.6.2 Labelling index data for the ileal crypts of control and guanethidine-treated 15-day-old rats. Each point represents the mean of three rats

Guanethidine treatment depresses the rise and slows the fall in I_s, which may be related to a slower rate of migration from crypt to villus in sympathectomised rats (367, 368). In Figure 2.6.3 I_m is plotted against time of day and

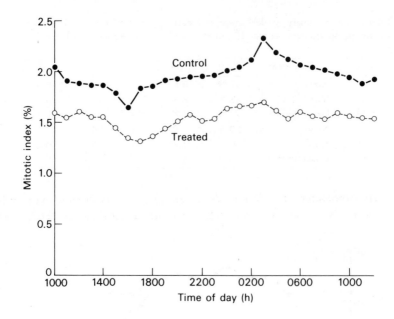

Figure 2.6.3 Circadian rhythm in mitotic index in the ileal crypts of control and guanethidine-treated 15-day-old rats. Each point represents the mean of 3 rats

demonstrates a circadian periodicity with an amplitude of 37 percent of the mean in controls; this is reduced to 20 percent in the guanethidine-treated rats. The pattern of the mitotic circadian rhythm is similar in phase to adult rats for both control and guanethidine-treated groups, although the amplitude of the rhythm is reduced in both 15-day-old groups (373).

2.6.3.2 MORPHOMETRY AND PROLIFERATIVE INDICES

Figures 2.6.4 to 2.6.9 describe the pattern of I_m, I_s, k_B, crypt depth, villus height and the ratio of villus height to crypt depth from days 15 to 23 after birth. The proliferative indices and the birth rate increase at 18 days and continue to increase during the remainder of the period of growth in this study. The number of cells in the crypt is fairly constant from 15 to 18 days, but begins to increase significantly on the 19th day. The size of the crypt doubles (over day–15 values) by between day 20 and 21 and is increased almost threefold

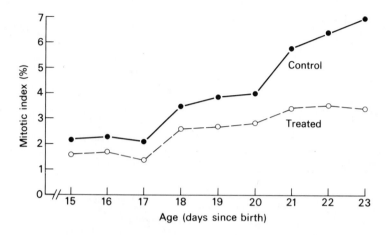

Figure 2.6.4 Mitotic index data in pre- and post-closure ileum of control and guanethidine-treated rats. Each point represents the mean of 4 rats

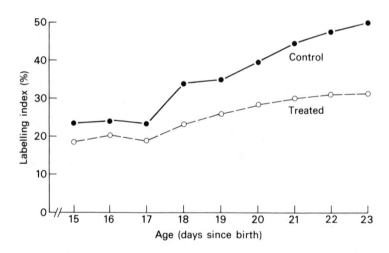

Figure 2.6.5 Labelling index data in pre- and post-closure ileum of control and guanethidine-treated rats. Each point represents the mean of 4 rats

by day 23. The height of the villus increases from 15 to 23 days, but only by about 36 percent. The ratio of villus height to crypt depth is greater in sympathectomised rats, while all other indices are reduced.

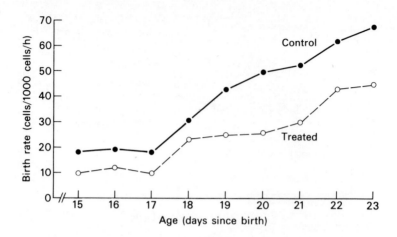

Figure 2.6.6 Cell birth rate in pre- and post-closure ileum of control and guanethidine-treated rats, from the stathmokinetic experiments

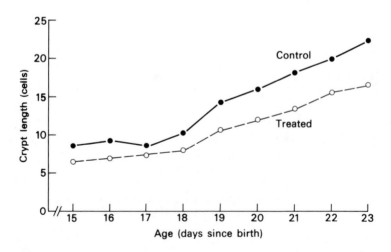

Figure 2.6.7 Crypt depth in pre- and post-closure ileum of control and guanethidine-treated rats. Each point represents the mean of 4 rats

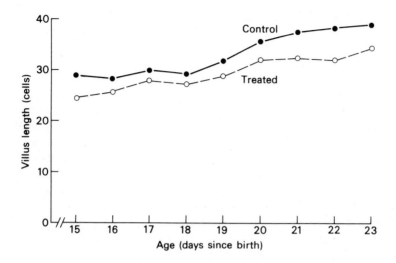

Figure 2.6.8 Villus height in pre- and post-closure ileum of control and guanethidine-treated rats. Each points represents the mean of 4 rats

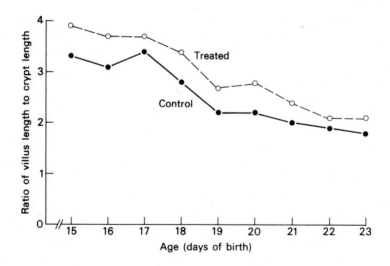

Figure 2.6.9 Ratio of villus height to crypt depth in pre- and post-closure ileum of control and guanethidine-treated rats. Each point represents the mean of 4 rats

2.6.4 DISCUSSION

2.6.4.1 NORMAL PATTERN OF ILEAL CRYPT CELL PROLIFERATION

Cell proliferation in the ileum has previously been shown to increase at the time of closure to macromolecules. The FLM data for 15-day old rats are compared with previous data from the same laboratory in Table 2.6.1. The ileal epithelium of 15-day-old rats has a slightly longer T_c than 8-day-old rats, with a longer t_{G_1} which may be related to the gradual differentiation of cells in the upper portions of the crypt. The situation may be similar to that in developing rat parotid gland where between 8 and 15 days after birth there is an elongation of t_{G_1} as differentiation and amylas synthesis progresses (368). Comparison of the ileal cell cycle of 8-day old rats with 28 and 45-day-old rats indicates a shortening of T_c (primarily in t_{G_1}) after closure, but a slight lengthening of T_c and t_{G_1} between 28 and 45 days of age. The results corroborate the findings of several laboratories indicating a slower rate of cell division in the small-intestinal epithelium of suckling rats (118, 729). The results differ from data (708) demonstrating an increase in T_c from 15 to 18 hours between infant mice (10 days old) and young adult mice (30 to 70 days old). These differences may represent species variation in development between rats and mice.

Similarly, the developmental pattern of neonatal crypt cell division appears to differ in suckling mice and rats. A fairly constant rate of mitosis in the mouse duodenum has been demonstrated (503) with two periods of reduced mitotic activity: from day 19 of gestation to day 2 after birth and from day 13 to day 19 after birth. This contrasts with data from rats in which the mitotic or labelling index in duodenum (829), jejunum (316, 729), and ileum (367, 729) is reduced in suckling rats and increases during the third week after birth. In the present study, there is a sudden increase in I_s, I_m and k_B at the 18th day after birth (at the time of closure) and a gradual increase until the 23rd day (during the early post-closure period). This burst in proliferative activity has been demonstrated in rat duodenum at 18 to 19 days and may be related to hormonal (829) and other factors, such as the switch from liquid to solid diet, which occur at about the time of ileal closure (567, 568). However, this increase in activity does not occur in the neonatal mouse (503) although a three-fold increase in the rate of extrusion does occur between days 15 and 21, with growth of villi and crypts resulting from the low rate of extrusion in the early neonatal perod. Although the temporal sequence or mechanism of increased renewal may differ in the rat, there must be a similar shift from growth to cell renewal as the number of crypt cells and the crypt-villus ratio increases (20).

The rate of cell division in the ileum of 3-week-old rats (days 21 to 23 after birth) is higher than that of adult rats (373, 531) as has been demonstrated previously in the jejunal epithelium (729). Most of these dividing cells appear to be added to the crypt which more than doubles in depth between day 15 and day 23 after birth. Some of the cells produced may also be used for expanding the villi, which grow by 36 percent between the 15th and 23rd day, and increasing the number of crypts (828) (which was not measured in the present study). The rapid growth of the crypt in the rat contrasts with the growth pattern in the mouse where 60 percent of villus and crypt height is attained by 15 days after birth (503).

Values for mitotic index and birth rate in 15-day-old rats are slightly higher than those obtained for 5-day-old rats (729). Tutton (729) determined the jejunal crypt cell turnover time in 5-day-old rats to be 79 h using a colchicine-induced stathmokinetic technique. Using his method our colchicine data may be extrapolated to obtain a turnover time of 37 h. A similar conversion of Tutton's data to cells/1000 cells/h results in a value of 8.8 which is about half of the present value of 18.7 cells/1000 cells/h. The differences could be due to variation in strain of rats, intestinal segment (jejunum versus ileum), or circadian variation, although circadian rhythm of mitosis may not be present in tissues during the early neonatal period (260, 371). The low rate of mitotic accumulation and the resulting long cycle time in Tutton's experiments may also be related to the ineffectiveness of colchicine in producing a linear accumulation of mitotic cells in young rats (648). Colchicine apparently becomes effective in metaphase arrest during postnatal development since linear accumulation of mitoses was induced in the present study of 15 to 23-day-old rats and in previous studies in other laboratories (20).

2.6.4.2 EFFECTS OF SYMPATHECTOMY ON NEONATAL ILEAL CRYPT CELL PROLIFERATION

The effects of sympathectomy on adult rat intestinal cell proliferation have been investigated by immunosympathectomy (190), chemical sympathectomy (369, 370, 373, 745) and surgical sympathectomy (382, 489, 745). These investigations have demonstrated a decreased rate of cell proliferation and migration (190, 369, 370) and an inhibition of the crypt cell circadian rhythm after sympathectomy (369). The present FLM study of the ileal epithelium of 15-day-old rats demonstrates an elongation of T_c, t_{G_1}, and t_S (primarily t_{G_1}). This pattern is similar to that seen in the intestinal crypts of adult rats treated with guanethidine in the neonatal period (369). The reduction of mitotic and labelling indices and the inhibition of the circadian rhythm in cell proliferation are also similar to those found in adult rats (369, 370, 373). Sympathectomy reduces crypt cell proliferation between 15 and 23 days after birth, and, although there is still increased activity in the post-closure ileal epithelium, crypt depth and villus height are also reduced. Sympathectomy delays, but does not permanently prevent, the post-closure acceleration of proliferative activity in the ileum since adult rats (neonatally sympathectomised) have normal compartment size (190), but retain a slower rate of crypt cell proliferation (190, 369, 370, 373).

The mechanism for autonomic nervous system regulation of cell division may involve either direct or indirect pathways. These mechanisms include alteration of visceral blood flow and gut motility (190) or more direct regulation through the intestinal plexuses and their 'diffuse neurohumoral synapse' (190, 325). Noradrenaline levels are lowered by 80 percent in the intestine after guanethidine treatment (351). The depletion of noradrenaline may be directly responsible for the inhibition of the crypt cell circadian rhythm in mitosis (Figure 2.6.3) and for the reduction of mitotic activity which occurs in sympathectomised rats. It has previously been suggested that noradrenaline plays a role in the normal regulation of circadian rhythms and the stimulation of mitotic activity during the nocturnal hours (368, 370, 373, 729, 745).

Sympathectomy also delays the removal of vacuolated pre-closure cells from the villus as these cells are absent by 20 to 21 days in control rats, but are often present on the villi of 23-day-old guanthidine-treated rats. This delay in neonatal ileal crypt cell proliferation appears to be similar to the prolongation of T_c and decreased cell proliferation induced by neonatal administration of the β-adrenergic stimulant, isoprenaline (367). However, the effect of sympathectomy is not a permanent inhibition of the redifferentiation of the intestinal epithelium from the suckling to adult-type as occurs after hypophysectomy (480, 828). After hypophysectomy at 6 days, the duodenal crypt cell labelling index at 22 days is lower than in 6-day-old control rats and the cell cycle time is similar to that of 6-day-old rats (828). In the absence of the hypophysis, ileal closure fails to occur by 24 days (828) and the villus epithelium remains heavily vacuolated with a juvenile morphological appearance (829).

The intestinal deficiencies produced by hypophysectomy may be overcome by treatment with thyroxine or cortisone (829). The glucocorticoids and thyroxine also play an important role in intestinal development (831). Adrenalectomised or thyroidectomised rats show depressed crypt cell mitotic activity which may be restored to control levels by relacement hormone therapy with cortisone and thyroxine respectively (831). Glucocorticoids have been implicated in the neonatal differentiation of the rat pancreas (164), parotid gland (567), and intestine (479, 831), and many of the developmental changes in these tissues occur together with alterations of plasma corticosterone levels (567). The closure of the ileum at 18 to 19 days after birth and the concomitant acceleration of crypt cell proliferation take place during the rise in plasma corticosterone levels from 12 to 25 days after birth (4, 12, 283, 567). In the adult rat, the synthetic glucocorticoid prednisolone shortens the jejunal crypt cell cycle (730, 744) while adrenalectomy prolongs it (730). The inhibition of cell division produced by adrenalectomy is only partially reversed by hormone replacement with prednisolone, indicating that the adrenal medulla and the catecholamine hormones may also be involved in the regulation of crypt cell proliferation in the intestinal epithelium (730). In this respect, norepinephrine has been shown to have a stimulatory effect on crypt cell mitotic activity, while epinephrine has an inhibitory effect (745), and although the role of the adrenomedullary hormones and their receptors have been analysed in the adult rat, their possible role in the acceleration of proliferation and other events involved with closure have not been investigated. However β-adrenergic stimulation with isoprenaline (367) has been shown to inhibit crypt cell proliferation in both pre- and post-closure ileum, indicating that adrenoreceptors and catecholamines may function in a similar manner in the neonatal and adult rat intestinal epithelium. Future experiments will analyse the effects of sympathectomy and the role of the adrenomedullary hormones on the alterations of morphology, enzymatic activity, and macromolecular absorption which occur during ileal closure and subsequent intestinal development.

2.6.5 SUMMARY

This study was designed to analyse ileal crypt cell proliferation before and after neonatal closure to macromolecular absorption, and to determine the effects of guanethidine-induced sympathectomy on cell proliferation. Previous studies have demonstrated that ileal crypt cell proliferation before closure (8 days) is significantly slower than in the post-closure period (28 days). The present experiments were designed to investigate ileal crypt cell division by the FLM technique at 15 days after birth (immediately before closure), to calculate I_m, I_s, k_B, and to measure crypt depth and villus height on days 15 to 23 after birth. In addition, the effects of the sympathetic nervous system on crypt cell proliferation were analysed by guanethidine-induced sympathectomy.

Guanethidine treatment resulted in a substantial reduction in superior cervical and coeliac perikarya at 15 days after birth, and FLM measurements of ileal crypt cell proliferation in 15-day-old rats showed that T_c was increased from 18 h to 23 h. Mitotic and labelling indices were significantly lowered and the circadian rhythm of crypt cell proliferation was depressed. Daily measurements of I_m, I_s and k_B from 15 to 23 days after birth demonstrated a sudden acceleration of activity on day 18. The birth rate increased from day 18 to day 23 with 3-week-old rats demonstrating a faster rate of ileal crypt cell proliferation than adult rats. The ileal crypt depth more than doubled between 15 and 23 days while the height of the villus column increased slowly but steadily during the period of this study. Cell division is inhibited by guanethidine-induced sympathectomy although there is still an acceleration of proliferation in the post-closure period. Sympathectomy also delays the progressive removal of the immature hydropic epithelial cells from the villi of the ileum. The possible role of the sympathetic neurotransmitter norepine-phrine and the adrenomedullary hormones in ileal closure and the post-closure acceleration of proliferation have been discussed and compared to effects of adrenocortical and other hormones.

ACKNOWLEDGEMENTS

The author would like to thank Charles A Brownley of CIBA-Geigy, New Jersey, USA for the gift of guanethidine sulphate, Susan Whitney for her excellent technical assistance, Joan Rome for typing the manuscript, and Drs John Clancy and Thomas Marino for proofreading it. This research was supported by NIH grant #DE 04557 and Anatomy Department Fletcher Endowment Fund.

2.7 The Stimulatory Effect of Butyrate on Epithelial Cell Proliferation in the Rumen of the Sheep and its Mediation by Insulin; Differences between In Vivo and In Vitro Studies

Takashi Sakata, Kazuo Hikosaka, Yoko Shiomura and Hideo Tamate

2.7.1 INTRODUCTION

The domestic hervibores or ruminants (cattle, sheep and goats) are of economic importance because they can utilise high-fibre low-protein diets by means of efficient intraruminal microbial fermentation (569). A multi-compartmented forestomach is the anatomical structure concerned with the utilisation of fibrous diets, and the rumen is its most capacious compartment able to accommodate up to 200 l in cattle (774). The inner surface of the rumen is lined by stratified squamous epithelium.

It is an organ for the storage of bulky diets while they undergo an efficient process of continuous fermentation (127, 343). The main products of ruminal fermentation are short-chain fatty acids (SCFA), such as acetic, propionic, and butyric acids, which are absorbed across the ruminal wall (25, 171), and also partly metabolised by the epithelium into lactate and such ketone bodies as acetoacetate and hydroxybutyrate (26, 173). The SCFA absorbed from the rumen account for approximately 50 to 60 percent of the digestible energy intake by the adult ruminant (26), so that blood glucose levels are always relatively low (570). The ruminal epithelium also absorbs inorganic ions (361), and urea diffuses into the lumen (340).

The stratified squamous epithelium of the rumen, unlike the simple protective epithelium of the oesophagus and forestomach of other animals (607), is extremely active metabolically. In the cells of the basal and transitional layers numbers of mitochondria, and high activities of lactate, malate, succinate and butyrate dehydrogenases and carbonic anhydrase are seen (398). Thus, the ruminal epithelium is exceptional in that important functions are carried out presumably by immature cells in the proliferating population. As in the oesophagus the function of protection of the mucosal surface is carried out by mature cornified cells.

The internal surface area of the rumen is increased up to 7 times by the presence of papillae in domestic cattle or goats (631), and from 22 to 30 times in some wild ruminants (330). A papilla is so vascular that it can be compared to an intestinal villus (632, 764).

Most of the adult structural features of the rumen, such as papillation of the mucosa, have developed by the time the young ruminant is weaned (774). Functional development of the organ (469) depends on enormous morphological changes very different from the postnatal development of the forestomach in other mammals (612). The high blood glucose level in young 'pre-ruminant' animals falls to adult levels in this period (477). Thus the nutritional advantages of the ruminant are acquired by post-natal development of the rumen, principally a gross enlargement of the organ and a modification of the mucosa to form papillae. It is clear that this development of the ruminal mucosa is stimulated by SCFA as a result of solid food intake and microbial fermentation (614, 699).

The shape and size of the ruminal papillae which determine the size of the epithelial cell population in the rumen are also influenced by nutritional changes both in domestic (218, 606, 698) and wild ruminants (330). The influences of the level of feed intake in general, and of high cereal diets in particular, have been most intensively studied.

There has been an excellent series of studies using breeding ewes, which eat 5 times more feed during early lactation than at maintenance (218). In these animals the weight and total DNA content of the ruminal mucosa relative to body weight or relative to central nervous system weight are closely and positively correlated with feed intake. Also the degree of propionate metabolism in the mucosa and the activities of the key enzymes are increased in absolute terms but remain relatively constant when expressed per unit weight of tissue. It has been suggested that the rumen of the breeding ewe adapts to the increased feed intake, morphologically and functionally, by means of hyperplasia of the ruminal epithelium. However, changes in the mitotic index (I_m) of the ruminal epithelium were not found during these periods (218).

High cereal diets sometimes result in parakeratosis of the ruminal epithelium (350) or rumenitis (217, 507), and histological observations suggest that these disorders are associated with a disturbance in epithelial cell proliferation (697). Most studies have focused on regulation of cell production, and only one study has been directly concerned with cell loss from the epithelium (696).

All the circumstances mentioned above, viz. weaning, hyperphagia, and use of high cereal diets, stimulate the development of the ruminal epithelium and are accompanied by an increased intraruminal production of SCFA. Therefore it was considered that the resulting higher concentration of SCFA in the rumen stimulates epithelial cell proliferation.

We have undertaken to demonstrate the stimulatory effect of SCFA on epithelial cell proliferation in the rumen of adult sheep by infusing SCFA directly into the organ. First we used butyric acid, since it is most effective in stimulating papillary growth in the rumen of the weanling calf (699).

Castrated male sheep were used in order to avoid any possible influences of the oestrus cycle. The SCFA solutions were administered via a ruminal fistula and samples of the ruminal mucosa were taken from the atrium ruminis via the fistula. The accuracy of the sampling site was later confirmed by post-mortem examination of the organ. The mitotic index of the basal layer cells, calculated as previously described (608), was used as the measure of the proliferative activity of the epithelium; because of variation within individuals repeated biopsies from the same animal were required.

2.7.2 THE EFFECTS OF BUTYRATE ON RUMINAL EPITHELIAL CELL PROLIFERATION IN VIVO

Fasted adult sheep were given n-butyrate into the rumen once daily at noon in amounts equivalent to the estimated total daily production level. In order to avoid undue changes in the pH of the contents of the rumen a 10 percent aqueous solution of sodium n-butyrate was used.

The dose was given rapidly over a period of 10 seconds. A second group of animals was given the same dose of the solution slowly over 20 to 24 h commencing at noon every day for 3 to 6 successive days. The intention was to simulate two different intraruminal fermentation rates by these two different rates of administration. Control animals were given the same volume of 2.65 percent saline which has the same molarity as the butyrate solution, or 0.9 percent saline (609).

Rapid administration of butyrate involved significant increases over control values in the I_m of ruminal epithelium on the day after the initial administration (Figure 2.7.1) (609). High values were seen on days 1 and 2, then they tended to decline even though the daily administration of butyrate was continued. Neither sheep given the same amount of butyrate slowly nor either of the saline controls showed any significant fluctuations in I_m throughout the 6-day experimental period.

Further observations showed that the stimulatory effect of butyrate first became obvious within 6 to 12 h of the initial administration, while the sheep given butyrate slowly showed no great change in I_m during the 24 h of infusion (Figure 2.7.2).

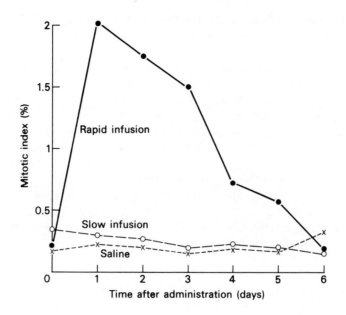

Figure 2.7.1 Mitotic index of the rumen epithelium of sheep given daily infusions of 18 mmol/kg butyrate, rapidly (10 sec) or slowly (20–24 h). Results are compared to those for rapid infusions of 0.9% or 2.65% saline, which were indistinguishable

2.7.3 THE EFFECTS OF ACETATE AND PROPIONATE ON RUMINAL EPITHELIAL CELL PROLIFERATION IN VIVO

The other two major SCFA produced in the rumen, acetate and propionate, were also investigated for their effects on ruminal epithelial cell proliferation, using the same techniques.

Doses of 18 mmol per kg of either sodium acetate or sodium propionate were administered rapidly into the rumen once daily at noon. Both caused an increase in I_m but only after 2 or 3 days of administration; thereafter values tended to decline although daily administration of the acids continued (Figure 2.7.3). The stimulatory effect of these acids was considered to be less than that of butyrate (611).

2.7.4 THE EFFECTS OF BUTYRATE ON CULTURED CELLS

Short-chain fatty acids are used as antimicrobial food additives by the food industry. They have been considered not to have any gross animal or human

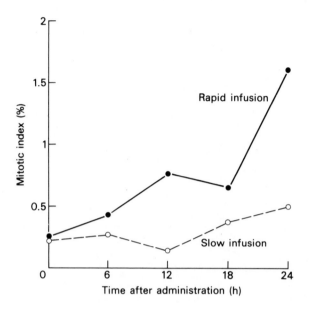

Figure 2.7.2 Mitotic index of the rumen epithelium of sheep after a single rapid infusion of 18 mmol/kg butyrate, compared to that during slow administration of the same dose

toxicity at the concentrations which are currently used (253). However, it has been demonstrated that butyrate at concentrations of between 0.1 and 100 mM inhibits the growth of a wide variety of cultured eukaryotic cells both of mammalian and of avian origin (445, 484, 554, 692). Other fatty acids (acetate, propionate, hexanoate, octanoate, decanoate) also inhibit the proliferation of these cells in vitro (253).

In addition to its inhibitory effect on cell proliferation butyrate reversibly alters the morphology of a number of cultured established cell lines of epithelial origin, changing them into a dendritic form (253, 445, 484, 692). In contrast, it does not alter the shape of cells of mesenchymal origin (253). The morphological influences of butyrate have been shown to be mediated through changes in DNA and protein synthesis (253).

Another notable effect of butyrate in vitro is its stimulatory effect on surface ganglioside localisation and on sialyltransferase activity, both of which are important for receptor function (231, 654). However, these two effects were considered to be unconnected.

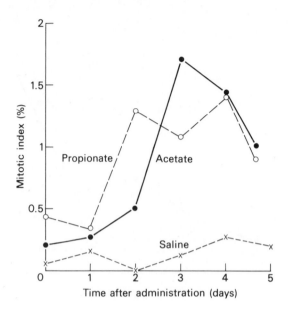

Figure 2.7.3 Mitotic index of the rumen epithelium of sheep given rapid daily doses of 18 mmol/kg propionate or acetate. Results are compared to those for rapid infusion of 0.9% saline

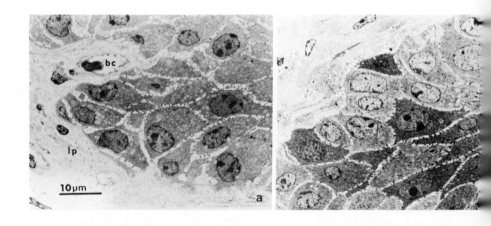

Figure 2.7.4 Rumen epithelium of sheep (a) before and (b) after 2 days' rapid infusion of 18 mmol/kg butyrate. The scale shows 10μm

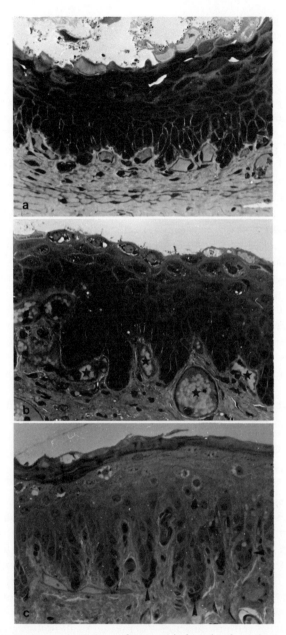

Figure 2.7.5 Rumen epithelium of sheep (a) before, (b) after 2 days' and (c) after 6 days' rapid infusion of 18 mmol/kg butyrate. Note the dilated subepithelial venules (stars) in (b) and degenerating epithelial cells (arrows) in (c)

2.7.5 THE INFLUENCE OF BUTYRATE ON THE MORPHOLOGY OF THE RUMINAL MUCOSA; IN VIVO OBSERVATIONS

We have shown (610) that the influence of butyrate in vivo on ruminal epithelium is entirely different from the in vitro effect. The cells of the basal layer of the epithelium are altered into rounded-up and swollen forms with a reduced number of cytoplasmic projections (Figures 2.7.4 and 2.7.5). The cytoplasm becomes electron-lucent, with many well developed mitochondria and clustered ribosomes, as well as a large euchromatin-rich nucleus.

Futhermore, the epithelium itself shows hyperplasia with some accentuation of the projections into the lamina propria within a few days of butyrate administration (18 mmol per kg per day); the cornified layer is shed, exposing nucleated immature epithelial cells to the lumen (Figure 2.7.5b). This is one of the early diagnostic features of rumen parakeratosis. We have shown (609) that abnormally increased cell proliferation of the ruminal epithelium triggers this disorder, as had been suggested by other workers (507, 697).

However, basal cells produced after butyrate application cornify much more rapidly than normal, so that the ruminal epithelium is again covered by a cornified layer within a few days (Figure 2.7.5c).

Under the present experimental conditions, the epithelial cell population, having increased, tends to revert to its initial size by a reduction in I_m (Figure 2.7.1) and by an increase in the number of degenerating basal cells (Figure 2.7.5c), so reducing the size of the mitotic pool and the rate of cell proliferation. Thus the ruminal mucosa seems to have a self-regulatory mechanism which maintains the normal state of the epithelium.

2.7.6 THE STIMULATORY EFFECT OF INSULIN ON RUMINAL EPITHELIAL CELL PROLIFERATION

The differences between the effects of butyrate on cell proliferation in vivo and in vitro suggest the existence of a system of hormonal mediation. In ruminants only two hormones, insulin and glucagon, are known to be released by SCFA (356, 450, 451). Insulin is important in mammalian cell proliferation in vitro (306, 504). Its level in the blood varies during the day, and seems to be influenced by feeding pattern (37), just as is proliferative activity (608). Thus it is possible that insulin is the mediator involved in SCFA-stimulated epithelial cell proliferation in the rumen. This suggestion is supported by the observation that oral epithelial cell proliferation is depressed in alloxan-treated diabetic rats (286). Therefore, we have performed experiments to investigate the effects of insulin on I_m in the rumen of adult sheep (605).

Two adult male castrated sheep were used in eight perfusion experiments under fasting conditions. In five experiments insulin (0.125 U per kg per h) was infused intravenously, together with glucose (300 mg per kg per h) to prevent hypoglycaemia. In two experiments the glucose only was infused. The same volume of physiological saline was administered in a control experiment. The period of infusion extended over 6 h in all cases.

Infusion of insulin-plus-glucose and of glucose alone both stimulated epithelial cell proliferation (Figure 2.7.6). Both treatments also resulted in

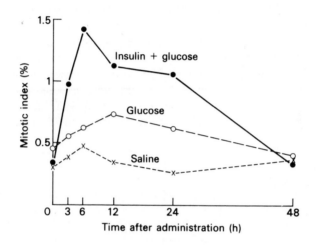

Figure 2.7.6 Mitotic index of the rumen epithelium of sheep following infusion for 6 h of 300 mg/kg/h glucose, with or without simultaneous infusion of 0.125 U/kg/h insulin. Results are compared to those for 6 h infusion of 0.9% saline

higher levels of plasma immunoreactive insulin (IRI) and plasma glucose during the infusion. Insulin-plus-glucose infusion resulted in higher I_m, higher IRI and lower plasma glucose than did glucose infusion. This suggests that stimulation of the I_m was due to the increased plasma IRI during the infusions, since the higher the plasma IRI the higher was the I_m.

The increased I_m resulting from the insulin-plus-glucose infusion was comparable to that occurring after intraruminal administration of sodium butyrate described earlier. Furthermore, increased plasma IRI levels during the insulin-plus-glucose infusion were about 50 percent of those after the intravenous administration of butyrate (2.5 mmol per kg) (450). Thus it is postulated that the stimulatory effect of butyrate on cell proliferation in vivo is mediated at least in part by insulin released by the acid.

2.7.7 THE EFFECT OF SHORT-CHAIN FATTY ACIDS ON CELL PROLIFERATION IN OTHER GASTROINTESTINAL EPITHELIA

The large intestine is similar to the rumen in that fermentative processes take place there. Recently the influence of SCFA on the colonic epithelium has been examined. Briefly, a SCFA solution (acetate 75 mM, propionate 35 mM, butyrate 25 mM, pH 6.1, 360 mosm), planned to simulate rat caecal contents, was injected into the lumen of segments of rat colon isolated by ligature. Small sections of the colon were taken from areas thus exposed to the solution ('exposed') and from neighbouring areas not so exposed ('unexposed'). Control animals were exposed to a SCFA-free but otherwise similar solution.

The I_m of the colonic epithelium was significantly increased within 1 h of the injection of the SCFA solution in both exposed and unexposed areas; there was no significant difference in the I_m between the two areas (Table 2.7.1). The I_m of both areas was significantly higher than that of the controls injected with the SCFA-free solution.

Table 2.7.1 Mitotic index (%) in the crypts of proximal and distal colon which were exposed or unexposed to solutions containing short-chain fatty acids or to SCFA-free solutions

	Proximal colon		Distal colon	
	Exposed	Unexposed	Exposed	Unexposed
SCFA	2.6	1.7	1.9	1.6
No SCFA	0.4	0.5	0.6	0.4

Thus SCFA increase I_m in colonic epithelium directly exposed to them and since adjacent unexposed epithelium was also affected, the effect of butyrate is not locally restricted. This supports the idea of mediation by humoral factors in a way similar to that found in the rumen (605). The blood vessels of the mucosa were dilated by SCFA only in the directly exposed sections.

It has been shown that some factors which evoke development of ruminal mucosa also stimulate development of other digestive organs (216). In lactating ewes for example, the weights of the reticulum, omasum, abomasum, small intestine, and liver were closely correlated with the level of feed intake, whereas the weights of other organs such as skeletal muscle, spleen, and central nervous system were not.

2.7.8 THE STIMULATORY EFFECTS OF CHEMICAL SUBSTANCES OTHER THAN SHORT-CHAIN FATTY ACIDS ON THE RUMINAL EPITHELIUM

The substance 1,2-propanediol (PD) also stimulates ruminal papillary growth in growing goats, even when administered into the glandular stomach, or abomasum (284). When radioactively labelled PD was administered into the abomasum of kids, activity was observed in the liver, ruminal mucosa, leg muscle, and in plasma, suggesting that PD is readily absorbed from the abomasum or small intestine, and is distributed to these tissues. Activity remained in the plasma for up to 4 h after administration of PD. Tritiated thymidine uptake by the basal cells of the ruminal epithelium was twice that seen in controls, and the possibility of direct stimulation of DNA synthesis by PD has been raised, as distinct from its gluconeogenic effect (285).

2.7.9 THE MECHANISM OF STIMULATION BY SHORT-CHAIN FATTY ACIDS OF EPITHELIAL CELL PROLIFERATION IN THE GASTROINTESTINAL TRACT

Several mechanisms accounting for the stimulatory effect of SCFA on the development of the ruminal epithelium have been suggested. That most frequently put forward is a direct effect of SCFA on the epithelium (217, 218, 614, 694, 699); SCFA or their metabolites are thought to be in the substrate for the biochemical reactions accompanying proliferation and migration. However, the results from the ligated rat-colon study (see Section 2.7.7) demonstrate that some effects of SCFA appear in unexposed epithelium. Intraruminal administration of SCFA also results in the development of abomasal, glandular-stomach, mucosa (700). These findings show that SCFA can stimulate epithelial cell proliferation indirectly.

Since SCFA stimulate blood flow to the rumen (172, 640, 723), this may play a part in promoting epithelial development (614, 774), but it is unlikely to be the prime modulator since intra-ruminal administration of 2.65 percent saline also leads to sub-epithelial capillary congestion but does not increase I_m (609, 610). Furthermore, capillary congestion was restricted to exposed regions of ligated rat colon, but both exposed and unexposed regions showed the change in I_m (Table 2.7.1).

Several groups have suggested humoral mediation in the action of SCFA (127, 218, 608), and we have found that insulin at least is one of the mediators involved (605).

The proposed pathway of hormonal mediation can be summarised: SCFA in the lumen are absorbed by the ruminal mucosa (and possibly by other gastrointestinal mucosae). Considerable amounts will be metabolised in the epithelium to lactate, acetoacetate, and hydroxybutyrate (26). The absorbed SCFA and possibly their metabolites in the blood stimulate the release of hormones (insulin for example) which, directly or via intermediary substances, stimulate gut epithelial cell proliferation. This idea of hormonal mediation is consistent with the stimulatory effect of SCFA on epithelium not directly exposed. Tissue specificity to the stimulus of intraluminal SCFA could be explained by the different sensitivity of the tissues to the hormone.

Hormonal mediation would also explain the results of studies with PD (284, 285). Possible pathways are either direct stimulation of hormone release by PD, or stimulation of gluconeogenesis in the kidney and liver (107, 204), with subsequent increase in plasma glucose resulting in increased insulin release.

Other hormones which could stimulate epithelial cell proliferation in the rumen include gastrin, which is released by the stimulus of oral food intake and causes insulin release in the ruminant. It is also a promoter of epithelial cell proliferation in the gastrointestinal tract. Glucagon, which is also released by SCFA in the ruminant (450) is another possible mediator, since this hormone stimulates gastric epithelial cell proliferation (194).

2.7.10 THE INFLUENCE OF NUTRITIONAL STATUS ON THE LONG-TERM DEVELOPMENT OF THE RUMINAL EPITHELIUM

Fasting influences cell proliferation and morphology of the ruminal epithelium (698). Therefore, since we used fasted sheep, it is possible that we have underestimated the stimulatory effect of butyrate, due to the preexisting depression of epithelial proliferation.

In animals maintained on a high cereal diet development of the ruminal epithelium continues for several months (Figures 2.7.7 and 2.7.8). The ruminal papillae become large, and the mucosa tends to form several ridges and furrows on the side of the papilla. The increase in population size and proliferative activity can be maintained for long periods, and the nutritional status of the animal is probably the major factor in this. Blood vessels in the papillary core are usually well developed (Figure 2.7.7), a feature also seen in animals adapted to an abundant supply of feed (300). It is suggested that the higher nutritional level promotes vascular development, which in turn supports the increased population of epithelial cells and the increased proliferative activity (Figure 2.7.8). In places the cornified layers appear to invaginate the central part of the epithelial peg (Figure 2.7.7), suggesting that maturation is influenced by the nutritional microenvironment around the cell, an environment determined by the amounts of nutrients supplied by the blood stream,

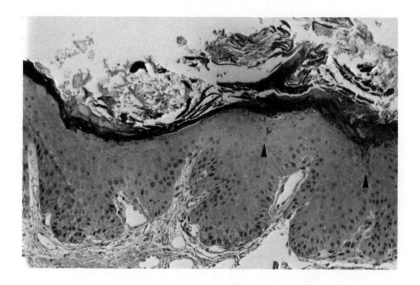

Figure 2.7.7 Rumen epithelium of a calf fed high cereal diets for 7 weeks.
Note the start of cornification at the centre of the epithelial pegs (arrows),
and the well-developed blood vessels

and by the distance of the cells from the blood vessels. It is likely that, once a cell moves out of this 'nourishing radius', it begins to cornify.

Thus the vascularisation of the ruminal mucosa seems to be essential in determining the pattern of long-term development of the epithelium. This concept is supported by the fact that the regional variation in papillary size closely correlates with regional variation in blood vessel density and in blood flow (774).

It has been suggested that there is a special period in which the stimulus of solid food intake, resulting in SCFA production, has a particularly marked effect on ruminal development in the growing animal (695). Lactating ewes, eating at 5 times maintenance, show relative resistence to the development of rumenitis (218). These two observations indicate that the sensitivity of the regulatory system of ruminal epithelial cell proliferation may be influenced by general physiological considerations such as age and reproductive status. According to the concept of hormonal mediation, the sensitivity of cell proliferation to dietary stimuli may be determined by the sensitivity of endocrine cells to stimulation by SCFA or their metabolites, and by the sensitivity of epithelial cells to hormones. The finding that there are age-dependent differences in the hormonal responses to feed intake supports this concept (37).

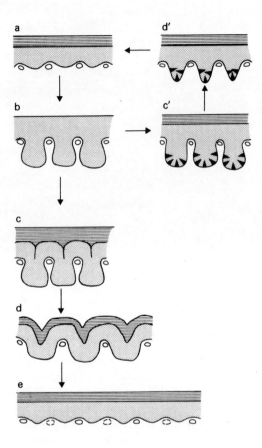

Figure 2.7.8 Schematic representation of rumen epithelium adapting to increased SCFA production: (a) is the unstimulated state; in (b) the epithelium develops downwards towards the lamina propria and upwards towards the luminal surface by means of stimulated cell production; cornified layers are usually dislocated and the number of proliferating cells increased. Under an enriched nutrition (c) the cell numbers are maintained, the surface is recovered by cornified cells and cornification begins at the centre of epithelial pegs. The invasion of cornified layers (d) results in the folding of the epithelium and the enlargement of the surface area, and when the development of the submucosa and vascular system (e) follows, the epithelium is flattened again, accompanying the total growth of the papilla. Under poor nutritional conditions (c') single cell death in the epithelium becomes more frequent, and (d') the epithelium is reduced to its initial mass

2.7.11 THE SIGNIFICANCE OF GUT FERMENTATION IN EPITHELIAL CELL PROLIFERATION IN THE GASTROINTESTINAL TRACT

Symbiosis with anaerobic microbes is common in many mammals, and hind-gut fermentation can be regarded as universal. Usually dietary fibre is the main substrate and SCFA are the main products (342, 477). Gut fermentation is the only strategy which mammals have developed to utilise dietary fibre, and studies of the significance of dietary fibre, of gut fermentation, and of SCFA should be integrated whenever possible.

Such integration should make it easier to understand the significance of oral food intake, the role of which has been studied by the comparison of oral with parenteral nutrition (193, 309, 418). The latter usually results in atrophy of gut epithelium, although total body weight remains almost constant. Because of the lack of substrate there would be little production of SCFA in the gut, and this would be expected to depress epithelial cell proliferation. Low levels of gastrin and possibly other factors may also be involved.

In the extreme case of the germ-free or gnotobiotic animal, which has no microflora in the gut, proliferative activity of the gastrointestinal epithelium is lower than that of conventional animals fed the same amount of the same diet (1, 261). The absence of gut fermentation, and consequently the absence of SCFA, may well be the reason for this. It is of interest that the caecum, which is the main site of SCFA production in conventional animals, shows the most marked alteration of all the gastrointestinal organs in gnotobiotic animals (261). The reduced proliferative activity in other parts of the gastrointestinal tract can be explained by reduced hormone release and reduced blood flow, both due to the absence of SCFA production.

ACKNOWLEDGEMENT

We thank Dr I D Hume for his advice on the manuscript. We also thank Ms U Nolda for her assistance in the illustration. We are very grateful to Dr T Hamada, Dr Y Sasaki and Mr H Ernst for their valuable information. Figure 2.7.4 has appeared in the Proceedings of the National Academy of Science (253), Figure 2.7.5 in the Japanese Journal of Zootechnical Science (610), and Figure 2.7.7 in the British Journal of Nutrition (605). We thank the editors of these journals for their kind permission to reproduce these figures.

SECTION 3

STEM CELLS

3.1 Stem Cells in Small-Intestinal Crypts
C S Potten

3.1.1 INTRODUCTION AND DEFINITIONS

The relevant definition of the word *stem* from a variety of English dictionaries is: 'the stock, ancestry or main line of descent from which the branches of a family are offshoots.' In fact, a recent edition of the Concise Oxford Dictionary (6th Edition 1976) defines a *stem cell* as 'an undifferentiated cell from which specialised cells develop.' This simple general definition obviously applies to all stem cells from the zygote through to adulthood. A more comprehensive definition for stem cells in adult tissues might be: 'the cells ultimately responsible for all cell replacement, ie, of both specialised cells and themselves, throughout adult life: the long-lived 'fixed' or 'anchored' cells that are the ancestors of any recognisable or hypothetical cell lineages within tissues.' Because they have greater division potential than other cells they are probably the only long-term repopulators of damaged tissue.

It might therefore be reasonable to examine tissues for cells that are some, or all, of the following: (a) precursors for specialised cells, capable of self-replication, long-lived, permanent, and fixed or anchored in the tissue; (b) cells at the origin, or responsible for the maintenance, of any cell lineages or cell migration pathways, ie, cells at specific positions within the tissue; and (c) regenerative or clonogenic cells.

Since differentiating or maturing cells may be capable of a limited number of divisions during maturation or further differentiation, thus amplifying each stem cell division, stem cells would also be: (d) distributed sparsely amongst the proliferative pool of cells; and (e) progressing through the cell cycle slowly in relation to the majority of cells in the proliferating pool, ie, spending protracted periods in G_0.

Other properties that might be associated, more or less exclusively, with stem cells are: (f) the evolution of special mechanisms to conserve the integrity of their DNA, for example special repair mechanisms (543), and possibly the selective retention of the older 'template' DNA strands that would largely be free of replication errors (86); (g) the possession of characteristic thymidine pools or thymidine metabolic pathways (532); and (h) susceptibility to systemic or local factors whose concentrations vary with a circadian rhythm, resulting in a high degree of synchronisation of stem-cell DNA-synthetic or mitotic activity (537).

The only situation where the ability to divide, enter DNA synthesis, or pass through the cell cycle, identifies a stem cell is the purely theoretical situation where specialised cells lacking any cell division capabilities develop directly from the stem cell population.

It is clear that those features after (c) cannot be used in isolation to identify stem cells, but they may be useful in suggesting where stem cells might be expected.

Before considering the intestinal crypts it is advisable to define two other terms that will be used in this paper. *Differentiation* of a cell is defined as the activation of a previously repressed region of the genome or a redistribution of the repressed–depressed gene pool resulting in the appearance of new transcriptional products and subsequently new cellular constituents (proteins), or other recognisable changes in the cell and its membranes. It is thus a qualitative change in the cell, the detection of which, in its earliest stages, depends on the sensitivity of the techniques used. *Maturation* of a cell is defined by the changes in the amount, concentration, or configurational pattern of these novel cellular constituents and is thus a quantitative term.

3.1.2 THE SMALL-INTESTINAL CRYPT

3.1.2.1 CRYPT CELL TYPES AND TURNOVER TIMES

The small-intestinal crypt of the mouse ileum contains about 250 cells in total (Figure 3.1.1), arranged as a sheet, one cell thick, moulded into a flask-shaped structure. At the base of the crypt there are 20 to 30 mature Paneth cells which have a long life expectancy in the crypt with a turnover time of 2 or 3 weeks (100, 104). The evidence as to whether maturing Paneth or goblet cells can undergo division is conflicting (80, 709, 725). The crypt may contain a very few enteroendocrine cells, the origin of which is slightly obscure; our observations indicate that not all crypts do in fact contain these cells and those that do usually only have one or two. They will not be considered further in this review; neither will intra-epithelial lymphocytes, whose origin is outside the crypt.

The crypt also contains a few mature mucus-secreting goblet cells. These are rarely seen at low cell positions and the mature cells migrate on to the villus with the columnar cells, possibly 'carried' by the same mechanisms. Our observations suggest that there are about 5 goblet cells per crypt, ie, 2 percent of the crypt cells excluding Paneth cells. The goblet cells have a turnover time of between 2 and 3 days (80, 99).

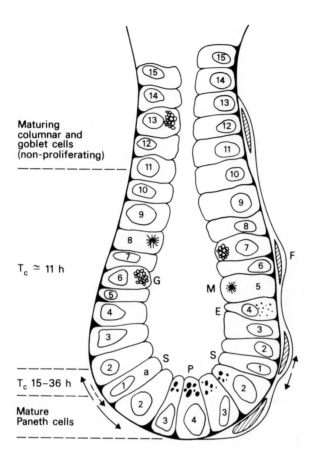

Maturing
columnar and
goblet cells
(non-proliferating)

$T_c \simeq 11$ h

T_c 15–36 h

Mature
Paneth cells

Figure 3.1.1 Schematic representation of a small-intestinal crypt showing Paneth cells (P), goblet cells (G), enteroendocrine cells (E), pericryptal fibroblasts (F) and mitoses (M). The cell position (1) immediately above the Paneth cells is the presumed stem-cell (S) position. Cell division is uncommon above cell position 10. It is suggested that a hypothetical focal point (a) for stem cells occurs at position 1. Cells displaced upwards from this position have a shortened cell cycle time and a higher probability for differentiation (543)

The great majority of the crypt cells (210 to 225 out of 250) are columnar cells displaying little or no evidence of differentiation. The cells in the top 4 or 5 cell positions do not normally show DNA-synthesis or mitotic activity, and movement onto the villus can be demonstrated by labelling experiments with tritiated thymidine (^{3}HTdR). They are probably, therefore, maturing or fully differentiated cells. The ten cell positions beneath this, comprising 150 to 200 cells, contain cells that are progressing rapidly through the cell cycle, with cell cycle time (T_c) of about 10 to 12 h, and, since the S-phase occupies about half the cycle time, these cell positions usually show a labelling index (I_S) of approximately 50 percent. These cells account for the cell production rates of 200 to 300 cells per crypt per day.

Fraction of labelled mitoses, stathmokinetic (6, 7) and continuous labelling experiments (542) show that the lowest cell positions, those just above the Paneth-cell region, have cycle times longer than the cells in the mid-crypt region, with T_c in the range 15 to 36 h.

3.1.2.2 RESIDENCE TIME OF CELLS IN THE CRYPT

It is clear from these values that the sojourn of any cell in the uppermost cell position of the proliferation compartment cannot last more than a few hours, after which it will be pushed, or pulled, or will actively migrate to the upper part of the crypt and then onto the villus. The sojourn of cells in each successively lower cell position will increase, and in the lowest cell positions might be as long as one day. The total life-span of many new-born intestinal columnar cells is no more than 2 to 4 days, after which they are lost from the villus tip.

The cells in the upper cell layers of the proliferation compartment can neither be regarded as capable of self-replication since they produce cells that no longer divide, nor as long-lived fixed cells; therefore they do not satisfy two of the important criteria for stem cells. This is largely true also for the cells at lower cell positions (2 to 10 in Figure 3.1.1). Cells at position 8 for example cannot be regarded as long-lived fixed cells, since their life expectancy in the crypt is short, and they divide to produce cells that are likely to be in cell position 9. The transition from position 10 to position 11 is commonly regarded as the boundary between proliferating and non-proliferating (differentiating) cells.

By this line of reasoning the only cells that are likely to remain for long in the crypt and to be 'fixed' are those at the origin of this cell movement, at position 1. These cells comprise a ring of 15 to 20 and may be 'anchored' in some way, or simply not be subject to displacement by any other cells. These few cells can also be seen to have long cell cycles, which can be greatly reduced if regeneration is initiated. Nevertheless not all of these cells need be stem cells: there may be fewer than 15 to 20 'anchorage points' in the ring. In that case the migratory pathway of the differentiating migrating cells may at first be circumferential.

3.1.2.3 PLURIPOTENCY AND STEM CELLS

Cheng and Leblond (103) have reported the results of a series of ingenious experiments indicating that at least three different cell types, Paneth, goblet and columnar, originate from cells situated at or near the crypt base. These experiments involved the use of ^{3}HTdR at low doses to kill some cells in the crypt base where radiosensitivity is greatest. The dead cells were rapidly phagocytosed by neighbouring cells which then contained ^{3}HTdR-labelled cytoplasmic markers (phagosomes). The distribution of these phagosomes, which were initially only in undifferentiated crypt-base cells, was followed. Cells of all three types were seen with labelled phagosomes after intervals equivalent to the turnover times for each of the cell types. These experiments could only be done because there are cells with an extreme radiosensitivity in the crypt base, the presumed site of the stem-cell population. This permitted a fairly specific labelling of cells early in the cell lineages. The experiments indicate that all crypt cells originate from some 20 cells in this region. The results also suggest that some pluripotency is associated with the stem cells: that the stem cells may produce cell lines that ultimately differentiate and mature in different ways, into Paneth cells, goblet cells, and columnar cells. This pluripotency is further suggested by the observation that the regenerated crypts after severe irradiation depopulation contain all cell types. Similar conclusions have been drawn from other irradiation experiments (788).

These, and the strategic or topographic conclusions, suggest that the number of stem cells is not more than 20 per crypt.

3.1.3 CRYPT REGENERATION

3.1.3.1 CLONAL REGENERATION STUDIES

Clonal regeneration techniques are the only experimental means available for the study of stem cells. There are, however, some limitations that have to be accepted for these studies in epithelial tissues. Some regenerative foci may originate from cells that are not true stem cells but cells early in the transit population. These clones, colonies, or foci would have a limited life-span and would lack further clonogenic capacity. This problem is complicated by the fact that some clones may 'bud' to form further clones or crypts (85). However, it is concluded that these 'transitory clones' do not contribute significantly since the number of clones per area or length of intestine does not vary greatly with time; repeated irradiation experiments, for example with three or more days between doses, show exactly the same shape of dose-response curve. Furthermore, studies conducted at 3 to 4 days (on microcolonies) provide the shoulder and early exponential portion of a dose-response curve, while studies conducted later

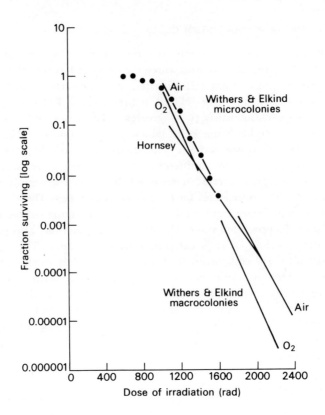

Figure 3.1.2 Crypt survival curve (black circles) obtained from measurements made on 460 mice (see Figure 3.1.3 for details). The curve is
compared with Withers and Elkind's data (809) for micro- and macrocolonies and data from Hornsey (337). These micro- and macro-colony data
appear to form part of a single exponential response curve

after irradiation (on macrocolonies), when some transitory clones might have
died out, provide the high-dose exponential part of the same curve (337, 809)
(Figure 3.1.2), and these two curves can be joined by a single straight line.

A review of the published micro- or macro-colony data reveals that although
all the curves clearly show a large shoulder, in fact almost a true threshold, the
final slope, usually based on only a few points, varies from experiment to
experiment.

Figure 3.1.3 illustrates the spread of values that has been obtained, using
similar animals, irradiation and scoring conditions, within our own laboratories
over several years. There has been some suggestion that these curves, rather
than having an exponential portion, have a continual curvature (461, 827).

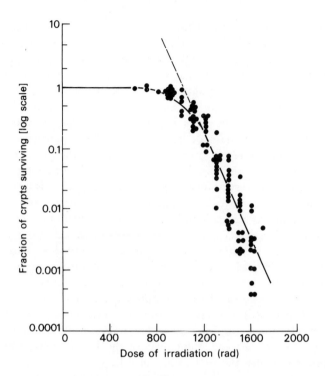

Figure 3.1.3 Data collected over a period of about 3 years from 460 mice. Each point represents at least 4 mice from which 5–10 intestinal circumferences were scored (600–1000 crypts at risk per mouse). The considerable scatter is obvious. There is a slight suggestion that the dose-response curve continually curves downwards, if equal weight is placed on each individual point. However, the average surviving fraction at each dose (influenced strongly by the high survival values (827)) provides a crypt survival curve that appears to have an exponential portion and is characterised by an extrapolation value of 2400 and a D_0 of 125 ± 14 rad. D_0 is the increase in dose required to decrease the proportion of crypts surviving by a factor of e^{-1}, ie 0.37)

However, this is contradicted by the facts that the micro- and macro-colony results lie on the same line and the overall means of data such as that shown in Figure 3.1.3 provide values that lie on a straight line.

3.1.3.2 CLONOGENIC AND CRYPTOGENIC CELLS

The question that concerns us is whether it is possible from this type of data to make any deduction concerning the number of clonogenic stem cells per crypt. The common interpretation of mammalian survival curves is that the shoulder region is largely a consequence of the number of sites per cell that have to be 'hit' by the irradiation and the fact that cells can repair some of the damage if given time. Such curves as that illustrated are crypt-survival curves and so contain an extra complication in that each crypt may contain many cells, the survival of any one of which is sufficient for the survival of the entire crypt. Once the exponential portion of the curves is reached, at about 900 to 1100 rads, then the survival of the crypt depends only on the survival of the last clonogenic cell, in fact the last hit in the last cell. The question is how many cells have to be killed to reach this exponential part of the curve, eg, is it 149 out of 150, 19 out of 20 or some other figure? This problem can be investigated by determining the recovery or repair capacity of intestinal cells by experiments involving administration of two separate doses or irradiation (*split-dose experiments*). The assumptions are made that: firstly the shoulder of the crypt-survival curve comprises two components only, cell number and cell recovery potential; secondly the recovery potential measured in a split-dose experiment is representative of previously unirradiated cells; and thirdly survival of crypt-colony-forming cells, cryptogenic cells, is independent of survival of any other cell. Initial studies based on these assumptions indicated that the number of clonogenic cells per crypt was less than the total number of proliferating cells, in fact about 80 clonogenic cells per crypt (314, 540). These experiments stimulated further studies and unfortunately the situation has since become more complicated. Since the probability of observing a regenerative focus in sections depends on its size, which, unlike the control crypts, is increasing rapidly with time after irradiation, it is necessary to correct the observed counts for any differences in the size of the regenerative foci compared to the control crypts. It has been assumed that the regenerative foci retain radial symmetry while increasing in size, and that the control crypts also possess radial symmetry. The latter may not in fact be the case. Omission of any size-correction factor indicates that virtually all crypt cells are clonogenic which is in conflict with the conclusions in Section 3.1.2.2.

3.1.3.3 SURVIVAL STUDIES AFTER CHANGES IN CRYPT SIZE

Several subsequent experiments have determined crypt survival curves under conditions where the overall size of the crypts differed. The rationale here is that if clonogenic and proliferating cells were the same, changes in numbers of proliferating cells should be reflected in changes in the size of the shoulder of the crypt-survival curve. A simple approach is to use a phase-specific cytotoxic agent before irradiation, such as hydroxyurea (HU), cytosine arabinoside (ara-C) or doses of ^{3}HTdR that kill S-phase cells by internal irradiation. The situation with these experiments is very confused. Hydroxyurea kills many cells in the proliferation compartment since about half are in S at any time. Because there is a circadian fluctuation in the number of cells in S, the time of day when the experiments are done should be carefully controlled. Tritiated thymidine, on the other hand, kills fewer cells, and has a greater specificity for cells in the lower regions of the crypt (Figure 3.1.4). Similar data for ara-C are not available

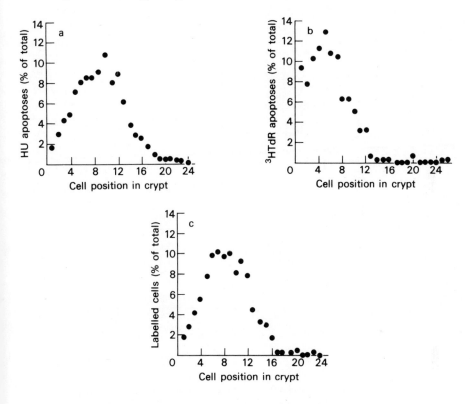

Figure 3.1.4 Distribution in the crypt of the number of histologically identifiable dead or dying cells or cell fragments (apoptoses), following (a) HU or (b) a high dose of ³HTdR. Each distribution was obtained by counting at least 200 dead cells. For comparison (c) the distribution of cells in DNA synthesis is also shown

but it has been assumed that it acts like HU. Initial experiments with ³HTdR and ara-C gave similar results and showed a change in the size of the shoulder of crypt survival curves (50). Thus it appeared that many clonogenic cells were in S, and it was assumed that at least some of these were in the proliferation compartment. Subsequent experiments with ³HTdR and colcemid have not produced the same result (Section 4.2), and the conclusion in this case would be that few if any clonogenic cells are normally in S. Other recent experiments with ^{3}HTdR have not shown any evidence of clonogenic-cell killing. We have recently conducted several experiments with HU which showed that, even though the number of S-phase cells varies with time of day, no circadian difference could be seen in survival curves for animals pretreated with HU,

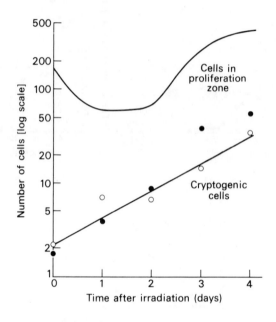

Figure 3.1.5 Changes in the number of clonogenic (cryptogenic) cells per crypt at various times after a dose of 900 rad γ-irradiation. Open circles are values obtained using independent D_0 values; black circles are values obtained using a common D_0. Also shown is a schematic representation of the changes in the total number of cells in the region of the crypt where maximum labelling is observed (540)

generated at the times of highest and lowest labelling index. If the HU was given 1 h before irradiation a similar effect could be seen at both times of day; the effect was particularly evident on the shoulder portion of the curve, ie, with high doses of irradiation it was minimal. If 6 h elapsed between HU and irradiation no effect could be detected at either time of day, ie the crypt survival curves were identical whether or not HU was given. The conclusions drawn from these experiments are that HU kills many S-phase cells and it is known to block most G_1 cells. If given shortly before irradiation it alters the shape of the survival curve, having a marked effect on the shoulder but less effect at high doses of irradiation. If cells are allowed to recover partially from the G_1 block then their radiosensitivity does not differ from cells irradiated without pretreatment with HU. In general, the effect of killing half the proliferating cells does not have a corresponding effect on the survival curve. To what extent changes in sensitivity due to cell cycle phases complicate these experiments is unclear.

Several experiments have been performed where the crypt size was altered by prior treatment with irradiation. It can be arranged that at the time of the survival curve the proliferation compartment is either smaller or larger (540) than the control unirradiated crypts. In these experiments the results are clearer because in no case does the size of the proliferation compartment reflect the size of the clonogenic compartment. Here the observations are consistent whether or not a size-correction factor is applied. When the crypts are small only a few cells are clonogenic, and the growth curves for clonogenic cells and proliferating cells (or total cells) have a different shape (Figure 3.1.5) (313). When the crypts are almost twice normal size, either 3 to 4 days after a single priming dose of irradiation or after repeated two-weekly doses, the number of clonogenic cells is similar to, or less than, that in control crypts. This means that there is no correlation between the size of the proliferation compartment and the size of the clonogenic compartment.

Although some confusion exists, partly due to differences in the strains of mice used, in the age of the mice, in the time of day the experiments were conducted, and in the mode of action of the various agents used, changes in the number of proliferating cells by a factor of two either way do not have a corresponding effect on the crypt survival curves. This indicates that the survival curves which measure clonogenic cells are unaffected by changes in the size of the proliferating population, so that only part of the proliferation compartment is clonogenic. However, the numbers of clonogenic cells cannot be determined accurately by these techniques at present.

3.1.3.4 CRYPT SURVIVAL AFTER DRUGS

Crypt survival curves after single doses of various cytotoxic drugs tend to have small shoulders and thus low extrapolation numbers (483). Many of these agents induce damage that cannot be repaired, so that they act like 'one-hit' agents. Thus the extrapolation values would be expected to be close to the actual number of clonogenic cells. These curves usually extrapolate to values less than 10 and often less than 5 cells per crypt. How these cells, which represent the drug-resistant clonogenic population, relate to the irradiation-resistant clonogenic population remains unclear.

3.1.4 GENERAL CONSIDERATIONS

One hypothesis which might explain some of the difficulties and inconsistencies in these results is the incompleteness of the original assumption that the shoulder of the crypt survival curve is due largely to multiplicity of stem cells and to recovery. It is possible that a third component which might be termed 'helper function' or 'anchorage' is involved. This component imparts an additional recovery or survival capability and is radioresistant and drug-sensitive. Attempts to define and characterise this are in progress.

Although it may not be possible to define the clonogenic population precisely it is clear in some circumstances that not all proliferating cells are clonogenic. Thus the crypt can be regarded as containing at least two types of proliferating cell. It can also be shown to contain at least two types of cell with differing responses to irradiation. Within the lower third of the crypt there are three or four cells which are exquisitely sensitive to irradiation (535). These

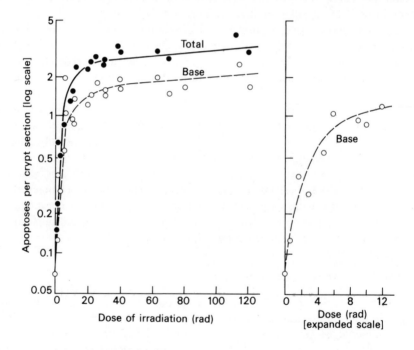

Figure 3.1.6 Dose-response curves for histologically identifiable dead cells (apoptotic fragments) in the whole crypt and in the crypt base. These curves are characterised by a steep initial region showing an extreme sensitivity (D_0 about 10 rads) and a 'plateau' where the number of dead cells does not increase greatly as the dose is increased (535)

appear as histologically identifiable dead cells within 3 to 6 h (Figure 3.1.6); at doses of more than 900 rad, which sterilise more than 99 percent of the crypt clonogenic cells, there are not many more dead cells recognisable histologically. Furthermore, many cells persist and enter S apparently normally (538); cell migration continues after these doses, and villus depopulation is not significant until 2 or 3 days after irradiation. This indicates that cell production must continue for a time, even though clonogenic cell kill has been extensive. At 1200 rads the situation differs little from that at 900 rads.

It has been suggested (86) that epithelial stem cells might selectively sort old and new DNA strands at division, eliminating the error-prone new strands to daughters destined for loss via differentiation and migration. There is some evidence (541) that between 1 and 5 cells per crypt might in fact behave in this way. If this is taken as an identifying feature of stem cells the number per crypt is small, but this population may represent only a special sub-class of stem cells (543).

3.1.5 A MODEL FOR CRYPT CELL ORGANISATION

The following model can be proposed for crypt proliferative organisation under steady state conditions (Figures 3.1.1 and 3.1.7). The crypt contains a ring of

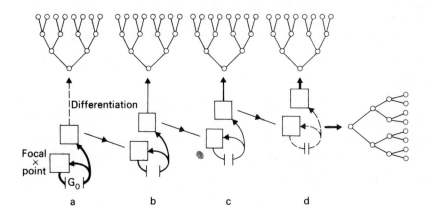

Figure 3.1.7 Schematic representation of the stem cells with their transit populations (lineages) at different positions ('shells') (b–d) in relation to the focal point (a). As the stem cell daughters are displaced from the focal point their cycle kinetics speed up and the differentiation probabilities increase (543)

15 to 20 stem cells at a position immediately above the Paneth cells. Three or four of these are extremely sensitive to irradiation and these may selectively segregate their DNA. They may also have other mechanisms for ensuring the integrity of their DNA, be situated in specific positions in the crypt, and cycle slowly (543). They produce daughters which are displaced slightly from the focal stem-cell positions. These 'displaced' cells may be radioresistant under normal conditions, because they possess further specialised repair mechanisms, and may also be aided by 'helper' cells or by a particular anchorage that enables them to persist in a damaged environment long enough to repair their own damage. Above this ring of stem cells there is a second ring of cells which possess a greatly reduced self-replicating capacity, a faster cell cycle time, and a greater probability of loss from the crypt. With each successive layer or ring, the self-replicating capacity falls, and the chance of loss from the crypt increases. The tolerance to irradiation may increase with increasing cell position because progressively less of the genetic pool is required as the options for differentiation and potential for proliferation are restricted. Initially the genes responsible for vital metabolism, reproductive potential, and the various differentiation options, are the major sensitive components of the gene pool. For a few vital, long-term, pluripotent cells, a considerably greater fraction of the pool may be critical, resulting in a sensitivity similar to that of germ or embryo cells (535). As the cells progress up the crypt their differentiation genes may be repressed as a particular pathway is adopted, reducing the sensitive-gene-target size. Finally, even the genes for reproductive potential may become repressed as the cells reach the higher levels of the crypt; this further reduces the sensitive-gene-target size and increases the overall radioresistance.

ACKNOWLEDGEMENTS

This work was supported by grants from the Medical Research Council and the Cancer Research Campaign. Besides my continued gratitude to Irene Nicholls, Caroline Chadwick, Joan Bullock and Dorothy Robinson for technical assistance, I am particularly grateful to Drs Hendry and Moore for many constructive discussions on the topics presented in this report and to Drs Hendry and Hume for permission to use their unpublished results. Figures 3.1.1, 3.1.5, 3.1.6 and 3.1.7. are redrawn from previous articles published respectively by Elsevier/North Holland, Taylor & Francis, Macmillan, and Elsevier/North Holland.

3.2 The Stem-Cell Zone of the Mouse Small-intestinal Epithelium

H Cheng and M Bjerknes

3.2.1 INTRODUCTION

3.2.1.1 IDENTIFICATION OF SMALL-INTESTINAL EPITHELIAL STEM CELLS

By the mid 1960s a general model of the small-intestinal crypt was emerging. Basically the epithelium was thought to consist of three separate compartments: a functional compartment, primarily the villus; a proliferation compartment, the lower two thirds of the crypt; and an intermediate region at the crypt top, in which maturation of the cells produced by the proliferation compartment takes place (404, 412). There was said to be a steady flow of cells out of the proliferation compartment into the maturation zone and thence onto the villi. Cell loss occurred from the villus tips (406). The most widely accepted model of the proliferation compartment is that of Cairnie, Lamerton and Steel (83, 84), in which the crypt epithelium is viewed as a steady-state proliferative system. Cells in the base of the proliferation compartment comprise an exponentially growing cell population with every mitosis yielding two proliferating cells; mitoses in the middle of the proliferation compartment have, corresponding to their distance from the base, an increasing probability of yielding non-proliferating cells; and all mitoses in the top of the proliferation compartment yield only terminally differentiating cells. Double labelling autoradiographic studies, which measured the flow rates of cells into and out of S-phase in the lower and upper crypt, are in general agreement with this model (74).

In addition to the villus compartment, most authors also recognised the existence of a second functional, or terminally differentiated, compartment: the Paneth-cell zone in the crypt base. It is important to emphasise that the Paneth-cell zone was not considered to be part of the proliferation compartment. Only Paneth cells were thought to reside in the crypt base and for this reason column counts often began by assigning position 1 to the cell immediately above the Paneth cell zone (555, 556, 557, 801).

Stem cells are those cells within a renewing system that have the capacity to proliferate throughout life and whose proliferation gives rise both to stem cells and to cells that go on to differentiate fully (403). The consensus was that the stem cells of the small-intestinal epithelium were found in the bottom of the proliferation zone, just above the Paneth-cell zone; this view is still held by some (536). A new cell type has since been described, a primitive cell with proliferative abilities, situated within the Paneth-cell zone and thought to be the specific progenitor of the Paneth cell population (39, 80, 104, 291, 725).

In 1974, however, Cheng and Leblond in a series of papers (99–103) elaborated and provided evidence for what they described as the 'unitarian theory of the origin of the four epithelial cell types.' First, in studies of the proliferation of each of the four epithelial cell lines, using both single injections and continuous infusion of tritiated thymidine (^{3}HTdR), they demonstrated that each of the cell lines undergoes renewal. By comparing the turnover times derived from these two methods, they demonstrated that mucous, Paneth, and enteroendocrine cell lines were not capable of maintaining their own rates of renewal whereas columnar cells were overproducing. They concluded that in the columnar cell line were the progenitors of all epithelial elements.

Within the crypt column there is a constant upward flux of cells towards the villus (83, 84, 405, 406, 557). As the cells migrate they also mature, resulting in a maturation gradient from the bottom of the crypt towards the top. It follows that the stem cells should be seen in the bottom of the crypt, and it was found that the most immature cells within the crypt were in fact those proliferating undifferentiated cells interspersed among the Paneth cells (101, 103). These cells were renamed the crypt-base columnar cells. Just above the Paneth-cell zone, cells were seen intermediate in appearance between the crypt-base columnar cell and mucous, enteroendocrine, and columnar cells Above this region there was a continuous gradient of increasing maturity along each cell line to the top of the crypt. It seemed that Paneth cells too were derived from the crypt-base columnar cells, because intermediate stages of differentiation between crypt-base columnar cells and Paneth cells had been found (104, 291, 725). Thus the crypt-base columnar cell appeared to be the common stem cell for all epithelial elements and this was confirmed by the following observations (103). Within six hours of an injection of 2 μCi of ^{3}HTdR per g body weight many crypt-base columnar cells died and were phagocytosed by neighbouring viable crypt-base columnar cells. This resulted in the presence of large labelled phagosomes 6 h after injection in many crypt-base columnar cells but not in any other cell type. At later times, labelled but more digested phagosomes began to appear in all of the other cell types and by 24 h after injection they were observed in well differentiated columnar cells at the top of the crypt. Crypt-base columnar cells must therefore have differentiated along each of the four cell lines.

3.2.1.2 MULTIPOTENTIALITY OF THE SMALL-INTESTINAL EPITHELIAL STEM CELL

Evidence in favour of a multipotential stem cell, as opposed to a morphologically homogeneous stem-cell pool which is in fact functionally heterogeneous, has come from a number of sources. Firstly, Cheng and Leblond (103) described cells containing two types of secretory granules, either both enteroendocrine and mucous granules, or both mucous and Paneth-cell granules and concluded that mucous, Paneth and enteroendocrine cells share a common multipotent precursor. Secondly, if it is assumed that neoplasms are derived from the transformation of one cell, then the observation of epithelial tumours containing more than one cell type supports the existence of a multipotential stem cell. Tumours have been found which contained both mucous and enteroendocrine cells (3, 317, 366, 684), and more rarely also Paneth cells (467, 671). If neoplasia does not alter their multipotentiality then it must once again be concluded that there is a common precursor for mucous, enteroendocrine, and Paneth-cell lines. Thirdly, after doses of irradiation strong enough to result in the survival of what is believed to be no more than one cryptogenic cell per crypt, columnar, mucous and Paneth cells are all present in the regenerated crypts (805, 806, 809). Finally, we have observed that all cell types do not appear simultaneously during development. The first cells to appear are columnar cells, then mucous cells and finally Paneth cells. Unless there are non-cycling precursors for the non-columnar cell types, this staggered appearance means that the precursor for Paneth and for mucous cells has the ability to produce columnar cells. Even at late stages in development when all cell types are present, we have noted that the non-columnar cells are initially far less prevalent than are the columnar cells.

3.2.1.3 SELECTIVITY IN STEM-CELL DIFFERENTIATION

A portion of the stem-cell population differentiates daily. The survival of the stem-cell compartment as such necessitates a certain selectivity in the differentiation of the stem cells. This is particularly obvious when it is considered that interspersed among the stem cells are some of their differentiated offspring. Principal among these are the Paneth cells which have a distribution coextensive with that of the stem cells, occupying the first 4 or 5 positions of the crypt column. Paneth cells are derived from the common epithelial stem cell (100, 103) and there must be some mechanism whereby one stem cell is induced to differentiate while its neighbour is not.

3.2.1.4 RESTRICTION OF STEM-CELL DISTRIBUTION

Columnar cells found within the Paneth-cell zone, and in particular in positions 1 to 4, are less well differentiated than columnar cells just above this region (101, 177). The proliferating cells within the Paneth-cell zone are selectively sensitive to ^{3}HTdR (103). As a group, cells in positions 1 to 4 have cell-cycle parameters that differ significantly from those of the proliferating cells higher in the crypt (6, 7, 9, 78, 83, 813, 814). Proliferating cells above position 4 have a strong circadian rhythm, whereas cells in positions 1 to 4 show no signs of variation throughout the day (9). In view of these differing characteristics it is likely that the two groups, cells in positions 1 to 4 and cells in positions 5 to 8, belong to different cell populations. Since the lower group has been shown to contain the common stem cells (103), it follows that the stem cells are probably limited to the first 4 or 5 positions.

3.2.2 HYPOTHESES FOR THE STEM-CELL DISTRIBUTION

The main facts as described above are explicable on the basis of two hypotheses.

3.2.2.1 THE SELECTION HYPOTHESIS

Basically, this hypothesis postulates a mechanism that selects one stem cell for in situ differentiation, into for example a Paneth cell, while allowing neighbouring stem cells to continue as stem cells. This process, taking place throughout the stem-cell distribution, would explain the intermingling of stem cells and their differentiated offspring. Complicating factors include the requirements for mechanisms capable of restricting the distribution of stem cells, for selecting particular stem cells for differentiation, and for controlling the direction of such differentiation.

3.2.2.2 THE STEM-CELL ZONE HYPOTHESIS

In this hypothesis we propose that stem cells in the first 4 or 5 positions receive no inducement to differentiate; only those that move to higher positions receive and respond to the signal to differentiate. If there is no stem-cell differentiation in positions 1 to 4 then there is no need for a selection process. Because of the absence of differentiation-inducing signals within the stem-cell zone the stem cells can exist indefinitely. The restricted location of stem cells can be explained because any that migrate above the stem-cell zone are induced to differentiate and cease to be stem cells. Finally, the intermingling of stem cells and differentiated offspring can be explained by the downward migration of differentiated cells from above the stem-cell zone, rather that by in-situ differentiation.

It appeared therefore that the most direct way to distinguish between alternative hypotheses was to determine the point of origin of the differentiated offspring of the stem cell. The following sections summarise our attempts to do so. The detailed results will be published separately.

3.2.3 TESTING THE STEM-CELL-ZONE HYPOTHESIS

3.2.3.1 ORIGIN AND MIGRATION OF PANETH CELLS

Selectivity predicts that formation of Paneth cells occurs throughout positions 1 to 4 whereas the stem-cell zone hypothesis predicts that it is restricted to the region above the stem-cell zone. If the latter is correct then the population of Paneth cells at the top of the Paneth-cell distribution should consist predominantly of cells formed more recently than those at the bottom. It was found that the smallest Paneth cells containing the smallest granules were located in positions 6 and 7, and the largest ones containing the largest granules were in positions 1 and 2. Similarly, death of Paneth cells was less prevalent in positions 4 and above than it was in position 1. Since these features are indicators of Paneth-cell age (100, 104), it can be deduced that there is an age gradient with the youngest cells at the top and the oldest at the bottom.

Direct evidence that formation is restricted to the top of the distribution was provided by autoradiographic studies using [3]HTdR. Although Paneth cells are renewed, they do not divide (80, 100, 104, 291, 405, 725) and so will not incorporate [3]HTdR. After several days labelled Paneth cells derived from labelled stem cells will begin to appear (103, 403), and so [3]HTdR incorporation can be used as a marker for newly formed Paneth cells and the distribution of such labelled cells can provide data on the site of Paneth-cell formation. Invariably, the first labelled Paneth cells to appear following a single injection of [3]HTdR were those highest in the crypt column. Measurements of granule size demonstrated that these cells were immature. Similarly, following continuous infusion of [3]HTdR, the first labelled Paneth cells observed were also the highest in their crypt column.

After two days' infusion, all Paneth cells in positions 5 to 7 were labelled, and since stem cells are localised to the lowest 4 or 5 positions of the crypt, it seems that the newly formed Paneth cells in positions 5 to 7 first appeared above the stem-cell zone. These combined morphological and autoradiographic data show therefore that induction of differentiation of Paneth cells in most crypts is restricted to the region above the stem-cell zone. It follows that all

Paneth cells found below position 4 must have arrived there as the result of downward migration and this was confirmed by appropriate gradients in cell size, granule size, and cell death. Conclusive evidence that these cells migrate downwards was provided by serial ^{3}HTdR-incorporation studies. The first labelled Paneth cells observed following a single injection of ^{3}HTdR were found exclusively at the highest levels of the Paneth-cell distribution. With the passage of time, labelled Paneth cells began to appear in lower positions and eventually in position 1. Following continuous infusion of ^{3}HTdR, the highest positions quickly acquired labelled Paneth cells; positions 3 and 4 followed, and positions 1 and 2 were last. At any one time there was always a decreasing proportion of labelled Paneth cells from positions 5, 6 and 7 towards position 1 indicating a downward migration of the labelled cohort.

3.2.3.2 STUDIES IN NEONATAL ANIMALS

In the jejunum of the adult mouse formation of Paneth cells is restricted to position 5 and above, and we have taken this as evidence for the stem-cell zone hypothesis. However restriction of formation to regions of low concentration would also be consistent with the observations, and since there is a Paneth-cell concentration gradient in the adult mouse this possibility must be investigated. The fact that in mice formation of Paneth cells does not begin until the seventh day after birth (471) provides an opportunity to distinguish between the alternative explanations for the positional restriction of Paneth-cell formation. The stem-cell zone mechanism predicts that in the neonatal animal, before the appearance of Paneth cells and the establishment of a Paneth-cell concentration gradient, the formation of these cells would nonetheless be restricted to the region above the stem-cell zone. On the other hand, if a mechanism dependent on Paneth-cell concentration were responsible, then this formation would initially be unrestricted as there would be no concentration gradient at that stage. Under either mechanism, the Paneth cell's propensity for downward migration would lead to the establishment of a concentration gradient and the adult distribution. The development of these cells in neonatal mice was studied in an attempt to differentiate between the two mechanisms.

On the first day of neonatal life, all Paneth cells were at the crypt-villus junction, which is roughly equivalent to position 5. This distribution persisted on day 2 with the exception of one Paneth cell found at position 3. On day 3 most were still at position 5 although they were becoming more prevalent in the lower positions. On days 4 and 5 the proportion in the lower positions increased steadily, and by day 10 an essentially adult distribution of Paneth cells was established.

As an indication of the age of Paneth cells in these neonatal animals, granule size was again used. The mean granule diameter in the lower positions was larger than in the higher positions, indicating that the cells in the lower positions were indeed older cells.

We take this as evidence against a role for the Paneth-cell concentration gradient in restricting the location of Paneth-cell formation and as further evidence in support of the stem-cell zone hypothesis.

Incidentally, our studies show that the stem-cell zone in the neonate seems to be of the same size as in the adult even though the crypt height in the neonate (<10 cells) is much shorter than that in the adult (32.5 cells).

3.2.3.3 ORIGIN AND DOWNWARD MIGRATION OF MUCOUS CELLS

Maps of the mucous cell distribution reveal that immature mucous cells first appear in large numbers in position 5 (99, 101). Most of these immature mucous cells undergo perhaps two mitotic divisions as they migrate upwards towards the villus (403) before they begin to mature into goblet cells. However some mucous cells do occur within the stem cell zone (99, 101) and we would expect this group of mucous cells to have originated and migrated like Paneth cells.

One hour after a single injection of ^{3}HTdR, labelled mucous cells were never observed below position 5. Only later did they begin to appear in the lower positions, and not until 4 days after injection were they observed in position 1. It is evident that a downward migration of labelled mucous cells occurs from position 5 to position 1. This observation is further supported by the fact that mucous cells found inside the stem-cell zone are more mature than those found at position 5; although they never attain the goblet shape, their mucous mass becomes large and the nucleus becomes condensed. Most upward-migrating mucous cells will undergo one or two divisions before terminal differentiation (403), but those that have migrated into the stem-cell zone do not take up ^{3}HTdR or divide, and may ultimately die there. It is concluded that such mucous cells as are found within the stem-cell zone originated in positions 5 and above, and then migrated downward.

3.2.3.4 ORIGIN AND DOWNWARD MIGRATION OF ENTEROENDOCRINE CELLS

Detailed positional studies as performed for other cell types were not feasible because of the small numbers of labelled enteroendocrine cells which appear after a single injection of ^{3}HTdR, but the results confirm that enteroendocrine cells are also formed above the stem-cell zone, and that most migrate upwards However, a few do migrate downwards and these show the typical spindle-shape of mature enteroendocrine cells; they have large round nuclei and many small dense granules in the basal region. Like the mucous and Paneth cells found within the stem-cell zone they do not divide.

3.2.3.5 ORIGIN AND DOWNWARD MIGRATION OF COLUMNAR CELLS

There is no obvious marker of mid-crypt columnar cells to distinguish them from the stem cells. That differentiation of the columnar cell population occurs at about position 5 can, however, be inferred. When cell cycle parameters were determined a clear transition was evident between positions 1 to 4 and 5 to 8 (6, 7, 9, 78, 83, 813, 814). Since columnar cells form well over 90 percent of the proliferating population (101) they must be responsible for the major component of the shift in cell cycle time. There is a similar transition between positions 4 and 5 in the morphological maturity of the cells (101, 103, 177), in the sensitivity of the cells to cytotoxic agents (103, 538) and in the circadian variation in the proliferative indices (9, 813). This provides some evidence that the stem-cell-zone mechanism applies to columnar as well as to mucous, enteroendocrine, and Paneth-cell production, but it gives no information about whether they migrate down into the stem-cell zone. This lack of information is of great concern because the presence of downward-migrating mid-crypt columnar cells in the stem-cell zone could give rise to serious misinterpretation of data from experiments aimed at investigating the stem-cell populations.

Mid-crypt mucous cells proliferate (99, 403), but those that migrate downwards into the stem-cell zone do not. Furthermore, mucous cells found within the stem-cell zone are well differentiated even though they never attain the goblet shape. That newly formed mucous cells, with the potential for one or two mitotic divisions, lose their proliferative ability upon entry into the stem cell zone suggests to us that this zone may not permit proliferation in non-stem cells. On entry into the stem-cell zone, any differentiating cell would respond to the microenvironment of the stem-cell zone by halting proliferative activity. This makes it possible to demonstrate whether or not downward migration of mid-crypt columnar cells occurs.

Immediately following a single injection of ³HTdR, heavily labelled columnar cells should be found throughout the lower regions of the crypt. Migration towards the villus will subsequently remove heavily labelled columnar cells from above the stem-cell zone, and cell division will dilute the label both within and above it. If some time after a single injection of ³HTdR, a population of heavily labelled mid-crypt columnar cells does enter the stem-cell zone from above, and if they do lose their proliferative ability on entry, then they should be the most heavily labelled columnar cells in the zone, because the labelled stem cells would have diluted their label. The suggested sequence of events described above is in fact realised.

One hour after a single injection of ³HTdR the most heavily labelled cells within the crypt are those in the crypt base (534, 538). However, we found that by 30 h after injection, heavily labelled columnar cells were no longer observed in the first four cell positions. The label present in the stem cells had presumably been diluted through cell division. In contrast, heavily labelled columnar cells were present at positions 5 and above. By 66 h heavily labelled columnar cells were found throughout the stem-cell zone, and must have arrived there by downward migration. At this time there are no longer any heavily labelled columnar cells above position 5, which indicates that they must have been dissipated by both upward and downward migration. Heavily labelled columnar cells are still observed 72 h after injection, but only in small numbers, and only deep within the stem-cell zone. There are two possible explanations: either they are migrating back out of the stem-cell zone or they are dying in situ. If they were migrating, heavily labelled columnar cells should have been present in positions 5 to 9 at later times, but none were seen. Since columnar cells migrating towards the villus normally live for no more than 3 to 4 days (83, 101, 405, 557), the disappearance of heavily labelled cells at the crypt base about 72 h after the injection corresponds to their expected life span. Labelled degenerating cells were observed 66 and 72 h but not 30 h after the ^{3}HTdR injection. Furthermore, unrecognisable degenerating cells can normally be seen in the stem-cell zone and may represent the remains of dead columnar cells. These observations strongly suggest in-situ death as the fate of columnar cells entering the stem-cell zone.

The possibility that the heavily labelled columnar cells are immature stages of enteroendocrine, mucous, or Paneth-cell lines is highly unlikely. The cells migrate too quickly to be enteroendocrine cells, and immature enteroendocrine and mucous cells are too rare to have contributed significantly to the large number of heavily labelled cells observed. In the same way and for the same reasons the possibility that they are immature Paneth cells can be dismissed.

3.2.3.6 PROLIFERATION IN THE STEM-CELL ZONE

Paneth, mucous, and enteroendocrine cells do not proliferate in the stem-cell zone. To determine whether the heavily labelled columnar cells found in the stem-cell zone 66 h and 72 h after ^{3}HTdR were undergoing cell division, labelled mitotic figures within the stem-cell zone were studied. None could be classified as being heavily labelled, and we conclude that the heavily labelled columnar cells of the stem-cell zone do not proliferate. The only cells in the stem-cell zone with proliferative abilities are the stem cells themselves.

3.2.3.7 STEM-CELL POTENTIAL OF MID-CRYPT COLUMNAR CELLS

Our results also have some relevance to the question of the stem-cell potential of mid-crypt columnar cells. Considerable interest has centred on this possibility, especially as it relates to the role of mid-crypt columnar cells in crypt regeneration following irradiation (534, 536, 540, 805, 809, 812). If these cells do have a readily available stem-cell potential then any that encountered a microenvironment capable of supporting stem-cell behaviour, such as the stem-cell zone, might be expected to express it. But the results demonstrate just the reverse. On entry into the stem-cell zone, the mid-crypt columnar cells stopped proliferating and died. We conclude that the mid-crypt columnar cells capable of downward migration, and perhaps all mid-crypt columnar cells, do not possess stem-cell potential.

3.2.3.8 THE STEM-CELL POPULATION

From our results an estimate of the number of stem cells within the jejunal crypt of the mouse was made. Our model for the crypt base states that in positions 1 to 4 there are on average 46 cells. Twenty-one of these are recognisable Paneth cells, three are unrecognisable immature Paneth cells, and one could be either an enteroendocrine or a mucous cell, leaving 21 cells of undetermined nature. If the proportion of labelled columnar cells within positions 1 to 4 that are heavily labelled is any indication, roughly one third of the 21 will be mid-crypt columnar cells that have migrated into the stem-cell zone. This leaves us with a rough estimate of 14 stem cells which, at this stage of our knowledge, can be presumed to be identical to each other.

3.2.3.9 CHALONE-LIKE SUBSTANCES AND THE STEM-CELL ZONE

The isolation of extracts with chalone-like activity (62, 617, 728), and the evidence that the villus has an influence in determining the cut-off point of proliferation within the crypt (54–56, 78, 79, 384, 583, 585, 620), combine to make a strong statement that the villus is secreting something that causes terminal differentiation of committed progenitors in the crypt. Most stem cells which leave the stem-cell zone form columnar cell progenitors and migrate up the crypt column, dividing as they go, until they reach a region in the upper crypt where they are said to receive a signal from the villus that induces terminal differentiation. A similar phenomenon operates in those committed cells that migrate downwards into the stem-cell zone; they lose their proliferative abilities and undergo terminal differentiation. The behaviour of the committed cells that migrate downwards into the stem-cell zone is so similar to that expressed by the committed cells as they reach the upper crypt that it suggests to us that the signalling factors in the upper crypt and the stem cell zone are similar if not identical. The factors in the upper crypt originate from the terminally differentiated cells of the villus, and it is likely that terminally differentiated cells within the stem-cell zone are a major source of the factors there. However, it is also possible that the stem cells themselves secrete similar factors.

The hypothesis that we are proposing is that the cells in the stem-cell zone (the stem cells themselves and some of their terminally differentiated offspring) secrete a factor which, at high concentrations, supports the existence of stem cells and induces terminal differentiation of committed progenitors. At low concentrations, such as would occur immediately above the stem-cell zone, cells are induced to differentiate. If no other modifying signals are received, differentiation is to columnar cell progenitors. If however, while at position 5, the cell receives one of three proposed modifying signals the direction of differentiation will be changed and the cell will form a mucous, an enteroendocrine, or a Paneth cell. There are many obvious alternatives to this hypothesis but this seems to be the simplest that can explain all the observations.

3.2.4 CONCLUSIONS

We believe that what follows is a valid representation of the mechanisms controlling stem-cell differentiation. The micro-environment of positions 1 to 4 is free from signals which result in stem-cell differentiation. Above position 4, the micro-environment is somehow altered and contains such signals. Accordingly, stem cells are restricted to the lower 4 positions. Differentiation along all epithelial cell lines begins when a stem cell moves from position 4 into position 5 and receives the inducing signals. Nearly all the differentiating cells that are formed in position 5, including most of the columnar, mucous, and enteroendocrine cells, participate in an upward migration to populate the villi. However, all the Paneth cells, some columnar, and a few mucous and enteroendocrine cells migrate downwards into the stem-cell zone. It is downward migration of differentiated cells from position 5, and not in-situ stem-cell differentiation which results in the presence of differentiated offspring of the stem cell within the stem-cell zone. As differentiating cells migrate downwards into the stem-cell zone, they continue to mature, indicating that the stem-cell zone, although unable to initiate differentiation in stem cells, is permissive of the maturation process. In the stem-cell zone, only stem cells are able to proliferate; mucous and mid-crypt columnar cells that migrate into the zone lose their proliferative ability. In addition, the loss of proliferative ability among those mid-crypt columnar cells that enter the stem-cell zone has led us to conclude that these cells have no stem-cell potential. It was estimated that there are approximately 14 stem cells in the mouse jejunal crypt.

ACKNOWLEDGEMENTS

This work was done with the support of grants from the National Foundation—March of Dimes and the Medical Research Council of Canada.

3.3 Circadian Variation in Proliferation of 'Cryptogenic' and 'Amplification' Cells in Mouse Descending Colon; a Comparison of Two Inbred Mouse Strains

Elizabeth Hamilton

3.3.1 INTRODUCTION

Circadian (diurnal) variations have been reported in both the labelling index I_s, and mitotic index, I_m, of the mouse small intestine (537, 653) and colon (93). In both tissues the time of the peaks in I_m and I_s coincide. In the small intestine the crypt cell cycle times, measured from fraction of labelled mitoses (FLM) curves begun at the times of the highest and the lowest I_s, were significantly different (653). Although circadian variations give rise to erroneous values for the length of the various cell cycle phases calculated from FLM curves (478), the total cell cycle time should be estimated correctly. The results of Sigdestad and Lesher (653) therefore suggest that cohorts of gut cells, which become labelled at different times of day, cycle at different rates.

In the mouse colon Chang (93) found that the greatest circadian variation in I_s occurred among the proliferating cells nearest the top of the crypt. However, he recorded no diurnal changes in the size of the proliferating population. This may be because the crypts were 'normalised' (82): since the length of the proliferation zone changed with the length of the crypt, proliferative indices (I_s and I_m) up the crypt were recalculated on the basis of a mean crypt length. This allowed for separate analysis of proliferation and non-proliferation zones, but obscured changes in actual cell numbers. In this paper, as in a previous one (287) changes in colonic crypt length have been quantified and related to the diurnal variation in colonic cell proliferation.

The radiosensitivity of small-intestinal crypts has been reported to vary diurnally (312). Crypt survival was lowest when the proliferative indices were highest (537). Since S-phase cells in the crypt are relatively radioresistant and those in mitosis are more radiosensitive (276) the data of Hendry (312) suggest that cryptogenic cells are not distributed evenly through the proliferating population and that they cycle synchronously. The present work provides further evidence for the synchronous cycling of cryptogenic cells in the mouse colon.

3.3.2 DIURNAL VARIATION

3.3.2.1 MATERIALS AND METHODS

Two inbred strains of mice kept at two different institutions have been compared in this study. Mice of the C57Bla$_t$ strain have been bred at the Imperial Cancer Research Fund laboratories for many years. The strain was originally selected for its low incidence of spontaneous tumours, which means that 50 percent of the mice live for at least $2\frac{1}{2}$ years. Results for 3 to 4-month-old male mice of this strain were compared with those from male CBA mice, 4 to 5 months old. The latter were bred at the Middlesex Hospital Medical School using breeding stock originally transported from the Cancer Research Campaign Gray Laboratory at Mount Vernon. Mice of both strains were kept, 4 to a plastic cage, with food and water ad lib, in a 12 hour light–dark cycle. The light was turned on at 0800 h for the C57Bl mice and 0700 h for the CBA. The four-hourly sampling times were therefore one hour earlier for the CBA mice. The C57Bl mice were fed Dixon's diet GR/R/3EK and the CBA mice were given Labsure CRM diet. The C57Bl diet had 10 percent more protein and 25 percent more 'metabolisable energy' per kg. It was also much higher in salt and trace elements. The diet the CBA mice ate, however, had 8 percent more fat and 42 percent more crude fibre per kg than that fed to the C57Bl.

The mice were injected with 30 μCi tritiated thymidine (^{3}HTdR) 40 minutes before being killed. Sections, 5 μm thick, were cut perpendicular to the long axis of the colonic lumen, dipped in Ilford K5 emulsion, and stained lightly with haematoxylin. Two counts of at least 1000 cells were made for each of the four animals in a group; only axial sections of crypts were counted. The number of cells, divided by the number of columns counted (2 per crypt) gave a mean value for cells per crypt column. Each column included about four cells in the adjacent surface epithelium. The number of cells in the crypt circumference was also counted in 10 transverse crypt sections per mouse, and the mean of these counts was used to calculate the total cells per crypt. Fifty crypt cell columns from each mouse were scored for labelled and mitotic cells at each position up the crypt. In crypts of the descending colon there is no basal zone of low proliferative activity (98, 710), so the proliferation zone can be defined by its upper limit alone.

3.3.2.2 RESULTS AND INTERPRETATION FOR C57Bl MICE

Figure 3.3.1 shows the mean dry weight of faeces produced per mouse in successive four-hour periods by a group of four male C57Bl mice in a metabolism cage to which they had become accustomed, having lived in it for a month before the start of the experiment. Production of faeces was highest between 2000 h and 2400 h, at the beginning of the dark period which is the active part of a mouse's daily cycle. Minimum faeces production occurred between 1200 h and 1600 h, in the middle of the light period when most mice are asleep.

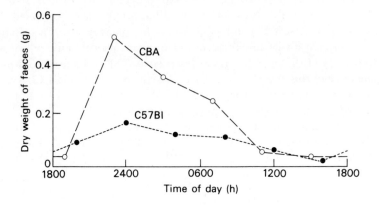

Figure 3.3.1 Mean weight of faeces per mouse collected from 4 male C57Bl mice, kept in a metabolism cage, at the end of successive 4 h periods, compared with that collected from 4 male CBA mice. The dark period for the C57Bl mice was from 2000 h to 0800 h, one hour later than for the CBA mice

Table 3.3.1 Morphometric and cytokinetic variables in colonic epithelium of C57B1 and CBA mice at different times of day. (CBA mice were studied 1 h before the times shown, but their light-dark cycle was also 1 h earlier than for the C57Bl mice)

Time of day (h)	Crypt length (cells)		Total cells per crypt		Mitotic index (%)		Labelling index (%)		Total S cells per crypt	
	C57Bl	CBA	C57Bl	CBA	C57Bl	CBA	C57Bl	CBA	C57Bl	CBA
20.00	27.1	31.7	311	366	1.84	0.82	8.98	6.19	29	23
24.00	26.5	32.5	305	378	1.88	0.52	9.29	5.49	29	21
04.00	28.3	35.9	331	425	1.64	0.44	12.11	10.63	38	45
08.00	26.9	35.4	312	418	1.73	0.89	11.88	13.89	35	58
12.00	38.0	34.4	438	404	1.98	1.43	15.98	9.70	68	39
16.00	33.5	31.4	390	362	1.01	1.91	9.30	8.21	29	30

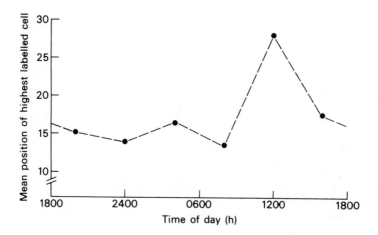

Figure 3.3.2 Diurnal changes in the mean position of the highest labelled cell in C57Bl mouse colonic crypts. The dark period for the C57Bl mice was from 2000 h to 0800 h

Table 3.3.1 shows that the maximum I_s is around 1200 h, rising at 0400 h from the low values of 1600 h to 2400 h. The length of the crypts, and therefore their total cell number, changes considerably throughout the day. The crypt columns are on average 11 cells longer at 1200 h than at all times between 2000 h and 0800 h. The position of the highest labelled cell (Figure 3.3.2) shows that most of the increase in crypt column length occurs in the proliferation zone. There is, however, a zone at least 10 cells long at the top of the crypt, where proliferating cells are not found at any time of day.

Figure 3.3.3 shows the changes in I_s within the proliferation zone of the crypt, the top of which is defined by the average position of the highest labelled cell. Comparison of this with Figure 3.3.1 and Table 3.3.1 demonstrates the sequence of diurnal changes in C57Bl mouse colon. The greatest production of faeces was between 2000 h and 2400 h; four hours before this the descending colon crypts lost their largest number of cells. Similarly, the greatest increase in cells per crypt was between 0800 h and 1200 h, four hours before the minimum faeces production. In C57Bl mice, therefore, cell loss from the descending colon appears to be associated with the passage of faeces through it, ready for excretion in the following four hours.

The I_s of the colon starts to rise from its trough at 0400 h eight hours after the greatest loss of cells from the crypts. The increase in S-cells per crypt occurs in two stages. Firstly the I_s of the proliferation zone rises to a maximum at

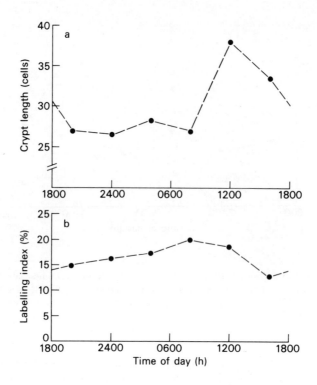

Figure 3.3.3 Circadian changes in (a) the crypt length and (b) the labelling index in the proliferation zone of C57Bl mouse colonic crypts. The dark period was from 2000 h to 0800 h

0800 h, then the size of the zone doubles at 1200 h. The total increase in S-cells may therefore involve two separate cohorts of cells.

The changes in I_s with position in the crypt are shown in Figure 3.3.4. The data have been averaged over groups of three cell positions; position 1 is at the base of the crypt. For all six times of day I_s was almost constant over the first nine cell positions. It then fell to zero within the next six to nine positions for every sample except that taken at 1200 h. At noon I_s was above 20 percent for a zone 18 cells long, and it fell to zero between positions 24 and 28. Between positions 9 and 28, therefore, there is a cohort of cells which enters DNA synthesis with a high degree of synchrony and is labelled only at one of the times studied, 1200 h.

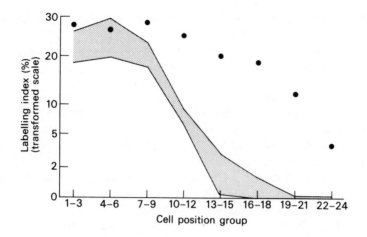

Figure 3.3.4 Labelling index distribution, in groups of 3 cell positions, at 1200 h in C57Bl mouse colonic crypts. The values at 1600 h, 2000 h, 2400 h, 0400 h and 0800 h all lie within the shaded area

3.3.2.3 RESULTS AND INTERPRETATION FOR CBA MICE

Faeces production in this strain of mice also varies diurnally. The rate of production is greatest in the four hours at the beginning of the dark period (1900 h to 2300 h) and least during the preceeding eight hours (1100 h to 1900 h).

Table 3.3.1 shows the circadian changes in I_s, I_m, and crypt size in CBA mouse colon. The greatest observed I_s is at 0700 h, and the highest I_m occurs eight hours later. The mean crypt length only changes by 4.5 cells over the 24-hour period. As in C57Bl mice the crypts are longest at the time of the highest I_s.

The labelling index rises most sharply between 2300 h and 0300 h, about eight hours after the crypts are at their shortest. It reaches a maximum at 0700 h, and by 1100 h it is again below the 0300 h value. The cells contributing to the peak must, therefore, move in and out of S-phase with considerable synchrony. The mitotic index rises about eight hours after I_s and is highest at 1500 h. These data suggest that the sequence of circadian changes in colonic crypts is the same in C57Bl and CBA mice: the crypts become shorter due to rapid cell loss, and eight hours later I_s starts to increase as a synchronous cohort of cells moves into S-phase. In CBA mice these cells are seen in mitosis 4 to 8 h later; a similar maximum I_m may have been missed by the four-hourly sampling in B57Bl mice (287). The correspondence between faeces production and cell loss from the colon is not as close in CBA mice as in C57Bl. In the CBA the colonic crypts lose most cells between 1100 h and 1500 h, eight hours before the maximum faeces production. The greatest increase in crypt cell number, probably due to the least cell loss, is between 2300 h and 0300 h, which is 8 to 12 h before the minimum faeces production.

The difference in the time between cell loss and faeces production in the two strains may be caused by a difference in their diets. In Figure 3.3.1 the weights of faeces produced by mice of each strain in successive 4-hour periods are compared. A CBA mouse produced 1.3 g of faeces in 24 h, while a C57Bl mouse produced only 0.6 g. Since the 'metabolisable energy' and protein per kg was less in the CBA than the C57Bl diet, CBA mice probably ate a greater weight of food per day. This may be why they produced twice the weight of faeces produced by C57Bl mice, even though there was only 42 percent more fibre per kg in their diet. It is uncertain why a higher residue diet should produce a greater time lag between colonic cell loss and faeces production. However, it is apparent that the higher dietary residue in CBA mice gives rise to much smaller changes in colonic crypt length. The greater faecal bulk in CBA mice apparently causes less cell loss.

Other differences between the colonic epithelia of the two strains may also be due to the difference in faeces production. As Table 3.3.1 shows, for most of the day I_s is higher in C57Bl than in CBA colon. This might be explained by a greater total cell production in C57Bl mice, to counter greater cell loss from the colon over a 24-hour period. Using the total number of cells per crypt and I_s, it is possible to calculate the mean number of S-cells per colonic crypt at each time. These values are also given in Table 3.3.1. On average there are two more S-cells per crypt in C57Bl than in CBA mice, which also suggests a higher total cell production in the former. However, the synchronised cohort of cells, which comes into S-phase eight hours after the maximum cell loss, is of a very similar size in the two strains. In C57Bl mice the mean number of S-cells per crypt increases by 39 and in CBA the number increases by 37 from the lowest to the highest value.

3.3.3 CRYPTOGENIC CELLS

The survival of cryptogenic cells in the colon of both strains of mice has been measured after whole-body X-irradiation. The animals were irradiated with 220 kVp X-rays at doses ranging from 600 to 1700 rad between 1000 h and 1200 h. Four and a half days later they were killed between 1500 h and 1700 h. Surviving crypts, seen as clumps of dark-staining cells, were counted in transverse sections of the colon stained with haematoxylin and eosin. Figure 3.3.5 shows the surviving crypts, expressed as a fraction of the number of crypts

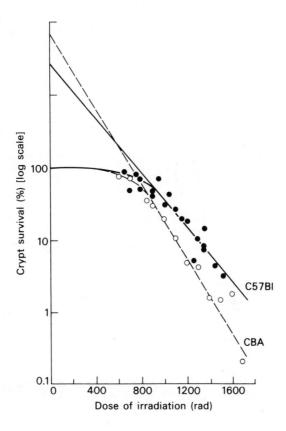

Figure 3.3.5 Crypt survival in the descending colon of male C57Bl and CBA mice, $4\frac{1}{2}$ days after a single exposure to whole-body X-irradiation

in comparable sections of unirradiated colon, in the two strains of mice. There is a slightly wider shoulder on the crypt survival curve for the C57Bl mice and, as can be seen, the slope is less so the D_0 value is higher; the curve for CBA mice has a higher extrapolation number, N (see Section 3.1).

The mice were also given split-dose whole-body X-irradiation. The first dose, 800 rad for CBA, 900 rad for C57Bl, was given between 1000 h and 1100 h, and the second dose was given six hours later. The animals were killed $4\frac{1}{2}$ days after the first dose. For each strain, the crypt survival after single and split-dose irradiation was fitted to a common D_0 value. The recovery factor (RF) and the number of cryptogenic cells per crypt were then calculated from the paired single and split-dose extrapolation numbers by the method of Hendry and Potten (314). The paired single and split-dose survival curves for the two

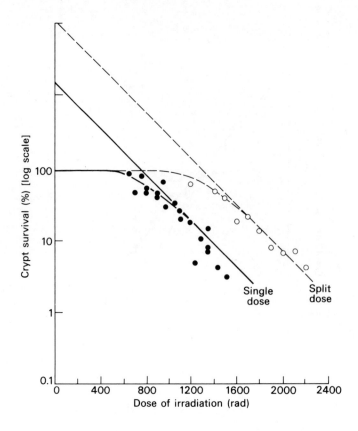

Figure 3.3.6 Crypt survival in the descending colon of male C57Bl mice, $4\frac{1}{2}$ days after single or split-dose whole-body X-irradiation

Table 3.3.2 The D_0 values, extrapolation numbers, recovery factors and numbers of cryptogenic cells per crypt, derived from fitting a common slope to single and split dose X-irradiation survival data on colonic crypts of C57Bl and CBA mice. The relative standard error for the number of cryptogenic cells per crypt, on the basis of this fitting procedure, is about 25%

		C57Bl	CBA
D_0 (rads)		272	193
N_1 (single dose)		15	28
N_2 (split dose)		104	277
RF	(N_2/N_1)	7.0	9.9
Cryptogenic cells (N_1/RF) per crypt		2.1	2.8

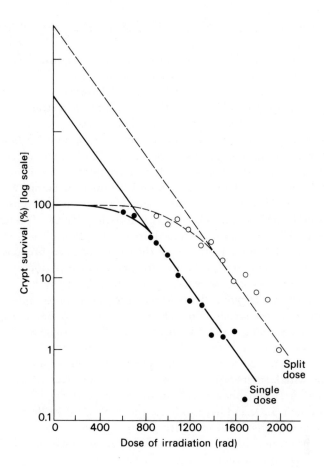

Figure 3.3.7 Crypt survival in the descending colon of male CBA mice, $4\frac{1}{2}$ days after single or split-dose whole-body X-irradiation

Table 3.3.3 The D_0 values and extrapolation numbers derived from fitting separate curves to single and split dose X-irradiation survival data on colonic crypts of C57Bl and CBA mice

	C57Bl		CBA	
	Single dose	Split dose	Single dose	Split dose
D_0 (rads)	225	316	164	260
Extrapolation number	28	38	78	46

strains are shown in Figures 3.3.6 and 3.3.7 and the parameters of these curves are given in Table 3.3.2.

The common D_0 value for colonic crypt survival is significantly higher in C57Bl than in CBA mice. The values for N and RF are lower, but not significantly so, in C57Bl than in CBA mice. However, the numbers of cryptogenic cells per crypt are virtually the same in the two strains: both types of mouse have 2 to 3 cryptogenic cells per colonic crypt.

The single and split-dose survival curves shown in Figures 3.3.6 and 3.3.7 diverge somewhat from the common D_0 values. Each survival curve was, therefore, fitted to an individual D_0 and their parameters are given in Table 3.3.3. As in Table 3.3.2, the D_0 values for C57Bl mice are significantly above those for the CBA. However, for both strains of mice the split-dose survival curve has a significantly higher D_0 than that for single doses. The reasons for this increase in D_0 have been discussed in detail (288). The most likely explanation is that the cryptogenic cells of the colon cycle synchronously. In an asynchronous population, only cells in a resistant phase of the cycle would survive the first dose of 800 or 900 rad, which kills nearly half the crypts (Figure 3.3.5). These resistant cells could then progress only to a more sensitive phase of the cycle for the second dose. The increase in D_0 during the split-dose irradiation suggests that all the cryptogenic cells have progressed to a more resistant phase of the cycle between 1000 h and 1600 h.

If this explanation is correct, then the cryptogenic cells cannot be a part of the population which enters S-phase 'on demand'. These latter cells are in DNA synthesis, a radioresistant phase (276), in the morning at the time of the first irradiation (Table 3.3.1), and have all left S-phase by 1600 h. If one postulates that the cryptogenic cells, because of their greater radioresistance at 1600 h, are in S-phase at that time, then they most probably lie somewhere in the bottom 12 positions of the crypt (Figure 3.3.4). An analysis of variance on the data for I_s at each position in the crypt showed that none of the positions 1 to 9 had a significantly different I_s at any time of day. Therefore, the cryptogenic cells may lie between positions 9 and 12 and cycle slowly, or they may lie amongst the bottom 9 cells and cycle at the same rate as the 'amplification' cells. A third, and the most likely, possibility is that the present techniques of analysis are inadequate to pick out a group of 2 or 3 cells in a crypt of between 300 and 400 cells.

3.3.4 CONCLUSIONS

The colonic crypts of C57Bl and CBA mice, therefore, have a similar proliferative structure. They contain 300 to 400 cells, the actual number of which varies diurnally. In the first nine cell positions, proliferation goes on at a constant rate over a 24-hour period. Between positions 10 and 18 a cohort of some 30 to 40 cells move into S-phase synchronously, at one particular time of day. The entry into S may be triggered by a decrease in the crypt length, as it occurs eight hours after the crypts are shortest. The cryptogenic cells also divide synchronously, but their position is uncertain, as there are only 2 or 3 of them. At the top of the crypt there is a zone, at least 10 cells long in C57Bl mice, where proliferation never occurs.

However, there are some interesting differences between the two strains. The cryptogenic cells of C57Bl mouse colon are unusually radioresistant, while those of CBA mice are not. The circadian changes in colonic crypt length and I_s are of a smaller magnitude in CBA than in C57Bl mice. This may be due to the CBA mice being fed a high residue diet. Some C57Bl mice are now being kept on this diet, and it will be interesting to see if the colonic circadian variation decreases and if diet affects the radiosensitivity of the cryptogenic cells of the colon.

ACKNOWLEDGEMENTS

Much of this work was carried out while I was on the staff of the Imperial Cancer Research Fund, Lincoln's Inn fields, London WC2. I would like to thank Dr L M Franks for his help and encouragement. I should also like to thank Mrs J Driscoll, Mrs T Barnes and Mr J Dobbin for their excellent technical assistance.

SECTION 4

RESPONSES TO CYTOTOXIC AGENTS AND OTHER STIMULI

4.1 The Intestinal Response to Cytotoxic Agents

Ronald F Hagemann

4.1.1 INTRODUCTION

The exposure of cell systems to cytotoxic agents may be considered in terms of the damage incurred and the response evoked. With the range of agents used in cancer therapy there are many modes of damage induction, with various outcomes at the cellular level (eg, sublethal injury, cell kill, cycle progression delays, etc.). This introductory section will focus on the response of normal tissue to damage, and particularly on those aspects of the response which are common to a number of cytotoxic agents.

The complex structural organisation of normal tissues such as the intestinal epithelium suggests, firstly, that defined intercellular spatial relationships help to maintain a constant production of differentiated cells, in order to ensure a level of cell production which will maintain a steady state with an adequate size of functional compartment. To accomplish this, mechanisms exist for monitoring either the functional compartment size itself, or the rate of loss of functional cells, or both. Secondly, the organisation suggests that both the capacity for damage recognition, and 'plans' for recovery from damage, exist. In this sense, damage may be considered as being a deviation from physiological steady state conditions. It follows that the 'plan' for recovery from damage is likely to be similar to, if not identical with, normal physiological control mechanisms. Thirdly, it is likely that a more or less set pattern of response to toxic agents exists; in other words the system can recognise damage in terms of only a limited number of consequences, possibly only one, and does not rely on the development of a separate stratagem for each type of injury encountered. And fourthly, it is reasonable to expect that a substantial degree of homogeneity exists both between individuals within a given species, and, with inevitable quantitative adjustment, between species differing markedly in other respects.

From an evolutionary stance, it seems likely that damage–response patterns in normal tissues have developed in response to naturally occurring environmental factors which challenge, to varying degrees of severity, the steady state of cell renewal. In the case of the intestinal renewal system, these factors may include both materials within the bowel lumen such as ingested abrasives, or heavy-metal ions which are directly toxic to villus cells, and crypt-active agents such as cycle-specific cell toxins. Thus we may anticipate that damage in this cell renewal system can be recognised at the level of both the crypt and the villus, and that once recognised, is responded to via the same cytokinetic adjustments responsible for the maintenance of the steady state.

Considered in the broad sense, the principal features of intestinal epithelial damage and resulting from such insults as irradiation, chemotherapy and physical agents (eg heat), either alone or in combination, and in single or multi-fraction exposures, are cell kill, fate of lethally damaged cells, and proliferation of surviving cells.

4.1.1.1 CELL KILL

This encompasses the usual considerations which affect reproductive integrity. Factors which determine the extent of cell kill include the inherent sensitivity of cells; the extent of repair of sublethal and potentially lethal damage; pharmacokinetic dilutions, inter- and intra-cellular detoxification; division dilution of cytotoxic drugs; the cell age distribution; the preferential stage of the cycle at which the agent has its effect; and multiplicity effects.

4.1.1.2 FATE OF LETHALLY DAMAGED CELLS

In the intestine, cells which have been rendered non-clonogenic may, for the most part, either remain viable and enter the functional compartment, or become functionally as well as reproductively incompetent and lyse in situ. Which of these two alternatives prevails in a given instance appears to be a qualitative property of the agent being applied. Whether the lethally damaged cells remain functional or lyse has a profound influence on the response of the tissue. Recognition of damage, for example, is earlier when cells are lost by lysis; the time until the subsequent proliferative response can be extended if cells enter the functional compartment, since potential epithelial denudation is delayed; and the usefulness of inter-fraction cell divisions in the case of multi-fraction treatment is affected; for if the resultant cells enter the functional compartment all such divisions are useful.

4.1.1.3 PROLIFERATION OF SURVIVING CELLS

Following repair of proliferative defects such as cycle-progression delays, surviving cells recognise that damage has occurred, and undertake accelerated proliferative activity. Operational properties include a decrease in cell cycle

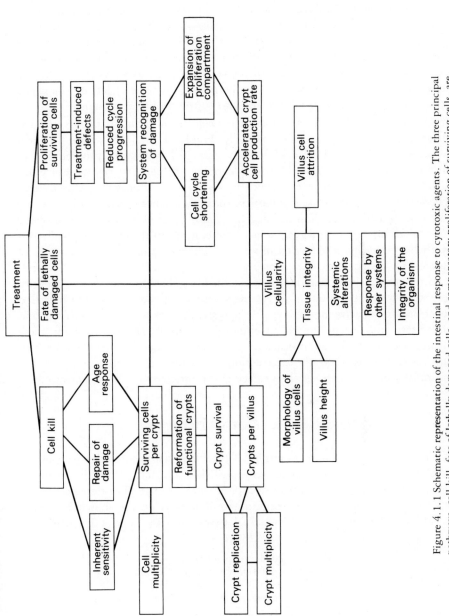

Figure 4.1.1 Schematic representation of the intestinal response to cytotoxic agents. The three principal pathways, cell kill, fate of lethally damaged cells, and compensatory proliferation of surviving cells, are illustrated

time, primarily due to a reduction in the G_1-phase, and a decreased probability of differentiation, which results in an expansion of the proliferation compartment; these changes are followed by an increased probability of differentiation and increased functional cell production. The extent and time of onset of hyperproliferative activity are dependent upon the extent of cell kill, the lifespan of cells in the functional compartment, the fate of lethally damaged cells, and the cellular capacity to respond to the proliferative signal.

The foregoing aspects of intestinal damage from cytotoxic agents and the subsequent response are summarised in Figure 4.1.1. The three principal features, viz. cell kill, fate of lethally damaged cells, and proliferation of surviving cells, are reiterated, as well as their confluence at the level of villus cellularity, the maintenance of which is the purpose of renewal in this system. The next level concerns tissue integrity, the maintenance of which is largely due to adequate cellularity. Tissue integrity is also affected by the response of the functional compartment itself, including alterations in the morphology of villus epithelial cells, and a reduction in villus height which decreases the amount of surface to be covered. Additionally, the aetiological factors in villus-cell attrition are likely to play a role in establishing the extent of tissue integrity following a given amount of cell damage. Reduced efficiency of the modified functional compartment may result in systemic effects such as nutrient and electrolyte imbalances, or bacteraemia, for example. To some extent these changes can be abrogated by other systems, as in the mobilisation of electrolytes and energy stores, and the destruction of bacteria by granulocytes, in the examples quoted above. In the balance is the integrity of the organism.

4.1.2 THE RESPONSES TO X-IRRADIATION

We may now turn to some examples of the intestinal proliferative response to cytotoxic agents, and how it relates to cell kill and fate of lethally damaged cells. Throughout, the data refer to experiments on mice. The responses of the jejunum to various levels of exposure to X-irradiation are shown in Figure 4.1.2, in terms of weight of intestinal tissue, and in Table 4.1.1 using the

Table 4.1.1 Number of proliferating cells per crypt 3 and 4 days after 500, 1000 or 1200 rad X-irradiation. Results are expressed as percentages of control values

| | Dose of irradiation (rad) | | |
	500	1000	1200
Day 3	190	240	180
Day 4	120	580	700

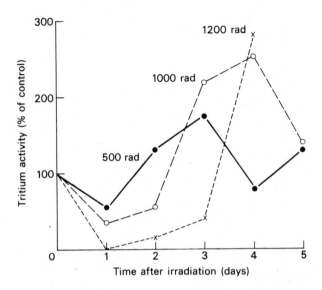

Figure 4.1.2 Thymidine incorporation per mg of jejunum, as a percentage of the control value, at different times after different doses of irradiation

intestinal crypt as a unit. At lower exposures which do not result in the complete destruction of any crypts, the compensatory response per crypt mirrors that per mg. However at the higher irradiation levels when the number of crypts per villus is reduced, cell production per crypt remains high, illustrating continued demand from a partially depleted functional compartment. This is illustrated in another fashion in Figure 4.1.3 wherein tritiated thymidine (^{3}HTdR) incorporation per crypt, and crypt survival (crypts per mg of wet weight of intestine), are plotted as a function of time after 1100 rad. Proliferative activity per crypt is highest when crypt number is least. As the crypt number is restored activity per crypt decreases. Thus there exists a balance between proliferative activity per crypt and the number of crypts feeding cells into the functional compartment.

The repopulation of individual crypts by means of enhanced cell proliferation after injury is very rapid, as is shown in Figure 4.1.4; this is in contrast with the relatively prolonged period taken to restore crypt numbers (Figure 4.1.3). For a limited time, essentially exponential repopulation of cells is seen, with a very short cell cycle time and a near zero probability of differentiation. It follows that the tissue can recover rapidly from high levels of cell kill provided that appreciable crypt loss has not occurred.

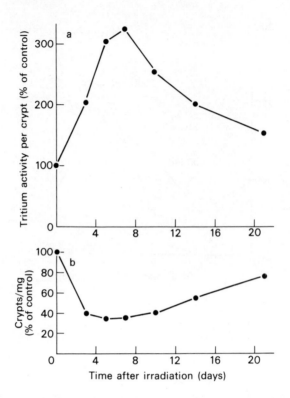

Figure 4.1.3 (a) Thymidine incorporation per crypt and (b) number of crypts per mg of jejunum, both as percentages of control values, at different times after a dose of 1100 rad X-irradiation

Figure 4.1.5 shows relative ^{3}HTdR incorporation during a 1-week course of fractionated X-irradiation (272). The fractionation schedules are indicated on each graph, and the results are expressed in terms of tritium activity per mg of jejunum as a percentage of control; for each schedule the integrated cell production, expressed as a percentage of control and representing the total area under the curve, is recorded. In the top 4 graphs a recognisable amount of damage has occurred and sufficient time has been allowed for the compensatory proliferative response. Integrated cell production levels for the 1 week period are close to control levels. In the case of 200 rad given for five successive days (Figure 4.1.5e) slight overall depression is seen which may be a reflection of the early damage being insufficient to be recognised and to evoke the compensatory response. Symmetrically distributed exposures do not provide sufficient time for an adequate proliferative response and overall proliferation is compromised.

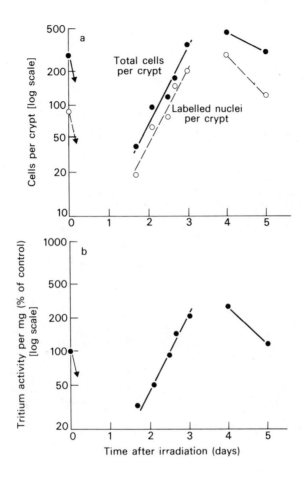

Figure 4.1.4 (a) The total number of cells per jejunal crypt, with the number of labelled cells, and (b) the thymidine incorporation per mg (as a percentage of the control value), at different times after a dose of 1000 rad X-irradiation

The data illustrated in Figure 4.1.6 are from animals in the 4th week of various schedules of regularly repeated X-irradiation therapy (272). In the case of 200 rad five times per week (Figure 4.1.6a) the damage from the previous weeks' therapy has now clearly been recognised, and proliferation is accelerated. The system functions well, judged by integrated cell production, when an adequate time for compensatory proliferative activity is permitted (Figures 4.1.6b and c), and poorly when it is not (Figure 4.1.6d).

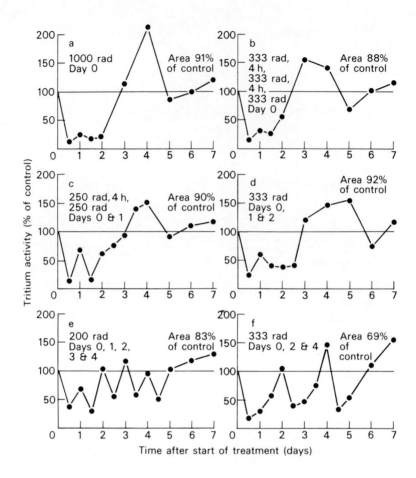

Figure 4.1.5 Thymidine incorporation per mg of jejunum, as a percentage of the control value, during a 1-week course of X-irradiation. A total exposure to 1000 rad was given as shown in each figure. The area under the curve indicates the integrated cell production over the period

4.1.3 CYTOTOXIC DRUGS WITH AND WITHOUT IRRADIATION

Hydroxyurea and vincristine are examples of cytotoxic agents which lyse proliferating intestinal crypt cells in situ, whereas irradiation and adriamycin permit entry of cells into the functional compartment. The influence of this important difference on the timing of the onset of heightened proliferative activity is shown in Figure 4.1.7. The fate of lethally damaged cells largely

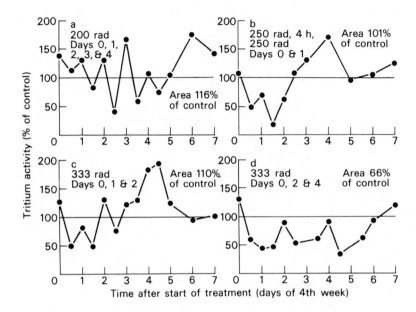

Figure 4.1.6 Thymidine incorporation per mg of jejunum, as in Figure 4.1.5, during the 4th week of treatment

determines when the signal for accelerated proliferation is given. This can be utilised to alter post-treatment proliferation kinetics as illustrated in Figure 4.1.8. Proliferation curves are shown for vincristine alone, irradiation alone and the two agents in combination. When vincristine is given prior to irradiation so that cells can be blocked in mitosis and subsequently lysed, the time course of the proliferative response for the drug plus irradiation is like that of the drug. and considerably earlier than that of irradiation only. This incidentally illustrates a second important point, namely that following irradiation only, accelerated proliferation could occur earlier than it does; in other words the irradiated cells are not unable to respond to an early proliferative signal, the signal is simply given later in the case of irradiation than in the case of a lysing drug.

We have already seen that the effect of a given fraction of irradiation is dependent upon the cellular conditions extant at the time it is given. Similar considerations can be applied to combinations of irradiation and drug therapy as shown in Figures 4.1.9 to 4.1.11. In these experiments a single large irradiation exposure of 1000 rad was given. Proliferative activity following this exposure was monitored and at subsequent times of low, high, and near control

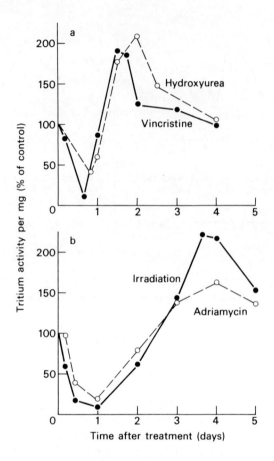

Figure 4.1.7 Thymidine incorporation per mg of jejunum, expressed as a percentage of the control value, at various times after (a) vincristine, or hydroxyurea, or (b) adriamycin, or X-irradiation. In the case of the first two agents most lethally damaged cells die and lyse in-situ; for the last two most enter the differentiated (function) compartment

levels of proliferation one of three chemotherapeutic agents was given. These agents were cytosine arabinoside, vincristine and adriamycin. The first two cause lysis of damaged cells in situ, whereas adriamycin does not. Animal survival following each type of treatment is shown as a percentage value against the appropriate curve. In Figure 4.1.9 the jejunal proliferative response is shown for the case where drugs were given when the proliferation compartment was small and just beginning to recover from irradiation. These conditions were

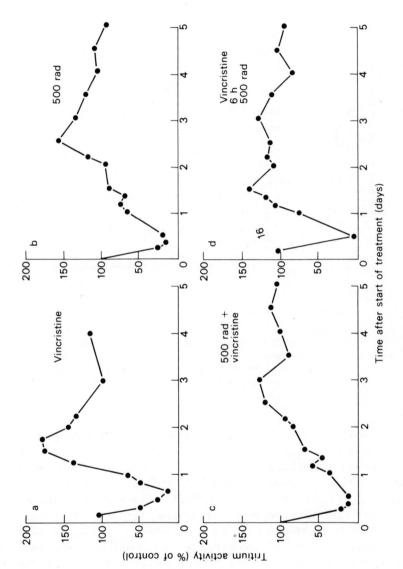

Figure 4.1.8 Thymidine incorporation per mg of jejunum, expressed as a percentage of the control value, at various times after (a) vincristine, (b) X-irradiation, or a combination of the two treatments given either (c) together or (d) with vincristine preceeding irradiation by 6 h

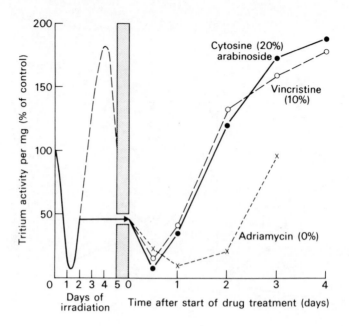

Figure 4.1.9 Schematic representation of the jejunal response to 1100 rad
X-irradiation, and the subsequent responses to cytosine arabinoside, vincristine, or adriamycin, given at the point indicated during the response to
irradiation. Results are expressed in terms of thymidine incorporation per
mg of tissue as a percentage of the control value. Percentages beside the
curves refer to animal survival

not well tolerated. The earlier proliferative response to cytosine arabinoside and
vincristine enabled a few animals to survive, but in the vast majority the drug
expedited denudation, and animal death occurred. This was despite the fact
that a large proliferative response was ultimately attained; it occurred, however,
too late to avert functional failure. In the case of adriamycin the proliferative
response occurred still later and no animals survived. Figure 4.1.10 shows the
consequences of giving these agents when the proliferative response to the
previous irradiation was near its maximum. In the case of cytosine arabinoside
the early proliferative response enabled all the treated animals to survive. More
also survived with vincristine; with this agent affected cells can accumulate over
a longer period of time and hence the total extent of cell kill is probably greater.
In marked contrast, the delayed response to adriamycin resulted in denudation
and death before sufficient new cells could enter the functional compartment.
When the agents were given after the cells in the greatly expanded proliferation

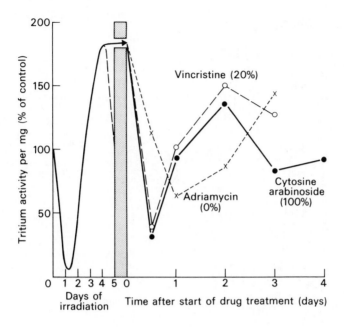

Figure 4.1.10 As Figure 4.1.9

compartment had entered the functional compartment (Figure 4.1.11) none induced sufficient intestinal damage to cause any deaths of animals, irrespective of whether the compensatory response occurred early, due to lysis of damaged cells, or later following entry of damaged cells into the functional compartment. Thus the various aspects of cell kill, fate of lethally damaged cells, and proliferation of surviving cells can provide adequate explanations for various treatment effects on the intestinal epithelium.

Some chemotherapeutic agents bind to sub-cellular components and hence provide the potential for delayed interactions, both in terms of cell kill and of cell proliferation. Figure 4.1.12 shows an interaction between actinomycin-D and X-irradiation in terms of cell kill. The drug was administered at zero time, and a single exposure to irradiation was given at various times thereafter. Cell kill was assessed by measuring crypt survival. Enhanced cell kill is observed when the irradiation is given as long as 5 days after the drug (274). Figure 4.1.13 illustrates the delayed toxicity of adriamycin, which is manifest as a progressive impairment of the tissue's capacity to undergo the compensatory proliferative response following injury. The highest curve shows the usual proliferative response to an abdomen-only exposure of 1000 rad; the others

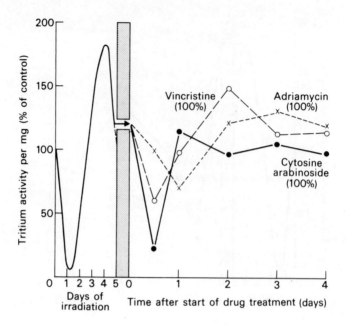

Figure 1.11 As Figure 4.1.9

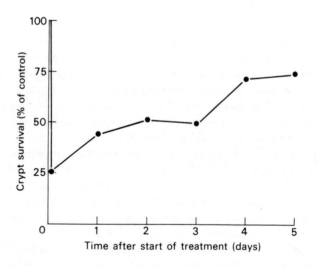

Figure 4.1.12 Jejunal crypt survival, as a percentage of the normal number of crypts per mg, at various times after treatment consisting of 500 μg/kg actinomycin D at time 0 and 800 rad X-irradiation on each of the 6 days

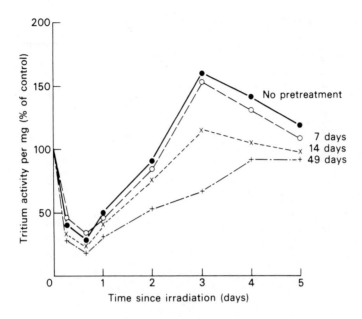

Figure 4.1.13 Thymidine incorporation per mg of jejunum, as a percentage of the control value, at various times after 1100 rad X-irradiation; adriamycin was given before irradiation at the intervals shown

indicate the proliferative response to 1000 rad when adriamycin at a dosage of 10 mg per kg had been given 7, 14 or 49 days prior to the irradiation. It should be noted that prior to the irradiation steady-state measures of proliferation were at control levels in all cases; only the ability to mount a compensatory response was affected by the drug. These findings raised the question of whether it was simply an addition of irradiation and drug damage which compromised proliferative capacity. In the colon, refeeding animals following a 3-day fast results in a burst of proliferative activity reaching about twice normal levels at 16 h after refeeding. This non-destructive induction of proliferation was then used in place of the 1000 rad irradiation exposure. The results are shown in Figure 4.1.14, in which graded doses of adriamycin were given 49 days prior to fasting and refeeding; proliferative activity in the colon was reestablished at control levels just prior to the fast. As shown in the figure, delayed toxicity was clearly seen, manifest as a dose-dependent failure of the colonic epithelium to enhance proliferation in response to refeeding. These results indicate that adriamycin results in a proliferative defect which is not manifest at steady-state levels of proliferative activity but is manifest when the system is called upon to respond to cellular damage.

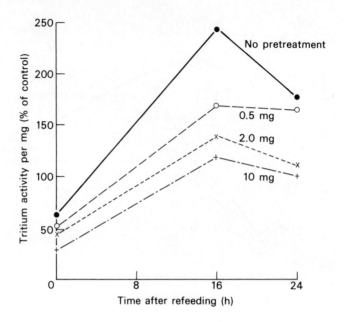

Figure 4.1.14 Thymidine incorporation per mg of colon, as a percentage of the control value, at various times after refeeding following a 3-day fast. Different doses of adriamycin were given 49 days prior to the fast

4.1.4 GROWTH CONTROL MECHANISMS

Studies of how in-vivo cell renewal systems are constructed, and how they respond to injury, provide insight into the mechanisms which have evolved to deal with situations which cause perturbations in steady-state conditions, and which, it would seem conservative to consider, also operate to maintain steady-state kinetics within rather narrow limits. The following partially speculative arrangement would seem compatible with available evidence. Proliferative activity, largely a function of the duration of the cell cycle phases and the size of the proliferation compartment, is directly influenced by cell density in the crypt. One could postulate mechanisms which would accomplish this; perhaps, as for cultured cells, there are defined concentrations of 'growth factors' required for proliferation, which in vivo would be provided by plasma. Exposure of crypt cells to these factors is thus quantitatively influenced by the surface area of the cell facing the source of these factors. If the capillary network is more developed towards the lower reaches of the crypt, proliferation will, in a steady state, be confined to this region. Damaging situations reduce crypt cellularity, resulting in a larger contact area between the now more spread-out surviving cells and the basement membrane, and hence a relatively greater exposure to plasma factors. Thus, both cell cycle shortening and upward expansion of proliferative activity might be expected. Both would be accomplished by a shortening of G_1 and a decision to undergo an additional round or rounds of DNA synthesis. As suggested at the outset, the signal mechanism should be the same both for the response to injury (at the level of both crypt and villus), and for the physiological maintenance of steady state. For the former, increased exposure to the basement membrane could result from decreased contact with neighbouring cells by virtue of reduced crypt cell content, either because of direct lysis of affected cells or at a later time because more cells which are reproductively incompetent enter the villus compartment than are produced by surviving cells in the crypt. The situation in the steady state is less dramatic but the same considerations could certainly apply. It has been pointed out by a number of investigators that the cell occupying the extrusion zone on the villus, though not yet extruded, is dead, perhaps due to cumulative exposure to cytoactive substances in the intestinal lumen. Shortly after physiological death, the cell loses contact with the basement membrane and, due to the unbalanced pressure exerted by its immediate neighbours, is forcibly extruded into the lumen. Its former neighbours then move slightly upward, with one (or several) now taking over the extrusion position. The cells immediately below, also experiencing less downward pressure than upward, move up slightly. This wave of transient reduction in the downward pressure exerted in the higher cell positions is translated sequentially to the crypt proliferation compartment. Since the basement membrane at the very bottom of the crypt is not free to move upward, as could the whole column of cells, those cells at the bottom of the crypt can only respond to the new unbalanced force on them by spreading out slightly, ie, by increasing the area of contact with the basement membrane. The situation in any given crypt would, of course, reflect extrusion from all of the villi on to which it feeds cells. Thus it is possible that cumulative exposure to the usual luminal conditions for a given species results in a characteristic rate of cell death at the villus apices. This could then be translated, as outlined above, to a given membrane surface area of cells in the lower crypt region facing the 'growth factors' responsible for governing the duration of the G_1-phase and the post-mitotic decision whether to enter a succeeding cycle of DNA synthesis. This, or a similar mechanism, could also provide a proliferative response to damage to the functional compartment per se, as may be anticipated from evolutionary considerations. Lastly, it would ensure a proliferative response proportional to the degree of injury encountered, irrespective of the site or mode of action of the injurious agent.

4.2 The Response of Small-Intestinal Stem Cells in the Mouse to Drug and Irradiation Treatment

Wayne R Hanson, Deborah L Henninger, R J Michael Fry, and Anthony R Sallese

4.2.1 INTRODUCTION

The cell renewal systems of epidermal and haemopoietic tissue are recognised to have a stem-cell population, relatively small in size, whose cells have long cell cycle times compared with the more rapidly proliferating cells in the amplification compartment (61, 105, 138, 446, 533). In the case of the intestine, the distinction between these two compartments has not been as clear. For various reasons some authors have considered the rapidly proliferating crypt cells to be clonogenic cells (50, 276, 278, 592, 807). Evidence in support of this view is based in part on the analysis of split-dose survival curves (461). This analysis resulted in an estimate of about 140 clonogenic cells per crypt, a number that is similar to the number of rapidly cycling cells per crypt.

Some authors consider that the rapidly cycling cells that survive injury from irradiation, from cytotoxic drugs, or from combinations of drugs and irradiation are capable of sufficient divisions to produce microcolonies (252, 278, 524). Further evidence that the rapidly cycling cells are clonogenic was provided by the results showing that the S-phase-specific agents, high specific activity tritiated thymidine (HSA-^{3}HTdR) and cytosine arabinoside (ara-C), markedly reduced the number of clonogenic cells (50). These results suggest that a large proportion of clonogenic cells are in the S-phase of the cell cycle. However, other evidence indicates that there may be a population of epithelial cells in the lower part of crypts with morphological and proliferative characteristics different from the rapidly cycling cells. Detailed electron microscopic examination of normal crypts shows a morphologically primitive cell towards the crypt base (101, 103) and continuous ^{3}HTdR labelling studies show that cells in this area take up label at a later time than cells farther up the crypts (542). The cell cycle times of cells in the basal region are longer than those of cells in the middle region (6, 83, 818). Data from split dose survival curves suggest that there are fewer clonogenic cells than rapidly proliferating cells (314) and other results have been interpreted as showing differences between cryptogenic and proliferating cells in post-irradiation recovery (540).

Further evidence that a true intestinal stem-cell population exists with proliferative characteristics that are different from those of the rapidly cycling cells comes from results showing that HSA-^{3}HTdR given 17 h or 1 h before irradiation killed about half the crypt cells but did not reduce the number of surviving clonogenic cells (294). Similarly, colcemid injections that reduced the proliferating cell population of the crypt by half did not change the microcolony survival curve. These results, indicating that very few of the clonogenic cells are in S-phase at any given time, are not in agreement with those outlined above (50). The reason for the difference in the results is not known but may be related to the use of different strains of mice, as has been shown in the haemopoietic system (123).

Hydroxyurea (HU), and S-phase-specific cytotoxic agent, has been used to synchronise crypt cells by its reported blocking effect at the boundary between G_1 and S. Upon release from the block, the clonogenic cells show marked cell-age-dependent radiosensitivity fluctuations. There is a greater sensitivity when the cells are in late G_1 or early S and comparative resistance when the cells are in mid to late S (166, 252, 276). These results have been interpreted as indicating that the stem cells are normally in rapid cycle (278).

An alternative view is that the stem cells are in a prolonged G_1 phase and in response to HU, and perhaps other cytotoxic agents, they enter DNA synthesis in a partially synchronised fashion and proceed thus around the cell cycle at least once (295). This interpretation is consistent with evidence for the effects of HU (726, 749, 750) and other cytotoxic agents (239, 240, 496, 497, 544) on the haemopoietic pluripotent stem cell. Shortly after irradiation the cells in the colony-forming units (CFU) enter S, suggesting that although these hemopoietic stem cells are in G_0 or G_1 they must be relatively close to the G_1 to S boundary (383).

This paper reports some investigations into the proliferative characteristics of intestinal clonogenic or stem cells and their response to various cytotoxic agents.

4.2.2 MATERIALS AND METHODS

Several cytotoxic agents were selected for their specific effects and phase-dependent specificity. Colcemid, an effective metaphase blocking agent, causes depletion of crypt cells through the loss into the crypt lumen of cells blocked in mitosis. The rate of crypt cell depletion is dependent on the rate of entry of cells into mitosis and therefore on the cell cycle time (T_c). HSA-^{3}HTdR and HU were used as S-phase-specific agents, and doses of both γ-irradiation and irradiation with fission spectrum fast neutrons (fn) were used as less phase-specific cytotoxic agents.

4.2.2.1 COLCEMID

Colcemid, (150 μg per 30 g mouse) was given intraperitoneally to male B6CF$_1$ mice, 110 to 140 days old, every 3 h for a total of 4 injections. To investigate whether the 3 h interval between colcemid injections allowed the drug titre to fall to such levels that cells escaped the metaphase block and subsequent killing effect, a further group of mice were given 5 μg per g intraperitoneally every 2 h for a total of 6 injections. Control groups of animals were injected every 2 or 3 h with an equal volume of saline, the solvent for the colcemid.

Three hours after the last injection of colcemid or saline (12 h from the first injection), the animals were subjected to doses of ^{60}Co γ-irradiation between 1000 and 2000 rad at 45 rad per min to construct dose-survival curves using the microcolony assay technique (809). Four to $4\frac{1}{2}$ days after irradiation exposure, the animals were killed by cervical fracture and pieces of proximal jejunum were excised, fixed in a solution of alcohol, formalin and acetic acid, and embedded in paraffin for routine histological sectioning. The numbers of microcolonies were counted in between 6 and 18 intestinal cross-sections per mouse per treatment group at each dose of irradiation. The results were plotted on a semi-log scale, the exponential segment being fitted by linear regression weighted by both variance and the number of animals per point. To determine the effect of the treatment on the proliferating cells in the crypt, autoradiographs of crypt squashes (802) were prepared from animals that had received colcemid or saline for 12 h. One hour before the end of the 12 h treatment with colcemid or saline, 4 animals of each group were given 25 μCi ^{3}HTdR, of specific activity 1 Ci per mM, and killed 1 h later by cervical fracture. Pieces of proximal jejunum were fixed in Carnoy's solution for later crypt microdissection. Crypt squashes were prepared (802), and slides with 15 to 20 of these were dipped in Kodak NTB emulsion, stored for between 15 and 20 days at 4°C, and developed in Kodak D-19 developer. The total number of cells per crypt squash, labelled cells per crypt squash, when appropriate, and mitotic figures were counted.

4.2.2.2 HIGH SPECIFIC ACTIVITY TRITIATED THYMIDINE

HSA-^{3}HTdR of specific activity 60 Ci per mM was given to male B6CF$_1$ adult mice, at a dose of 1 mCi per mouse in a single intraperitoneal injection, 17 h before being killed for the crypt microdissection procedure, or before ^{60}Co γ-irradiation to construct dose-survival curves using the microcolony assay as described above. In a similar experiment, animals were given 2 injections of 1 mCi each 17 h and 1 h before being killed or receiving ^{60}Co γ-irradiation. Data from these animals and from control animals that received saline in an equal volume were compared.

4.2.2.3 HYDROXYUREA

HU at a dose of 15 mg per 30 g mouse was given intraperitoneally 15 minutes before or 15 minutes after increasing doses of ^{60}Co γ-irradiation to construct dose-survival curves. Other groups of mice were given HU 2 or 6 h before increasing doses of irradiation. These times were chosen as the minimum and maximum respectively of post-HU clonogenic cell survival (252). Autoradiographs of crypt squash preparations were made from tissue taken at these two times so that the total number of crypt cells surviving the HU treatment, and the total number in the S-phase, could be related to the radiosensitivity of clonogenic cells.

4.2.2.4 HYDROXYUREA OR HIGH SPECIFIC ACTIVITY TRITIATED THYMIDINE IN COMBINATION WITH COLCEMID

HU, at a dose of 15 mg per 30 g mouse, or 1 mCi HSA-^{3}HTdR, was given intraperitoneally to groups of animals, and followed 3 h later by the first of 4 intraperitoneal injections of colcemid (150 μg per mouse) given three-hourly. Three hours after the last injection of colcemid, 4 animals from each group were killed for crypt squashes and 5 or 6 animals were given increasing doses of ^{60}Co γ-irradiation to construct dose-survival curves using the microcolony assay. Data from these two groups and from animals that received 12 h of colcemid given every 3 h were compared (293).

4.2.2.5 GAMMA OR FAST NEUTRON IRRADIATION IN COMBINATION WITH COLCEMID

A dose of 50 rad ^{137}Cs γ-irradiation was given to 120 B6CF$_1$ adult male mice. Immediately, one group of 10 mice was started on a course of 12 h of colcemid and another group of 10 was given saline every 3 h during the same 12 h period, after which 6 animals from each group were given 1100 rad ^{137}Cs γ-irradiation which results in clonogenic cell survival giving rise to an average of 40 ± 3 microcolonies per circumference in untreated animals. Six hours after the same initial dose of 50 rad γ-irradiation another group of 20 mice was divided into 2 groups of 10 each and started on the 12 h treatment of colcemid or saline as described above. The same procedures were carried out on 4 more groups, each of 20 mice, except that 12, 18, 24 or 30 h elapsed between the initial treatment and the initiation of 12 h colcemid or saline. An identical experiment was done with fission spectrum fast neutrons where 20 rad fn (average energy 0.85 MeV) was delivered to 120 adult mice in the Janus reactor at Argonne National Laboratory. At 6, 12, 18, 24, 30 or 72 h later, groups of 20 mice were started on 12 h of colcemid or saline treatment (to 10 mice each). To explore whether there might be a threshold dose of the initial irradiation below which there would be no effect on clonogenic cells, doses of 0, 13, 25, 38 and 50 rad ^{137}Cs γ-irradiation were given to 100 adult B6CF$_1$ mice (20 at each dose level). The animals not actually irradiated were carefully sham-irradiated, and handled identically to irradiated animals. Twelve hours after these small challenge doses animals were started on 12 h of colcemid or saline treatment. Four animals in each group were killed for subsequent crypt dissection to assess crypt cell parameters, while at the same time the remaining animals were given 1100 rad ^{137}Cs γ-irradiation to reduce clonogenic cell survival to a countable level.

4.2.3 RESULTS

The 12 h treatment of colcemid given every 3 h reduced the number of intact cells per crypt from a control level of 254 ± 11 to 156 ± 8. Blocked metaphases in crypts are lost into the lumen 2 to 3 h after arrest. Even though the number of cells per crypt was greatly reduced, the number of clonogenic cells which survived irradiation did not change from saline-treated animals (Figure 4.2.1) which suggests that the rapidly cycling cells are not the cells which form microcolonies. Nor when colcemid was given every 2 h for 12 h was there a change from controls. These results show that blocked clonogenic cells are not escaping from the block through metaphase in the 3 h interval between colcemid injections. The S-phase cytotoxic agent HSA-^{3}HTdR reduced the number of cells per crypt from 254 ± 11 to 142 ± 4 when samples were taken 17 h after one injection of 1 mCi. When two injections of 1 mCi were given, one 17 h and the other 1 h before death, the number of surviving cells per crypt was 132 ± 6. The cytotoxicity in this case is presumed to be due to β-irradiation from ^{3}H incorporated into newly synthesised DNA. Although the number of cells per crypt was reduced by both treatments of HSA-^{3}HTdR, the clonogenic cell survival remained the same as in controls (Figure 4.2.2). HU, which is also cytotoxic to cells in the S-phase of the cell cycle, although by a different mechanism, did not reduce the clonogenic cell survival when given 15 minutes before or after ^{60}Co γ-irradiation. When animals were irradiated 2 h after HU, the clonogenic cell survival curve was shifted to the left, but when 6 h were allowed between HU and irradiation the cell survival curve was

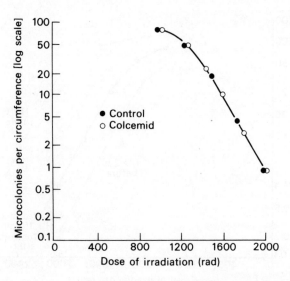

Figure 4.2.1 Microcolonies per intestinal circumference after different doses of ^{60}Co γ-irradiation in controls and after 12 h of colcemid given at 3 h intervals

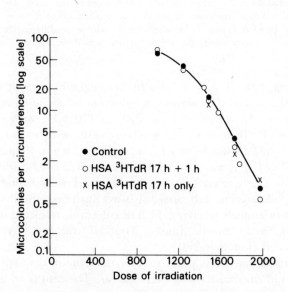

Figure 4.2.2 Microcolonies per intestinal circumference after different doses of ^{60}Co γ-irradiation in saline-injected controls or in animals 17 h or 17 h and 1 h after HSA-^{3}HTdR

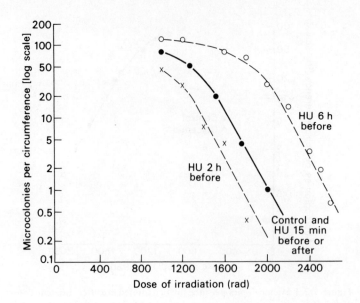

Figure 4.2.3 Microcolonies per intestinal circumference after different doses of irradiation in mice treated with 15 mg hydroxyurea 15 minutes before or after irradiation, 2 h before irradiation, or 6 h before irradiation. The values at lower doses of irradiation on the shoulder of the survival curves represent counts of what appear to be whole crypts which are different from the microcolonies counted at higher doses of irradiation

displaced to the right (Figure 4.2.3). Autoradiographs of crypt squashes from animals killed 2 h after HU showed a reduction in the number of cells from 254 ± 11 in controls, with 90 ± 6 labelled, to 170 ± 11, with 3 ± 1 labelled. Six hours after HU there were 142 surviving cells, with 79 ± 7 labelled.

When HSA-^{3}HTdR was followed 3 h later by 12 h of colcemid, the number of surviving intact cells was reduced to 94 ± 3 with 37 ± 2 mitotic figures per crypt. When similarly treated animals were exposed to increasing doses of ^{60}Co γ-irradiation, clonogenic cell survival was unaltered from saline-injected controls or from animals receiving 12 h of colcemid, resulting in 73 ± 4 cells per crypt and 53 ± 3 mitotic figures. After HU the cell survival curve was shifted to the left (Figure 4.2.4).

Gamma-irradiation is less phase-specific than the drugs used in the above experiment, and fn-irradiation is even less so. The results of giving a small challenge dose of 50 rad ^{137}Cs γ-irradiation followed at various times by 12 h of colcemid or saline are presented in Figure 4.2.5, and show that colcemid, which normally does not reduce clonogenic cell survival in untreated animals,

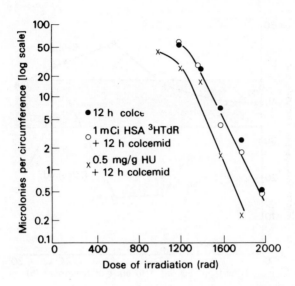

Figure 4.2.4 Microcolonies per intestinal circumference after different doses of ^{60}Co γ-irradiation after 12 h colcemid, 1 mCi HSA–^{3}HTdR plus 12 h colcemid, or HU followed by 12 h colcemid

reduced it when started 12, 18 and 30 h after the challenge dose. When colcemid was begun immediately or 6 h afterwards, however, there was little difference from control values, which was also true for animals started on colcemid after 24 h. The values for saline-injected controls 18 and 24 h after 50 rad γ-irradiation were above values obtained for saline-injected control animals not irradiated. Similarly, exposure to 20 rad fn-irradiation resulted in a marked increase in the effect of subsequent exposure to colcemid and 1100 rad ^{137}Cs γ-irradiation (Figure 4.2.6). The effect was more marked and more prolonged than after exposure to 50 rad γ-irradiation. After 6 h the number of micro-colonies in the group given 20 rad fn-irradiation plus saline plus 1100 rad γ-irradiation is slightly below the number after 1100 rad γ-irradiation alone. The D_0 (see Section 3.1) for crypt cells after exposure to fn-irradiation is 53 rad (264) and therefore it is likely that the 20 rad fn-irradiation reduced the number of clonogenic cells sufficiently for the reduction to be detected by the assay some 12 h later. At 72 h the number of microcolonies in this 20 rad fn-irradiation plus saline control group was higher than in the 1100 rad γ-irradiation group, which may result from the presence of an increased number of clonogenic cells due to an overshoot in recovery.

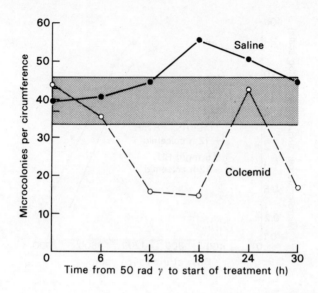

Figure 4.2.5 Microcolonies per intestinal circumference as a function of time between a challenge dose of 50 rad ^{137}Cs γ-irradiation and the beginning of a 12 h treatment of saline or colcemid, followed by 1100 rad. The shaded area indicates approximate 95% confidence limits for the value after either 1100 rad alone or 12 h colcemid plus 1100 rad

The greatest differences between irradiation plus colcemid and irradiation plus saline were seen when the interval between irradiation and treatment was 12 to 18 h (Figures 4.2.5 and 4.2.6). When this interval was held constant at 12 h, but the initial challenge dose of ^{137}Cs γ-irradiation was varied, there was no dose tested below which an effect was not seen, and the effects produced were similar (Figure 4.2.7). There was no difference between colcemid or saline-treated sham-irradiated controls although the number of microcolonies was lower than in the similar controls of most other experiments.

Cell counts of crypt squashes from animals receiving increasing challenge doses of γ-irradiation and killed 24 h later (after 12 h saline) showed a gradual decline from about 255 cells in sham-irradiated controls to 175 cells after 50 rad γ-irradiation (Figure 4.2.8). The number of mitotic figures per crypt increased from 7 in sham-irradiated animals to 26 after 50 rad γ-irradiation. The number of cells per crypt in colcemid-treated animals receiving increasing doses of γ-irradiation from 0 to 50 rad remained fairly constant at about 80 as did the number of about 50 intact mitotic figures (Figure 4.2.8).

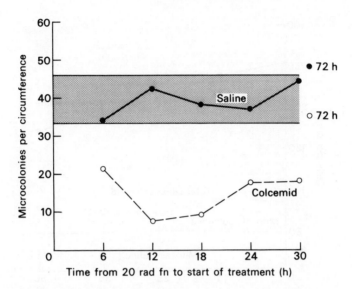

Figure 4.2.6 Microcolonies per intestinal circumference as a function of time between a challenge dose of 20 rad fn-irradiation and the beginning of a 12 h treatment of saline or colcemid, followed by 1100 rad ^{137}Cs γ-irradiation. The shaded area is as in Figure 4.2.5

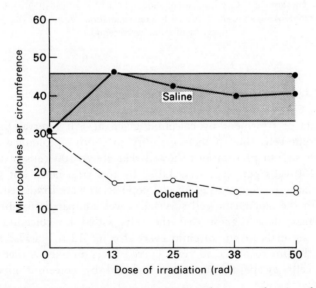

Figure 4.2.7 Microcolonies per intestinal circumference as a function of the challenge dose of ^{137}Cs γ-irradiation given 12 h before 12 h treatment of saline or colcemid followed by 1100 rad. The shaded area is as in Figure 4.2.5

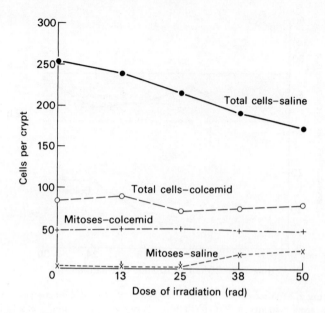

Figure 4.2.8 Total cells and numbers of mitoses per crypt squash after different doses of ^{137}Cs γ-irradiation followed by a 12 h treatment of saline or colcemid. Animals were killed 24 h after irradiation, 12 h after the first injection of saline or colcemid

4.2.4 DISCUSSION

Twelve hours of treatment by colcemid given at 3 h intervals kills small-intestinal crypt cells due to their inability to survive prolonged metaphase block. Crypt squash preparations showed that about 100 cells of the normal average of 250 cells per crypt were killed by this treatment, but when mice treated similarly to those assayed for cell population were irradiated, there was no change in the clonogenic cell survival curves compared to saline injected controls. These data suggest that the cells killed by colcemid were not clonogenic. Animals given colcemid every 2 h for 12 h likewise showed no change in the microcolony survival curve. It is unlikely, therefore, that clonogenic cells escape mitotic arrest induced by colcemid given at 3 h intervals.

HSA-^{3}HTdR, cytotoxic to cells in the S-phase of the cell cycle, reduced the number of crypt cells to about 140 when given 17 h, or 17 and 1 h before assay. This cytotoxic effect should affect predominantly the rapidly cycling amplification compartment cells since about half of these cells are the S-phase. Clonogenic cell survival data taken from these irradiated animals were unaltered from control values. HU, also cytotoxic to S-phase cells, did not alter clonogenic cell survival when given immediately before or after irradiation, and as it is unlikely that irradiation altered the enzyme-mediated cytotoxicity of the drug, these data also suggest that cells in the S-phase of the cell cycle are not clonogenic.

When animals were irradiated 2 h after HU, the clonogenic cell survival curve was shifted to the left. Autoradiographs of crypt squashes taken from similarly treated animals showed that about 80 cells were killed, in fair agreement with the estimate of 90 cells per crypt in the S-phase. The effectiveness of HU for blocking the entry of cells into S was shown by the finding of an average of only 3 labelled cells per crypt. When these same parameters were measured 6 h after HU, the total cell population was little changed, but the number of labelled cells was greatly increased to about 80, indicating that by this time the G_1 to S block was no longer effective and cells were undergoing DNA synthesis. When cell survival curves were constructed from animals irradiated 6 h after HU, the curve was shifted to the right. These results agree with those of others (166, 252, 276); however, it is possible to take an alternative view to the one which supposes that these data demonstrate that clonogenic cells are the rapidly cycling population (278). The change in radiosensitivity after HU suggests that the clonogenic cells are in rapid cycle after HU treatment, but if they were normally in rapid cycle, colcemid or HSA-^{3}HTdR should have killed some and thus shifted the survival curve to the left. The data suggest that HU rapidly recruits clonogenic cells from a G_0 or an extended G_1 phase of the cell cycle into DNA synthesis; this suggestion is similar to one that has been made concerning the action of HU on the haemopoietic system (749). Support for this interpretation is given by the experiments showing that more cells per crypt are killed by a 12 h treatment by colcemid when begun 3 h after HU than when the same colcemid treatment is given after HSA-^{3}HTdR. Further, HU followed by colcemid reduces the clonogenic cell survival either by shifting the cells to a more sensitive part of the cell cycle or, more likely, by recruitment of the clonogenic cells into rapid cycle where they are subsequently susceptible to colcemid block and cell death. HSA-^{3}HTdR followed by colcemid does not alter clonogenic cell survival. These data suggest that the mechanism of recruitment is not mediated through S-phase cytotoxicity, at least during the times investigated in these experiments, but is possibly a direct effect on the stem-cell population. An increased labelling index in the cells at the base of crypts in rats during recovery after HU treatment has been demonstrated (10). If the interpretation that HU recruits stem cells into rapid cycle is correct, then recruitment must be rapid since the clonogenic cells appear first to overcome a 3 to 4 h G_1 to S block, then proceed through a 6 h S-phase and a 2 h G_2-phase before entering mitosis where they are susceptible to colcemid. These data suggest that the clonogenic cells are predominantly in late G_1.

When 50 rad ^{137}Cs γ-irradiation is followed at various times by 12 h of colcemid or saline, the first observed difference in clonogenic cell survival after 1100 rad ^{137}Cs γ-irradiation is seen at 12 h. Our interpretation of these data is that 50 rad γ-irradiation recruits intestinal clonogenic cells into rapid cycle similarly to HU. The control animals received identical treatment except that saline was given at various times after 50 rad γ-irradiation instead of colcemid. The assay dose of 1100 rad was given to both colcemid and saline groups at the same time, but different groups were irradiated at various times of the day.

When a dose of 20 rad fn-irradiation was given in a similar experiment, differences between saline- and colcemid-injected animals were seen throughout the period from 6 to 30 h and were more marked than with 50 rad γ-irradiation. This difference is consistent with greater relative biological effectiveness (RBE) of fn-irradiation compared to γ-irradiation (264), but the relationship of RBE to the apparent recruitment effect is uncertain.

The methods of investigation of the intestinal stem cells reported in this paper are indirect and the interpretation of the results is complicated by a number of factors. The survival of clonogenic cells after irradiation is thought to show a circadian rhythm (312), and this may explain the variation in the number of microcolonies after exposure to 12 h of saline and 1100 rad ^{137}Cs γ-irradiation at different times after the 50 rad γ-irradiation challenge dose (Figure 4.2.5). However, it is unlikely that diurnal effects could account for the data from colcemid-injected animals since the saline-injected animals were irradiated at the same time and should reflect any variation. Treatment by 50 rad γ-irradiation or 20 rad fn-irradiation may cause a shift in the cell age distribution so that there is an increase in the number of clonogenic cells in more sensitive or less sensitive parts of the cell cycle depending on the time after challenge, but this variation in radiosensitivity should also be reflected in the values for saline-injected controls. A reduction of clonogenic cell survival after the challenge dose may not only be seen early in the saline-injected groups, but it may cause an increase in survival at 30 h and later, as a result of an overshoot during recovery.

Despite these various factors we believe that the marked reduction in clonogenic cells between 6 and 30 h after a challenge dose of 20 rad fn-irradiation followed by 12 h colcemid, and assayed with 1100 rad ^{137}Cs γ-irradiation, compared to the several appropriate controls (Figure 4.2.6), indicates that the challenge dose enhanced the effect of colcemid. The effect of the challenge dose is interpreted to indicate an increased rate of entry of clonogenic cells into mitosis, which is consistent with a shortening of the cell cycle.

Both 50 rad γ-irradiation and 20 rad fn-irradiation are low doses when considering acute effects on any in-vivo cell system, especially the intestine, but it is apparent that even lower doses have a similar recruiting effect. Although the saline-injected, sham-irradiated control value was lower than that normally seen in other experiments, 12 h of colcemid had no effect (Figure 4.2.7). However, a dose as low as 13 rad γ-irradiation appears to recruit stem cells into rapid cycle, thus making them susceptible to the effects of colcemid. There is no apparent difference between the degree of recruitment from 13 to 50 rad γ-irradiation even though cell counts from crypt squash preparations showed a decrease from 250 to 175 as the dose was increased from 0 to 50 rads (Figure 4.2.8). The lack of a dose-dependent response for clonogenic cell recruitment compared with the dose-dependent death of crypt cells might be taken as evidence that these two events are separately controlled. However, with higher challenge doses the reduction in clonogenic cells surviving the 12 h colcemid treatment is more prolonged than with lower doses and therefore the apparent lack of dose-dependency is misleading.

If it is correct that clonogenic or stem cells are recruited into rapid cycle, where they are vulnerable to colcemid, then the number of clonogenic cells should increase, and by 12 h nearly double, in saline-injected control animals if both daughter cells remain clonogenic. However, the number of clonogenic cells remains nearly constant, especially after 20 rad fn-irradiation. These results suggest a very sharp demarcation of proliferative characteristics between the two daughter cells of a stem-cell division. Apparently, one cell remains a clonogenic cell and the other becomes an amplification division cell without clonogenic capability. It is possible that this response is dose-dependent, and with higher doses and greater damage both daughter cells remain in cycle in the stem-cell compartment.

The results of these investigations suggest that in the B6CF$_1$ strain of mouse the intestinal stem cells are predominantly in a G$_0$ phase or in an extended G$_1$ phase of the cell cycle near the G$_1$ to S boundary. In response to treatments of HU, γ-irradiation, or fn-irradiation, these cells are recruited into rapid cycle.

4.2.5 SUMMARY

The normal kinetic state of the intestinal stem cells, assumed to be the same as the clonogenic cells of the microcolony assay (809), is an important consideration when assessing the effect of a single dose of phase-specific drugs or the less phase-specific effects of a single exposure to irradiation. Changes in the cell age distribution, through alteration of the initial kinetic state of the stem cells surviving drug or irradiation exposure, probably alter the effects of subsequent exposures, especially if the time between multiple treatments is short. Studies were done to try to understand both the initial kinetic state of intestinal stem cells and the altered state of stem cells surviving drug or irradiation exposure.

A phase-specific cytotoxic agent, high specific activity tritiated thymidine or colcemid, was given in regimens which killed about half of the rapidly cycling crypt cells. These treatments did not alter clonogenic cell survival after irradiation, suggesting that stem cells are not initially in rapid cycle. Furthermore, when irradiation was given 15 minutes after S-phase specific hydroxyurea, there was no change in clonogenic cell survival; however, the irradiation response of stem cells at various later times after HU treatment suggested that the stem cells may have responded by going into rapid cycle. The decreased clonogenic cell survival after HU and 12 h colcemid, given to block and kill rapidly cycling crypt cells in mitosis, contrasts with the lack of effect of 12 h of colcemid alone; this also suggests that HU recruits stem cells. However, such a recruiting effect is not seen after HSA-^{3}HTdR, at least not at the same time, suggesting that the recruiting mechanism is not related to S-phase cytotoxicity alone. To see if irradiation caused similar alterations in stem-cell kinetics, animals were subjected to small doses of fast neutrons or ^{137}Cs γ-irradiation. Results suggested that irradiation recruited stem cells into rapid cycle similarly to HU, a dose as low as 13 rads being sufficient. Furthermore, there was no difference in the magnitude of recruitment between 13 and 50 rads when colcemid or saline was started 12 h later; however, the time course of recruitment may be dose-dependent. The number of cells per crypt surviving 0 to 50 rad ^{137}Cs γ-irradiation declined from about 250 to 175.

These results suggest that a number of agents with different modes of cytotoxicity recruit surviving stem cells (apparently in G_1) into rapid cycle. The mechanism of recruitment does not appear to be completely dependent on the degree of cytotoxicity.

4.3 The Effect of Cytosine Arabinoside and other Phase-specific Cytotoxic Agents on Proliferation, Radiosensitivity, and Survival of Jejunal Stem Cells

T A Phelps

4.3.1 INTRODUCTION

The response of intestinal epithelial cells to irradiation can be greatly influenced by prior administration of cytotoxic agents, and the effects of phase-specific cytotoxic agents are of particular interest. From the clinician's point of view the responses to combination chemotherapy and radiotherapy are of interest because the majority of crypt cells are very sensitive to these agents, a fact which to a large extent limits their therapeutic use. From the point of view of the pure scientist, use can be made of such agents to answer fundamental questions about the size, proliferative status and radiosensitivity of the crypt stem-cell compartment.

Investigations have previously been made on the effects on jejunal crypt cells of the S-phase-specific agent cytosine arabinoside (ara-C), and on the response of cryptogenic cells to irradiation administered at various times after ara-C. Twelve hours after ara-C administration, irradiation resulted in a large increase in cryptogenic cell survival; a similar increase observed after multiple injections of hydroxyurea (HU) has been attributed to synchronisation of cells into a radioresistant cohort towards the end of the S-phase (252, 810). This paper is concerned with the mechanism and consequences of the radioresistance induced by ara-C. Use has been made of other phase-specific drugs including HU, which is specific for the S-phase, and the metaphase-arresting agents vincristine and colcemid.

4.3.2 MATERIALS AND METHODS

4.3.2.1 THE MICROCOLONY ASSAY

A modified version (50) of the microcolony assay of Withers and Elkind (809) was used for all intestinal cryptogenic cell experiments. The term 'cryptogenic cell' is used here to describe a cell which is capable of regenerating into a crypt-like structure by $3\frac{1}{2}$ days after high doses of irradiation. Such regenerated crypts are also known as microcolonies and this microcolony assay technique is based on three assumptions: firstly that doses of irradiation which reduce microcolony survival to the level of the exponential region of the microcolony survival curve are sufficiently high to result, on average, in the survival of only one cryptogenic cell per crypt; secondly that one cryptogenic cell is capable of producing a microcolony; and thirdly that cryptogenic cells survive independently of each other. Cryptogenic cells therefore represent a clonogenic population of cells, but this population may include cells which are not 'functional' stem cells (103). There is a large but imprecisely determined number of cryptogenic cells per crypt. The term 'multiplicity' is used to refer to the number of cryptogenic cells per crypt existing at any one time. Because of the large multiplicity in crypts of normal animals, it is necessary to use a high assay dose of irradiation to bring microcolony survival down to the level of the exponential part of the survival curve. The assay dose used here was 1300 or 1400 rad, and by giving a drug at various times before irradiation it is possible to determine whether altering this time interval influences the toxicity.

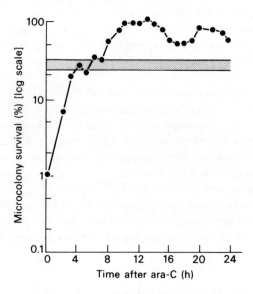

Figure 4.3.1 Microcolony survival after an assay dose of 1300 rad given at various times after administering 200 mg/kg ara-C intraperitoneally. The shaded area represents approximate 95% confidence limits for microcolony survival in the absence of ara-C

4.3.2.2 QUANTITATIVE HISTOLOGICAL METHODS

C57Bl female mice between 8 and 12 weeks old were irradiated with 60_{Co} γ-rays at about 50 rad per min, and microcolonies were counted $3\frac{1}{2}$ days later. Mice were given 20 μCi tritiated thymidine (^{3}HTdR) 30 min before being killed by cervical dislocation, and histological cross-sections cut from four 15 mm long portions of jejunum, starting distal to the ligament of Treitz, using a minimum of 5 mice per point. Autoradiographs were prepared to facilitate identification of regenerating crypts. The number of microcolonies per transverse section of jejunum was expressed as a simple proportion of the number of crypts visible in cross-sections of unirradiated mice. To determine labelling (I_s) and cumulative mitotic indices, mice were given vincristine, at a dose of 1 mg per kg for metaphase arrest, $1\frac{1}{2}$ h before death, and 20 μCi ^{3}HTdR per mouse 30 min before death. Ara-C was used at a dose of 200 mg per kg in saline, and HU at a dose of 900 mg per kg in saline. When vincristine was used as a cytotoxic drug it was given over a period of 12 h at 3-hourly intervals at a dose of 0.6 mg per kg per injection. Colcemid used as a cytotoxic drug was given at a dose of 1 mg per kg per injection over a period of 12 h as for vincristine.

4.3.3 RESULTS

4.3.3.1 MICROCOLONY SURVIVAL, LABELLING INDEX AND CUMULATIVE MITOTIC INDEX AFTER CYTOSINE ARABINOSIDE

To determine microcolony survival when the time between ara-C and irradiation was varied, mice were given 200 mg per kg of the drug intraperitoneally between 0 and 24 h before an assay dose of 1300 rad. The results are shown in Figure 4.3.1. When the drug was given within 5 min of irradiation, there was a much smaller microcolony survival (1.3 percent) than when 1300 rad alone was given (25 percent). As the time interval increased between ara-C and irradiation, microcolony survival rapidly rose to a maximum at 10 to 13 h, followed after a slight reduction at 16 to 19 h by a second peak at 20 to 23 h. The microcolony survival showed a cyclic pattern correlating well with labelling index except that microcolony survival rose before I_s did (Figure 4.3.2). The labelling index and the cumulative mitotic index (also shown in Figure 4.3.2) were determined 0 to 24 h after mice were given ara-C but no irradiation. The variation in I_s indicates that DNA synthesis ceased altogether for a period of at least 2 to 3 h. By 4 h the G_1 to S block was cleared and cells quickly resumed DNA synthesis, producing a partially synchronised cohort which was in the S-phase 10 to 12 h after ara-C administration. These cells then moved on to G_2, and a second peak of cells in S-phase was observed at about

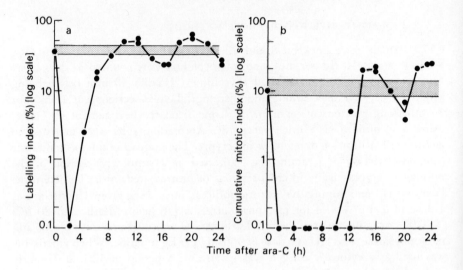

Figure 4.3.2 (a) Labelling and (b) cumulative mitotic indices at various times after intraperitoneal administration of 200 mg/kg ara-C. Shaded areas represent approximate 95% confidence limits for the values in control animals

20 h. The induced synchrony was only partial since I_s never fell below 20 percent after cycling resumed. The cumulative mitotic index shows that cell division started at 12 h and was maximal 14 to 16 h after drug administration. These data are similar to previous observations (11, 410) though no second peak in proliferative activity was reported. The correlation between the cyclic pattern of microcolony survival and I_s would be expected if the result of ara-C administration was a partial synchronisation of cells into a radioresistant cohort 10 to 12 h later, but the induction of radioresistance in late S-phase 10 to 12 h after ara-C does not explain the fact that microcolony survival began to rise before the appearance of labelled cells. It is possible that some of the radioresistance developed in late G_1, or there may have been some early repair of cell damage which accounts for the initial rise in microcolony survival.

4.3.3.2 MICROCOLONY IRRADIATION DOSE-RESPONSE CURVES AFTER CYTOSINE ARABINOSIDE

In order to investigate the nature of the protective effect, dose-response curves after graded doses of irradiation were obtained for normal animals and for mice irradiated immediately (0h) after ara-C or 12 h after ara-C. The three curves thus obtained are shown in Figure 4.3.3.

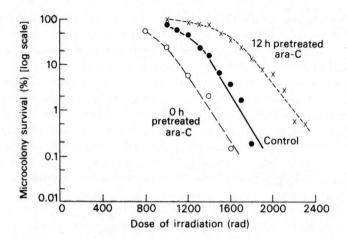

Figure 4.3.3 Microcolony irradiation dose-response curves for control mice, and mice pretreated immediately or 12 h before with 200 mg/kg ara-C

Comparison of 12 h-pretreated and irradiated control curves. Microcolony survival observed for 12 h-pretreated mice was much higher than that of irradiated controls. This large increase cannot be accounted for solely by synchronisation of cryptogenic cells into a radioresistant cohort in late S. This could only lead to an increase in numbers of late S-cells; it could not cause cells to take on more resistant properties, since the survivors of the irradiated control curve are already in the most radioresistant phase of the cell cycle, assumed to be late S. The maximum I_s achieved after ara-C is 50 percent compared to the normal I_s of 33 percent, so that one would expect a maximum increase of a factor of 1.5 in microcolony survival as a result of synchronisation of cells into late S. The actual difference observed was tenfold.

The microcolony survival curve for 12 h-pretreated mice was characterised by a much larger D_q (quasi-threshold dose, or shoulder) than the irradiated control curve (1520 rad versus 1050 rad). The D_0 (see Section 3.1) of the 12 h-pretreated mice rose slightly, but not statistically significantly, to 146 rad from the irradiated control level of 111. Because of the large shoulder of the microcolony survival curve, the assayable dose range for cryptogenic cells is at fairly high doses and it is only necessary to increase the D_0 of the irradiated control mice by 30 percent to account for the observed difference in microcolony survival between 12 h-pretreated mice and irradiated controls. The D_0 change observed, therefore, is sufficient to produce the microcolony survival obtained even if it is not large enough to be statistically significant. The rises in D_q and D_0 result in a dose difference of about 420 rad at the 10 percent microcolony survival level and about 500 rad at a survival of 1 percent. The microcolony survival for the 12 h-pretreated curve is not exponential at doses of less than 1800 rad. At lower doses any enhanced cryptogenic cell survival is therefore masked. For this reason use of 1300 rad as the assay dose in fact underestimates the true difference obtained at 12 h in Figure 4.3.1.

Comparison of immediately-pretreated and irradiated control curves. The 0 h curve in Figure 4.3.3 shows that when mice were given ara-C immediately before irradiation there was marked toxicity relative to irradiated controls, manifest as a one decade fall in microcolony survival. There is no apparent difference in D_0 values and the decrease in microcolony survival is consistent with killing of potential cryptogenic cells without a change in radiosensitivity. This has been interpreted as evidence that a substantial proportion of cryptogenic cells are sensitive to the S-phase-specific agent ara-C and are therefore rapidly proliferating (50). It should be pointed out, however, that the cells which survive irradiation to form colonies are the most resistant ones. If one accepts the assumption that cells in late S-phase are the most radioresistant ones in the normal crypt population, then the survivors of the irradiation-only curve as well as those of the 0 h-pretreated curve must be cells in late S-phase. This means that some at least of the S-cell population must survive the combination of ara-C and irradiation. In any case, the tenfold drop in microcolony survival is more than would be expected if ara-C were merely killing S-phase cells since I_s in the normal crypt is only 33 percent. Killing all the S-phase cells would result in only a threefold decrease in microcolony survival from that of the irradiated controls, although this decrease would be greater if the drug were available within the cell for longer periods of time. This suggests that in addition to the independent toxicity of S-cells caused by ara-C alone, there is an interaction between ara-C and irradiation when given together which results in further cryptogenic cell kill.

Comparison of 12 h-pretreated and immediately-pretreated curves. Comparison between mice pretreated at 12 h and 0 h, on the exponential region of the curves reveals a difference of over 2 decades in microcolony survival. Since both groups of mice received ara-C and irradiation, the very large increase in microcolony survival after 12 h must be due to a modification of irradiation effect brought about by the difference in time between drug and irradiation. Figure 4.3.2 indicates that there was no appreciable mitotic activity by 12 h after ara-C, so an increase in multiplicity through division could not have contributed to the increased survival.

The results suggest that slightly more than a tenfold increase in microcolony survival could be explained on the basis of synchronisation of cells; a further decade increase could occur as a result of the observed increase in D_0. Since the D_0 increase required is in addition to the effects of radioresistance in late S-phase, the involvement of a mechanism other than induction of synchrony is suggested.

4.3.3.3 MICROCOLONY SURVIVAL, LABELLING INDEX AND CUMULATIVE MITOTIC INDEX AFTER HYDROXYUREA

Experiments were done with HU to establish whether the effect on cryptogenic cells of this drug was similar to that produced by ara-C. If the two drugs produced the same correlation between microcolony survival and labelling index in terms of timing and magnitude it would be evidence that the ara-C-induced phenomenon was not unique.

To determine microcolony survival when the time between HU and irradiation was varied, mice were given 900 mg per kg intraperitoneally between 0 and 24 h before an assay dose of 1400 rad. The results are shown in Figure 4.3.4. When the drug was given within 5 min of irradiation, there was a

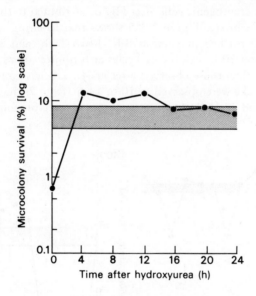

Figure 4.3.4 Microcolony survival after an assay dose of 1400 rad given at various times after administering 900 mg/kg hydroxyurea intraperitoneally. The shaded area represents approximate 95% confidence limits for microcolony survival in the absence of hydroxyurea

smaller microcolony survival (0.75 percent) than when 1400 rad alone was given (7.5 percent). As the time interval increased between HU and irradiation, microcolony survival rapidly rose to a maximum figure of 16 percent at 4 h, but this survival was only slightly above the irradiated control level, and it gradually decreased to that level by 16 h. These results are similar to those for ara-C in that there was an initial fall in microcolony survival when mice were irradiated immediately after HU, and that microcolony survival rose rapidly to exceed the irradiated control level by 4 h after HU. However, the remaining pattern of microcolony survival after HU was different from that obtained for ara-C. Not only was the rise in microcolony survival less, but there was no change in radiosensitivity with phase of the cell cycle. Radiosensitivity changes may not have been observed because the 4 h time intervals between points were not frequent enough. These differences in microcolony survival between ara-C-pretreated and HU-pretreated mice are not due to the different size of assay dose used. Figure 4.3.3 shows that if ara-C had been assessed using 1400 rad (as was HU) the differences between minimum survival at 0 h and maximum survival at 12 h would have been even greater than that shown in Figure 4.3.1 with an assay dose of 1300 rad. Nor can the lack of variation in radiosensitivity of cryptogenic cells after HU be attributed to the failure of this drug to induce synchrony. Figure 4.3.5 shows that labelling was resumed by 4 h after HU and reached maxima at 8 h, 14 to 18 h, and 24 h, with two minima at 12 h and 20 h, exhibiting cycles at 8 h intervals which were much more pronounced than those observed after ara-C. Likewise mitoses were first seen at 8 h and peaks were observed at 10 to 14 h, 18 to 20 h, and 24 h, with minima at 16 h and 22 h. Again the troughs were more pronounced than after ara-C.

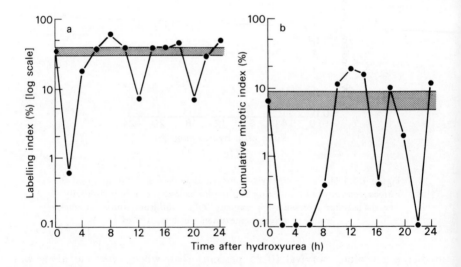

Figure 4.3.5 (a) Labelling and (b) cumulative mitotic indices at various times after intraperitoneal administration of 900 mg/kg hydroxyurea. Shaded areas represent approximate 95% confidence limits for the values in control animals

4.3.3.4 MICROCOLONY IRRADIATION DOSE-RESPONSE CURVES AFTER HYDROXYUREA

Figure 4.3.6 shows dose-response curves obtained after graded doses of irradiation for normal animals and for mice irradiated immediately after HU (0 h). The comparable microcolony survival curve 0 h after ara-C is shown for comparison. Irradiation immediately after HU results in a fall of microcolony

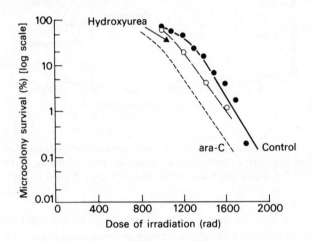

Figure 4.3.6 Microcolony irradiation-dose-response curves for control mice and mice pretreated immediately before with 900 mg/kg hydroxyurea. The corresponding curve for 200 mg/kg ara-C is also shown

survival which is again consistent with killing of potential cryptogenic cells in the absence of a change in radiosensitivity. But the toxicity of HU under the experimental conditions is only half of that observed for ara-C. One possible explanation for this difference is that the HU microcolony curve may represent only the killing of cryptogenic cells which were in S at the time of drug administration.

4.3.3.5 MICROCOLONY IRRADIATION DOSE-RESPONSE CURVES AFTER VINCRISTINE OR COLCEMID

Both of the S-phase-specific agents investigated have revealed a toxicity to cells which is consistent with the rapid proliferation of a significant proportion of cryptogenic cells, in which case other cycle-specific agents should reveal similar toxicities. Two metaphase arresting agents, vincristine and colcemid, were given at 3-hourly intervals over a period of 12 h. This schedule should be

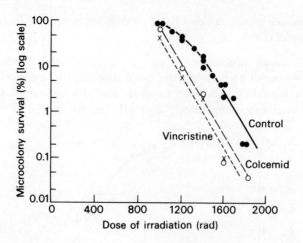

Figure 4.3.7 Microcolony irradiation-dose-response curves for control mice and mice irradiated immediately after the last injection of 1 mg/kg colcemid or 0.6 mg/kg vincristine intraperitoneally every 3 h for 12 h

sufficient to arrest all cells in mitosis for the duration of one cell cycle time. At the end of this time mice were given a range of irradiation doses; the results are shown in Figure 4.3.7. In combination with either colcemid or vincristine irradiation produced a tenfold decrease in cryptogenic cell survival compared to that observed with irradiation alone. This toxicity was equivalent to that produced by ara-C and irradiation. Only about 10 percent of cells which survived irradiation alone were able to survive the combination of irradiation with vincristine or colcemid. It may be that this 10 percent represents the proportion of cryptogenic cells which are not subject to metaphase arrest and are therefore slowly-proliferating.

4.3.3.6 REGENERATION OF CRYPT CELLS AFTER 1000 RAD γ-IRRADIATION

The regeneration of crypt cells after a test dose of 1000 rad was investigated by determining the cumulative mitotic index of crypts up to 24 h after irradiation. The results are shown in Figure 4.3.8. The crypt cells of mice pretreated with ara-C resumed mitosis 4 to 5 h earlier than the crypt cells of mice not so pretreated. The resumption of mitosis, which was quite sudden for both pretreated and irradiated controls, is consistent with a sudden removal of a premitotic block. There was a greater proportion of arrested mitoses (14 percent at its highest) in pretreated mice than in irradiated control mice (3 percent). This is to be expected since pretreated cells were partially synchronised by ara-C

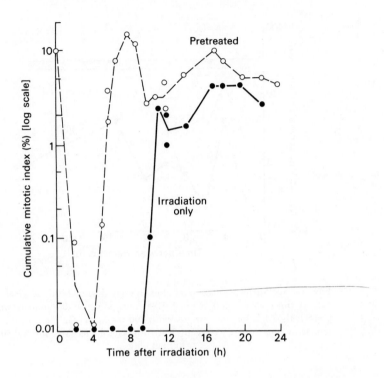

Figure 4.3.8 Cumulative mitotic index at various times after a test dose of 1000 rad. Some of the animals were pretreated 12 h before the test dose with 200 mg/kg ara-C

into a cohort of cells in late S-phase at the time of irradiation and then were further synchronised by the irradiation itself, which presumably spared cells in late S. The earlier resumption of mitosis in pretreated cells is discussed later (see Section 4.3.4).

4.3.3.7 REGENERATION OF CRYPTOGENIC CELLS AFTER 1000 RAD γ-IRRADIATION

Figure 4.3.9 shows the microcolony survival when cryptogenic cells were assayed at times up to 24 h after 1000 rad, using an assay dose of 1300 rad. The times correspond to the determinations of the cumulative mitotic index of crypts. If the cryptogenic cells follow the pattern of the crypt as a whole, differences in the age distribution of crypt cells should be reflected as cyclic changes in microcolony survival of cryptogenic cells. Pretreated mice had higher microcolony survival at most times, and both sets of mice exhibited

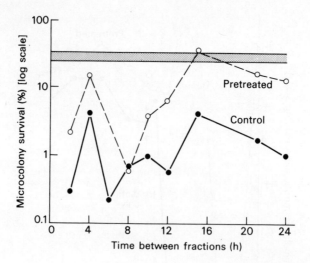

Figure 4.3.9 Microcolony survival after an assay dose of 1300 rad given at various times after a test dose of 1000 rad. Some of the animals were pretreated 12 h before the test dose with 200 mg/kg ara-C. The shaded area represents approximate 95% confidence limits for microcolony survival after 1300 rad only

cyclic changes in microcolony survival, which was lowest for pretreated mice at 8 h after 1000 rad, corresponding to the appearance of pretreated cells in the radiosensitive mitotic phase. Likewise, microcolony survival was highest at 4 and 15 h after 1000 rad, when cells are expected to be in S-phase. Until 4 h cells are presumed to be in S because they have not yet moved out of the radioresistant phase in which they were irradiated. The rise in microcolony survival between 2 and 4 h after 1000 rad probably represents repair of sublethal damage (201) which is complete in intestinal cells by 4 h after irradiation (808). The rise in microcolony survival after 8 h could be the result of an increase in the number of cryptogenic cells due to division, combined with movement of these cells into the radioresistant S-phase at the time the assay dose was given. Both pretreated and irradiated control mice exhibit cyclic changes in microcolony survival, which are probably related to the differences in age distribution observed for crypt cells.

Figure 4.3.10 shows the results of an experiment in which microcolony survival was assayed up to 7 days after 1000 rad to determine whether recovery of cryptogenic cells occurs more quickly in pretreated mice than irradiated controls. Once again the assay dose was 1300 rad, but in this case it was necessary to give 2×10^7 bone marrow cells per mouse intravenously after the

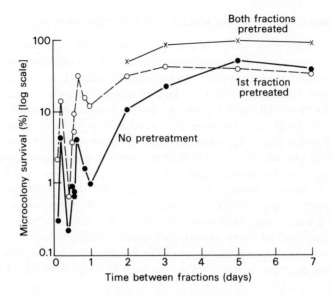

Figure 4.3.10 Microcolony survival after an assay dose of 1300 rad given at various times after a test dose of 1000 rad. Some of the animals were pretreated 12 h before the 1000 rad dose, and some 12 h before each dose, with 200 mg/kg ara-C

test dose of irradiation to allow survival of the mice throughout the experiment. The cyclic changes in crypt cell proliferation following irradiation and ara-C-induced synchrony are reflected by cyclic patterns of microcolony survival during the first 24 h. The rise in microcolony survival between 1 and 3 days after 1000 rad reflects the rate of regeneration of cryptogenic cells at these times after irradiation. There was no evidence to suggest that regeneration of cryptogenic cells occurred faster in pretreated mice; in fact, the slope of the curve is steeper between 1 and 3 days in irradiated control mice. Pretreated mice began with a higher initial cryptogenic cell population, however, since they were protected against a large amount of the 1000 rad test dose. For this reason the data may not accurately indicate the potential rate of regeneration of which pretreated cryptogenic cells are capable. For comparison, survival observed with a time interval of from 2 to 7 days, when both the 1000 rad test dose and the 1300 rad assay dose were preceded by ara-C, has been included (523). It is clear that pretreatment of both fractions resulted in the most rapid and complete intestinal cryptogenic cell recovery of the three regimens used.

4.3.3.8 ANIMAL SURVIVAL SIX WEEKS AFTER WHOLE-BODY IRRADIATION

Animal survival curves were obtained at 6 weeks after irradiation to show whether radioprotection of cryptogenic cells by ara-C pretreatment at 12 h also leads to improved animal survival in whole-body irradiated mice. 'Gut' death is widely accepted to occur within 5 days of irradiation, whilst 'bonemarrow' death occurs from 10 to 14 days or later. Previous experience indicates, however, that the division between 'gut' death and 'bone marrow' death is not clear-cut. For this reason the effects of three different treatments were assessed for improving animal survival: the first consisted of ara-C pretreatment 12 h before irradiation; the second, bone marrow reconstitution using 2×10^7 cells per mouse to prevent bone-marrow failure; and the third, administration of 350 mg neomycin per 100 ml drinking water for the duration of one week before and 2 weeks after irradiation. Neomycin is a non-absorbable antibiotic and this schedule of administration largely prevents endotoxic shock caused by the Gram-negative bacteria of the gut (755). Figure 4.3.11 indicates that bone marrow reconstitution is sufficient on its own to prevent much of the 'gut'

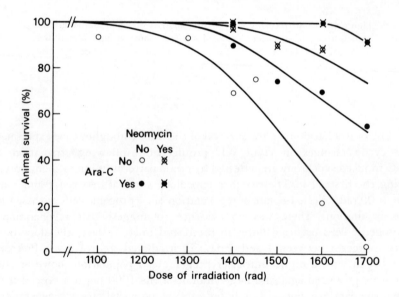

Figure 4.3.11 Animal survival irradiation-dose-response curves 6 weeks after whole body irradiation. Animals were given various combinations of ara-C, neomycin and bone-marrow treatment (see text). Results are shown only for those receiving bone-marrow transplants, as survival without bone marrow was virtually zero even at low doses of irradiation

death that would normally occur after doses greater than 1100 rad. Neither neomycin nor ara-C pretreatment alone were effective in preventing death at doses in excess of 1100 rad. When combined with bone-marrow reconstitution, however, it can be seen that ara-C pretreatment and neomycin treatment resulted in higher animal survival than bone marrow alone. The most effective schedule combined all three treatments and permitted survival of 90 percent of mice even at 1700 rad. Many of these mice survived to 6 months post-irradiation. Since 12 h ara-C pretreatment enhanced whole animal survival in these circumstances we conclude that increased cryptogenic cell survival leads to improved animal survival. This has also been shown by others (15, 337, 808), but the effect of compromising bone marrow was not considered in their reports. Our data show that endotoxic shock, insufficient numbers of cryptogenic cells, and compromised bone marrow all play a role in causing death after intestinal irradiation damage.

4.3.4 DISCUSSION

This paper is concerned with the mechanism and consequences of induction of radioresistance in cryptogenic cells after ara-C administration. Examination has also been made of the effects of HU, vincristine and colcemid. It seems clear that ara-C 'protection' is partly related to synchronisation of stem cells into a radioresistant cohort as a result of the G_1 to S block induced by this S-phase-specific agent. When the block is removed, cells continue to cycle in a partially synchronous fashion, and if they are irradiated in a radioresistant phase of the cell cycle this will lead to enhanced microcolony survival. It has been well documented that many single cells in vitro are most radioresistant in the S-phase, particularly in late S (784), and are most radiosensitive in G_2 and mitosis. The data in Figure 4.3.1 and 4.3.2 confirm that the characteristics exhibited by cryptogenic cells are probably similar to these reported for single cells in vitro. After ara-C a strong correlation was observed between micro-colony radiosensitivity and cell-cycle age of crypt cells in all experiments undertaken. This correlation is also shown in Figure 4.3.8 and 4.3.9 after the cyclic patterns of cryptogenic cells and mitosis were shifted in time by a test dose of 1000 rad.

Despite the higher microcolony survival which resulted when crypt cells were irradiated in the S-phase, it was shown that synchronisation of cells into the S-phase could not fully account for the tenfold rise in microcolony survival exhibited by 12 h pretreated mice; this would be expected to result in no more than a 1.5-fold increase in microcolony survival compared with irradiated controls. The remainder of the protective effect can be explained either by the D_0 increase observed, or, if this was an artifact, by an increase in capacity to repair sublethal damage. Some alternative is required in addition to the effects of radioresistance in late S-phase, however, to account for the size of change observed, and so the involvement of a mechanism other than induction of synchrony is suggested.

There was no evidence of HU-induced radioresistance comparable to that observed after ara-C, despite the apparent induction of synchrony by this drug. This is further evidence that much of the high microcolony survival seen 12 h after ara-C is unrelated to cell-cycle synchrony; the cyclic pattern may simply be superimposed upon an elevation of microcolony survival resulting from the non-cycle-related mechanism.

All the data obtained support the conclusion that quite a large proportion of the crypt population is cryptogenic, and that many of these cryptogenic cells are rapidly cycling. Figure 4.3.6 showed that only 50 percent of cryptogenic cells which survived irradiation alone were able to survive when HU was given immediately before irradiation; if ara-C was given immediately before irradiation cryptogenic cell survival dropped to 10 percent of the irradiated control level. When vincristine or colcemid was given over a period of 12 h before irradiation, cryptogenic cell survival was again only 10 percent of the irradiated control level. These experiments all suggest that the cryptogenic cell population is sensitive to phase-specific agents. Strong correlation has been demonstrated between radiosensitivity of cryptogenic cells and cycle-phase of the overall crypt population in ara-C-pretreated mice and in mice receiving ara-C or 1000 rad or both as a pretreatment.

Figure 4.3.8 showed that after a test dose of 1000 rad, mice treated with ara-C 12 h previously resumed mitosis 5 h earlier than did mice receiving 1000 rad only. The earlier entry into mitosis of crypt cells in pretreated mice could be due to an earlier removal of a G_2 to M block or, if pretreatment caused a shortening of cell cycle time, it could be due to faster movement of cells from S-phase into mitosis. If pretreated cryptogenic cells moved out of S more quickly due to a shorter cell cycle time, Figure 4.3.9 would have indicated an earlier drop in microcolony survival as pretreated cells moved into the radiosensitive G_2 and mitosis; this was not observed. If, on the other hand, both pretreated and irradiated control cells did not differ significantly in the rate of movement out of S, but a G_2 to M block was removed earlier from pretreated cells, one would expect little difference between pretreated and irradiated control microcolony survival curves. The comparative differences in radiosensitivities between pretreated cells in mitosis and irradiated control cells in G_2 would probably not be distinguishable since both of these phases are very radiosensitive. The sharp rises in mitosis for both curves in Figure 4.3.8 are consistent with the sudden removal of a mitotic block from G_2 cells poised for entry into mitosis. The experimental points determined at 6 to 12 h in Figure 4.3.9 did not permit precise fitting of the microcolony survival curve at these times; even so, the data are consistent with the interpretation that the shorter mitotic delay for 12 h-pretreated cryptogenic cells is caused by an earlier release from a G_2 to M block.

Investigation of animal survival showed that the occurrence of 'gut' death 5 to 7 days after whole-body irradiation could be prevented by combinations of bone-marrow reconstitution, administration of neomycin, and pretreatment with ara-C 12 h before irradiation. It is apparent therefore that bone marrow, endotoxins, and the number of surviving cryptogenic cells all play a role in irradiation 'gut' death.

4.3.5 SUMMARY

The effects of a single injection of cytosine arabinoside or hyroxyurea on crypt cell proliferation and cryptogenic cell radiosensitivity have been assessed. Labelling and mitotic indices indicate that synchrony was induced in crypt cells after administration of either of these S-phase-specific drugs. Only cytosine arabinoside produced a pattern of cryptogenic cell survival which corresponded to the presence of cells in S-phase. The magnitude of the radioresistance induced maximally 12 h after cytosine arabinoside was greater than that which could be accounted for by synchronisation of cells into a radioresistant late S cohort. Irradiation of crypts immediately following a 12 h period of mitotic arrest from vincristine or colcemid revealed a marked toxicity to cryptogenic cells compared with the irradiated controls. Toxicity was also observed when crypts were irradiated immediately after a single injection of cytosine arabinoside or hydroxyurea. These findings are consistent with the hypothesis that a large proportion of cryptogenic cells are sensitive to cycle-specific cytotoxic agents, and therefore are rapidly cycling. Animal survival experiments show that 12 h pretreatment with cytosine arabinoside also improved animal survival after whole body irradiation, and that bone marrow, endo-toxins, and intestinal cell survival all play a role in the prevention of 'gut' death.

ACKNOWLEDGEMENTS

I would like to gratefully acknowledge the technical assistance of Mrs Ann Pearson and Miss Sue Clinton, and the helpful discussions and advice of Dr N M Blackett. This work was partially supported by NCI grant No. 5 RO1 CA20519-03.

4.4 Relative Importance of Luminal and Systemic Factors in the Control of Intestinal Adaptation

Robin C N Williamson and Ronald A Malt

4.4.1 INTRODUCTION

The cell turnover of small-bowel mucosa exceeds that of any other healthy organ (400). Under steady-state conditions in the adult, the precise balance between the production of epithelial cells in the crypt and their extrusion from the villous tip may be maintained by an intrinsic feedback mechanism of control (793) (see Section 2). This kinetic equilibrium can be perturbed by several stimuli including surgical shortening of the gut. Following partial enterectomy more rapid replication and migration of crypt cells results; there is evidence that increased numbers of immature enterocytes populate the villus (179, 783).

Cells lining the alimentary canal are ideally placed for exposure both to substances present in the intestinal lumen and to those delivered by the bloodstream. Falling intraluminal concentrations of nutrients could readily explain the decrease in villous height normally seen between pylorus and ileocaecal valve, and the reversal of this gradient after ileo-jejunal transposition (21, 582). The small bowel and colon are peculiarly sensitive to decreased oral intake of food (18, 281, 511, 792), and adaptation to the loss of functioning small bowel is reduced or even abolished by total parenteral nutrition (215, 221, 419). Since fasting profoundly affects the secretory and hormonal output of the gut, food might also influence mucosal cell proliferation by indirect pathways. Bile, pancreatic juice and several different hormones have been implicated as tropic agents for enteric mucosa, ie, as exerting a stimulatory or permissive effect (17, 352, 782, 793).

The rapidity of onset of changes in the adapting gut (297, 298, 501, 502, 511) has facilitated our studies of the regulatory mechanisms described in the present review. Increased contents of RNA and DNA are detectable in ileal mucosa within two days of jejunal resection, while intestinal transection alone has a short-lived effect on the distal bowel. The initial response to proximal resection is greater than that obtained merely by delivering upper alimentary contents direct to the ileum. This response, together with data from cross-circulation studies and evidence of adaptation both proximal to the site of resection and in isolated intestine, supports the contention that systemic factors have an appreciable role in the control of intestinal adaptation.

4.4.2 MATERIALS AND METHODS

4.4.2.1 EXPERIMENTAL TECHNIQUES

Male Sprague-Dawley rats weighing between 170 and 250 g were used throughout. Animals were housed in groups of 4 to 6 in hanging cages with wire-mesh bottoms. Quarters were lit in alternate 12 h cycles. Rats received standard chow ad lib, except that food (but not water) was withdrawn overnight after operation. All operations were carried out between 0800 h and 1300 h. Light anaesthesia was produced with diethyl ether. The small bowel was measured from the ligament of Treitz to the ileocaecal valve by gently stretching against a ruler. The length of the entire jejunum and ileum so measured ranged from 90 to 100 cm. Intestinal anastomoses were fashioned using a single continuous layer of 6/0 silk sutures.

Rats were killed by cervical dislocation at varying postoperative intervals. One hour before death each animal received a subcutaneous injection of 50 μCi of tritiated thymidine (^{3}HTdR) of specific activity 6.7 Ci per mole. Immediately after death the intestines were excised, gently flushed with ice-cold saline solution and spread on a glass plate resting on crushed ice. Appropriate segments of small bowel were cut, opened longitudinally and gently stretched to an exact 5 cm length from which the mucosa was scraped between 2 glass slides. Specimens were frozen in liquid nitrogen within 5 to 10 min of death and were stored at $-70\,^\circ$C for later chemical analysis. Histological examination of the scraped muscularis revealed very few crypts left behind by this method, and no lymph follicles were removed. In certain experiments the internal circumference of the small bowel was measured with a ruler, and additional specimens of small bowel were fixed in 10 percent formalin for subsequent preparation of 5 μm-thick histological sections for morphometric estimations.

Amounts of RNA and DNA in thawed, homogenised mucosal samples were estimated (327, 636). Aliquots of the DNA fraction were counted by liquid scintillation spectrometry at 25 percent efficiency corrected by internal standardisation. The specific activity of DNA (total radioactivity divided by DNA content) thus represents the intensity of cell proliferation during the hour between labelling and death. Histological slides were coded to eliminate observer bias, and the lengths of 10 properly orientated villi and crypts were measured per slide, using an ocular micrometer.

Statistical significance was assessed by Student's t-test for paired or unpaired data as appropriate.

4.4.2.2 JEJUNAL TRANSECTION AND RESECTION

Fifty-five rats were randomised to receive either no operation (*controls*), laparotomy with delivery and handling of the small bowel (*sham controls*), *transection* and suturing of the jejunum just distal to the ligament of Treitz, or *resection* of the proximal one third (30 cm) of the combined jejunum and ileum with immediate anastomosis. Animals were killed 48 h after operation. Two contiguous 5-cm segments were cut from the centres of the middle and distal thirds of the small bowel for 'duplicate' assays of mucosal RNA and DNA. Mean values from contiguous specimens were used for comparisons between groups.

4.4.2.3 CROSS-CIRCULATION

Two hundred rats were matched in pairs by weight to within 10 g and were joined in free-running vascular parabiosis. Vascular parabiosis was established from the carotid artery of one parabiont through the jugular vein of its partner, and rats were securely sutured together from elbow to knee (481, 800). Each couple was able to move freely about the cage without restraint, to eat and to drink.

Control pairs (C-C) had no abdominal operation. In *transection* pairs (T-XT), 1 rat (T) undergoing jejunal transection was cross-circulated with a partner (XT) having an intact abdomen. Similarly in *resection* pairs (R-XR), 1 parabiont (R) undergoing jejunal resection was linked to a partner (XR) without laparotomy. Intestinal operations were performed as before. Cannulation and anticoagulation with heparin (35 u) were carried out before abdominal surgery, and a booster dose of heparin (40 u) was administered by subcutaneous injection after 24 h. Parabiotic pairs were separated at 47 h. Rats were individually labelled and killed, and specimens were taken as before.

4.4.2.4 RESECTION, BYPASS, PANCREATOBILIARY DIVERSION

One hundred and eighty-one rats were allocated to one of 4 operative groups (Figure 4.4.1). Jejunal *transection* was performed as a control operation. *Pancreatobiliary diversion* (PBD) was carried out by isolating a duodenal segment containing the papilla and restoring duodenal continuity by end-to-end anastomosis; the upper end of the papillary segment was then closed and invaginated and the other end was anastomosed end-to-side to the ileum, midway between the ligament of Treitz and the ileocaecal valve. *Bypass* of the

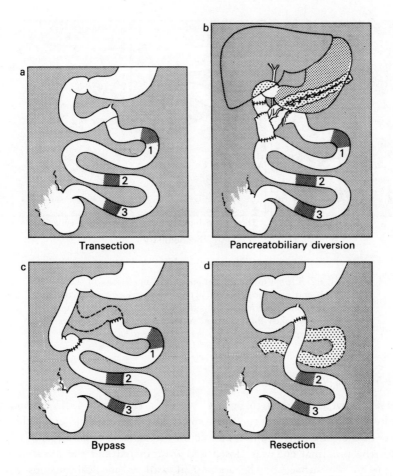

Figure 4.4.1 Schematic trepresentations of the operations of jejunal transection, pancreatobiliary diversion, 50% proximal small bowel bypass, and 50% proximal small bowel resection. Specimens were taken from (1) jejunum, (2) upper ileum and (3) lower ileum for biochemical analysis

proximal half of the small bowel was achieved by end-to-side jejunoileal anastomosis, leaving a long blind loop. *Resection* of the proximal half of the small bowel was followed by direct end-to-end anastomosis. Each animal received a subcutaneous injection of 4 ml of 0.9 percent saline solution at the end of the operation. Rats were killed 2, 7 and 30 days after operation. Mucosal scrapings for biochemical analysis were obtained from 5-cm segments cut from the centres of the first, third and fourth quarters of the combined jejunum and ileum. Adjacent specimens of jejunum and upper ileum were taken for histological measurements.

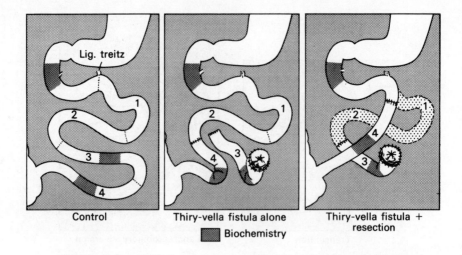

Control   Thiry-vella fistula alone   Thiry-vella fistula +
resection

■ Biochemistry

Figure 4.4.2 Schematic representation of the operations of Thiry-Vella fistula with and without resection. The fistula was created in the third enteric quarter, and resection, when performed, was of the first two quarters. Specimens were taken from duodenum, upper ileum (third quarter) and lower ileum (fourth quarter) for biochemical analysis

4.4.2.5 THIRY-VELLA FISTULAE

Ninety rats were assigned to one of 3 groups (Figure 4.4.2). *Controls* had laparotomy with handling of the entire small bowel. In a second group the third quarter of the combined jejunum and ileum was isolated as a *Thiry-Vella fistula* (TVF); the proximal end was closed and invaginated and the distal end was brought to the surface of the abdominal wall as an ileal mucous fistula. Intestinal continuity was restored by end-to-end anastomosis. In the third group, *TVF + resection*, creation of an identical TVF was accompanied by resection of the first and second quarters of jejunoileum. Rats were killed 2 and 7 days after operation. Mucosal scrapings were obtained from 5-cm segments of bowel cut from the centres of the duodenum, third quarter (upper ileum) and fourth quarter (lower ileum) of jejunoileum.

4.4.3 RESULTS

4.4.3.1 JEJUNAL TRANSECTION AND RESECTION (800)

Ninety-five per cent of the animals remained in good condition 48 h postoperatively. At this time controls had surpassed their initial body weight by 3.7 percent, while the other 3 groups remained between 0.5 and 3.3 percent below starting weight (p < 0.001). Weight loss was greatest in rats with jejunal resection.

The reproducibility of both the sampling technique and the biochemical assay was tested by comparing nucleic acid contents obtained from contiguous specimens of mid and distal bowel. The coefficients of variation were 3.6 percent for RNA and 4.9 percent for DNA. The true analytic error may actually have been lower because of the decreasing gradient of mucosal mass through the small bowel (18, 21).

The biochemical results in mid and distal bowel are summarised in Table 4.4.1. Mean RNA contents in controls and sham controls ranged from 2.00

Table 4.4.1 Nucleic acid contents, total radioactivity and specific activity of DNA per 5 cm mucosa in mid and distal small bowel 48 h after operation. Values significantly different from controls are indicated by *(p < 0.05), **(p < 0.01), or ***(p < 0.001). All variables show significant differences between transection and resection except DNA in the distal bowel

Location	Operation	Number of rats	RNA (mg)	DNA (mg)	Total radioactivity (dpm × 10⁻³)	DNA-specific activity (dpm × 10⁻³)
Mid small bowel	Control	12	2.25	1.69	174	104
	Sham	13	2.19	1.81	150	84*
	Transection	13	2.39	2.21***	166	78**
	Resection	14	3.31***	2.56***	336***	131*
Distal small bowel	Control	12	2.00	1.72	191	112
	Sham	13	2.22	1.96*	176	91
	Transection	13	2.20	2.16***	196	94
	Resection	14	2.54***	2.21***	297***	138*

and 2.19 mg per 5-cm mucosa and DNA contents from 1.60 to 1.96 mg, with virtually no differences between the two groups. Transection did not significantly alter the amount of RNA, but it did increase DNA content in both mid and distal bowel. Resection caused significantly greater increments than transection in RNA and DNA in mid bowel, and in RNA alone in distal bowel.

The mean total radioactivity incorporated into DNA of controls, sham controls, and rats with transection ranged from 150 to 196 × 10³ dpm per 5 cm mucosa, with no significant differences between the 3 groups. Radioactivity was substantially higher after resection than after any other treatment. The 25 percent reduction in DNA-specific activity of mid bowel after transection reflects dilution of the radioactive DNA by a greater amount of preformed DNA; since cell proliferation at 48 h is not increased, the hyperplasia following transection appears to be a temporary phenomenon. By contrast, specific activity 48 h after resection was increased despite a substantially higher DNA content, indicating persistent hyperplasia.

4.4.3.2 CROSS-CIRCULATION (800)

About a third of parabiotic couples in which satisfactory flow was obtained at the outset survived with patent cannulae for 48 h. Mean weight loss was between 6 and 14 percent in the 3 operative groups, being greatest in both members of resection pairs (p <0.01). Amounts of RNA and DNA in cross-circulated controls varied from 1.30 to 1.60 mg per 5 cm mucosa, and there were corresponding reductions in nucleic acids in transection and resection pairs, when compared with values obtained in individual animals. Nevertheless, in animals actually having abdominal operations (T,R), values were significantly higher than control values for RNA, DNA, total radioactivity and DNA-specific radioactivity in mid bowel, and also for total radioactivity and DNA-specific radioactivity in the distal bowel (Table 4.4.2).

Table 4.4.2 Nucleic acid contents, total radioactivity and specific activity of DNA per 5-cm mucosa in mid and distal small bowel 48 h after operation. In the parabiotic pairs T had jejunal transection and XT was the partner not undergoing transection; R had jejunal resection and XR was the partner not undergoing resection. Values significantly different from control pairs are indicated as in Table 4.4.1

Location	Operation	Number of rats	RNA (mg)	DNA (mg)	Total radioactivity (dpm × 10^{-3})	DNA-specific activity (dpm × 10^{-3})
	Control	10	1.30	1.39	103	74
	T	9	1.92**	1.76*	213**	120**
Mid small	XT	9	1.50	1.45	187**	134**
bowel	R	10	1.92***	2.09***	252***	123***
	XR	10	1.27	1.58	184**	117*
	Control	10	1.40	1.61	122	76
	T	9	1.83**	1.83	220**	122**
Distal small	XT	9	1.48	1.25*	208*	173**
bowel	R	10	1.45	1.70	195***	119**
	XR	10	1.28	1.42	175*	135**

The differences between transection and resection found in individual animals did not occur under vascular parabiosis, perhaps because of delayed adaptation due to stress.

The responding partners with intact abdomens (XT, XR) linked to parabionts with jejunal transection or resection showed no increase over control values for RNA or DNA. But in groups XT and XR, both total radioactivity and specific activity of DNA were substantially increased. A comparison of paired data between parabiotic partners showed that nucleic acid values were nearly always significantly higher in rats actually having abdominal surgery than in the intact partner; the direct response therefore exceeded the transmitted response.

4.4.3.3 RESECTION, BYPASS, PANCREATOBILIARY DIVERSION (795)

Yields of healthy survivors in the four operative groups varied from 74 to 90 percent at the time of death. Pancreatobiliary diversion (PBD) entailed the longest operation and caused the highest immediate weight loss and mortality rate. The gains in body weight were similar after all four operations, except that transection controls remained slightly heavier throughout, and rats with bypass weighed least at 30 days (91 percent of controls).

Throughout the intestinal tract in transection controls there was a gradual increase with age in the amounts of RNA and DNA, and in villous height and crypt depth; there was a corresponding reduction in DNA-specific activity, as proliferating cells were 'diluted' with greater numbers of mature enterocytes. In bypassed jejunum (Figure 4.4.3) this trend was reversed. Decreased amounts of RNA and DNA were detected after 48 h of intestinal exclusion, and by 30 days

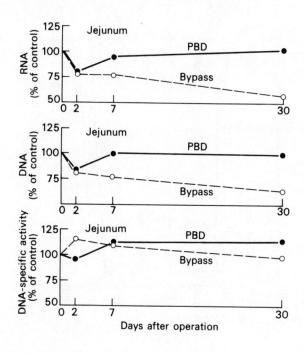

Figure 4.4.3 Nucleic acid content and DNA-specific activity of the jejunum 2, 7 and 30 days after pancreatobiliary diversion (PBD) or proximal enteric bypass. Results are expressed as percentages of values in transection controls. Mean values were obtained from between 11 and 13 rats per group using 5-cm samples of mucosa

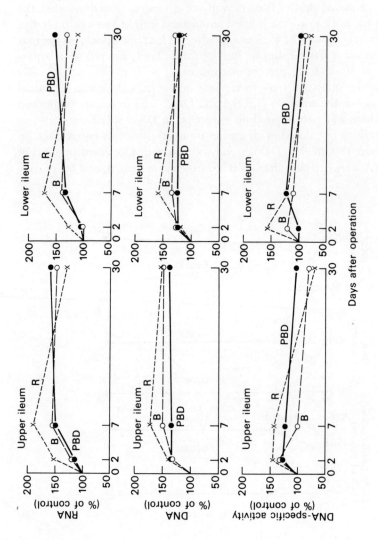

Figure 4.4.4 Nucleic acid content and DNA-specific activity of the upper and lower ileum 2, 7 and 30 days after pancreatobiliary diversion (PBD), proximal enteric bypass (B), or resection (R). Results are expressed as percentages of values in transected controls. Mean values were obtained from between 11 and 14 rats per group using 5-cm samples of mucosa

values relative to transection controls (including internal circumference) were even lower. There was a 14 percent reduction in villous height at this time (p < 0.05), but crypt depth and DNA-specific activity were unaltered. A normal proportion of epithelial cells thus appears to proliferate in atrophic intestinal mucosa.

Diversion of pancreatobiliary secretions from the jejunum caused transient but significant reductions in levels of RNA and DNA at 48 h which promptly recovered by 1 week and may simply have reflected the postoperative weight loss in these animals.

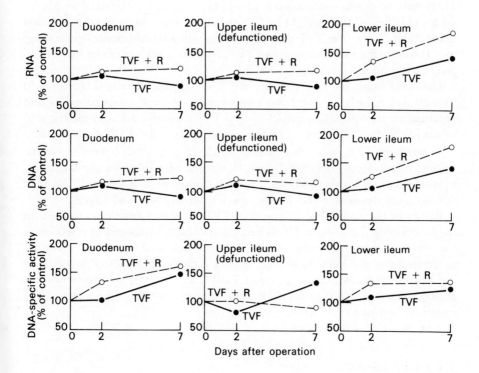

Figure 4.4.5 Nucleic acid content and DNA-specific activity of the duodenum and upper and lower ileum 2 and 7 days after creation of a Thiry-Vella fistula, either alone (TVF) or accompanied by proximal small bowel resection (TVF + R). Results are expressed as percentages of control values. Mean values were obtained from between 8 and 13 rats per group using 5-cm samples of mucosa

In the upper and lower ileum (Figure 4.4.4), resection, bypass and PBD were all followed by increased quantities of RNA and DNA 48 h postoperatively, and these increments persisted throughout the experiment. Resection caused the greatest rise in every variable at 2 and 7 days, including internal circumference, villous height and crypt depth (795). High specific activity at these times indicated the intensity of this early response to proximal enterectomy. By 30 days, however, values in animals with bypass or PBD equalled or exceeded those found after resection.

4.4.3.4 THIRY-VELLA FISTULAE (794)

There were no deaths in the control group; rats regained their initial weight by 48 h and increased their weight by 25 percent at 7 days. Body weight remained lower 2 and 7 days after TVF alone, and lower still after additional jejunectomy (p < 0.01). In the two groups with a TVF, 61 and 72 percent of rats survived in good condition until killed.

Duodenal values for RNA, DNA, and DNA-specific activity (Figure 4.4.5) were all significantly increased over control values at 2 and 7 days after TVF and proximal enterectomy. Creation of an ileal TVF alone did not alter nucleic acid values in the duodenum, but it increased specific activity of DNA at 1 week.

In rats with TVF alone, there was no evidence of mucosal hypoplasia in the isolated upper ileum even after 7 days. Compared with values in normal ileum, jejunal resection significantly raised 48 h contents of RNA and DNA in defunctioned ileum at 2 and 7 days; specific activity was unchanged.

Bypass of the upper ileum alone (as a TVF) increased nucleic acids levels in the functioning lower ileum by 40 percent at 7 days. Concomitant resection of the jejunum caused elevation of RNA and DNA at 2 days, and a further substantial rise at 7 days. Moreover, specific activity of DNA was increased by one third over control values at 2 and 7 days, and internal circumference was greatly increased after removal of three-quarters of the jejunoileum from intestinal continuity.

4.4.4 DISCUSSION

These studies provide cumulative evidence to support involvement of humoral substances in compensatory intestinal hyperplasia. Firstly, transient hyperplasia of the distal small bowel after simple division and repair of the jejunum seems more readily attributable to hormones than to alteration of luminal contents produced by the injury. The response to transection is dependent on the effects of laparotomy and intestinal manipulation. Secondly, the rapidity and uniformity of the enteric response to surgical stimuli shown in these and other experiments (297, 289, 501, 502, 511) are entirely consistent with a systemic mechanism of control.

A stimulatory hormone released by transection, and especially by resection, of bowel could explain increased uptake of thymidine in the enteric mucosa of parabionts with intact abdomens linked to partners with intestinal operations. Cross-circulated rats exchange at least 10 percent of their blood volume every minute (481); conflicting evidence from experiments using cutaneous parabiosis (365, 434, 714, 715) probably reflects inadequate intermingling of blood-streams in these preparations. Our data using vascular parabiosis are supported by a similar study in the pig (391). The validity of interpreting elevated specific activity of DNA (without alterations in DNA content) as an indication of early hyperplasia is considered in detail elsewhere (800). Stimulatory hormones might also account for the rapid hyperplasia found both in the duodenum, proximal to the site of jejunal resection, and to a more modest degree in the upper ileum, when isolated as a Thiry-Vella loop. Other reports confirm compensatory hyperplasia on both sides of a resected enteric segment (297, 298), in the ileum after colectomy (66, 811), in small bowel distal to the site of complete neonatal atresia (711, 722), in mucosal autografts (712) and in Thiry-Vella fistulae (299).

Inhibitory hormones might also contribute to the regulation of mucosal growth in the gut. Neither pancreatobiliary diversion nor jejunal bypass reproduces the intensity of cell proliferation seen during the first week after jejunal resection. Similarly, although bypass of the upper ileum (as a TVF) causes distal hyperplasia at 7 days, no changes are detectable at 2 days when post-resectional adaptation is generally present. These findings suggest the involvement of an extraluminal tropic factor in addition to food and alimentary secretions. Resection would immediately deplete levels of a hypothetical inhibitory hormone elaborated by functioning small-bowel mucosa, allowing regeneration of sufficient mass of tissue to restore original concentrations. Bypass, causing progressive mucosal hyperplasia, would produce a more gradual depletion of circulating inhibitor. The end result appears to be the same, but only resection seems to cause any compensatory growth in the colon (795). In the small bowel at least, post-resectional hyperplasia persists indefinitely (792).

Besides contributing to post-resectional hyperplasia, hormones seem likely to be among controlling elements in adaptive growth of the bowel during lactation, diabetes and hypothermia (793). No clearcut enterotropic hormone has been identified despite Loran's hypothesis of an 'intestinal epithelial growth hormone' transmissible between parabiotic rats (434, 435). Although gastrin exerts a tropic effect on the gastric fundus, duodenum and pancreas, and hypergastrinaemia occurs after small-bowel resection (352, 680), the evidence for a similar action on the remainder of the small bowel and colon is much less convincing (485, 793). In particular, we could demonstrate no differences in the degree of post-resectional hyperplasia or starvation-induced hypoplasia between rats with either gastric fundectomy or antrectomy, operations which alter serum gastrin levels by a factor of twenty (511). The combined administration of cholecystokinin and secretin has recently been shown to prevent the mucosal atrophy seen in dogs with total parental nutrition (341), but this observation may simply reflect increased pancreatobiliary secretion. Among other candidate hormones, enteroglucagon, anterior pituitary hormones, and mineralocorticoids may be tropic to the gut, whereas secretin, vasoactive intestinal polypeptide and glucocorticoids may conceivably be antitropic. The subject is reviewed in detail elsewhere (252, 793).

Although luminal factors cannot explain all aspects of the adaptive response, their dominant role in compensatory hyperplasia (179) is underlined by the experiments reviewed in this paper. The prompt, progressive and ultimately profound reduction in mucosal mass seen in bypassed jejunum has been confirmed by many other workers (792), though nucleic acid contents appear much more sensitive indices of reduced cell mass than morphological measurements. By contrast, defunctioned upper ileum shows no evidence of hypoplasia within a week of exclusion from the nutrient stream. Jejunum is more sensitive than ileum to the effects of either starvation or isolation as a TVF (18, 299). It is logical that the integrity of the jejunal mucosa should depend on the high nutrient concentrations to which it is usually exposed. In accordance with other investigators (17, 782), we have shown that pancreatobiliary secretions exert a strong tropic action on distal bowel mucosa. Pancreatic juice appears to have the more prolonged effect (796). The absence of pancreatobiliary secretions from the intestinal lumen diminishes compensatory hyperplasia but does not abolish it completely (642).

Intestinal adaptation seems to be maximal only when actions of topical and humoral agents coincide. Thus the response in functioning loops exceeds that in defunctioned loops, distal adaptation exceeds proximal adaptation, and hyperplasia is greater in parabionts actually receiving transection or resection than in partners with intact abdomens. The small bowels (and colons) probably undergo transitory hypoplasia during the first few hours after the stress of anaesthesia and surgery, with a burst or proliferative activity when feeding is resumed. Exogenous nutrients must affect the gut in part by indirect means, since isolated bowel remains sensitive to oral intake of food (115, 192) and ileal infusions of glucose stimulate jejunal growth (660). The presence of food in the bowel stimulates the release of hormones and endogenous secretions, both of which facilitate the digestion of that food and the production of monosaccharides and amino acids that may exert a direct trophic (ie, nutritive) influence on the intestinal epithelium.

4.4.5 SUMMARY

The mechanisms controlling intestinal adaptation have been studied by measuring nucleic acid contents, thymidine uptake and morphometric indices in rat small-bowel mucosa. Jejunal transection causes an ephemeral hyperplasia of the distal small bowel, as shown by ileal increments in DNA alone at 48 h. Greater elevations of RNA and DNA following jejunal resection at this time are accompanied by increased DNA-specific activity, adaptive hyperplasia is more intense and prolonged. Rats linked in free-running vascular parabiosis can transmit an agent that increases DNA-specific activity in the ileum of parabionts with intact abdomens that are cross-circulated with partners having jejunal transection or resection. Although distal diversion of pancreatobiliary secretions and proximal enteric bypass both cause prompt distal hyperplasia, the intensity of adaptive response is surpassed by that observed during the first week after enterectomy; this discrepancy disappears by 1 month. Jejunal resection causes limited hyperplasia both in the duodenum and in isolated loops of ileum (Thiry-Vella fistulae) after 2 to 7 days, but maximal changes occur in ileum remaining in continuity with the nutrient stream. The results argue strongly for an involvement of humoral factors in compensatory intestinal hyperplasia, and although the direct effect of food in the intestinal lumen remains a dominant influence, it may exert its tropic effect on the bowel in part by stimulating hormonal secretion.

ACKNOWLEDGEMENTS

The original work reviewed in this paper was supported by a grant (CA-17324) from the National Cancer Institute through the National Large Bowel Cancer Project and by the Shriners Burns Institute, Boston Unit. We are grateful to Dr F L R Bauer, Dr T W Buchholtz, Dr J E A Oscarson, Dr J S Ross and Mrs Rebecca Adjoyan for assistance. Original illustrations were kindly supplied by Mr G James, Medical Artist, and Miss Elizabeth Hurst, Superintendent Photographer, of the Department of Medical Illustration, Bristol Royal Infirmary, and we thank the Editor of the British Journal of Surgery for permission to use Figure 4.4.2.

4.5 The Effect of Oestrogens on Cell Population Kinetics in the Colonic Crypt of the Mouse

William W L Chang and Martin B Hoff

4.5.1 INTRODUCTION

Oestrogens are systemic modulators of cells proliferation, inducing in their target organs a growth-related response which involves the synthesis of RNA, protein and DNA (91, 262, 290). This response is initiated by interactions with cytosol receptors (91, 349, 719), and is eventually manifest by increases in DNA synthesis and mitotic activity, and by growth.

In some of the non-target organs, including the intestine, the cytosol receptors of oestrogens have not been identified. However, receptors have been demonstrated in other non-target organs such as pancreas (613), heart (683) and brain (468), and in cells such as fibroblasts (357) and eosinophils (704). The significance of the presence of oestrogen cytosol receptors in most of these non-target organs or cells is at present unclear.

On the other hand, specific oestrogen-binding sites have been demonstrated on the cell membrane of target organs (525) and these are lacking in epithelial cells of the intestine. However, neither the significance of the membrane receptors of oestrogen in relation to their specific action on the target cells nor the relationship between the membrane and cytosol receptors has been elucidated.

The mitotic activity of cells in many non-target organs, including various segments of the alimentary canal, has been shown to vary with the phases of the oestrous cycle in the mouse primarily due to the stimulatory effect of oestrogens (68, 69), and this view was confirmed in studies of corneal epithelium (207). By a double labelling technique, it has been demonstrated that the duration of the DNA-synthetic (S) phase and consequently the cell cycle time (T_c) became shortened in epithelial cells in four segments of intestine following oestrogen administration to ovariectomised mice (244), but neither the tritiated thymidine (^{3}HTdR)-labelling (I_s) nor the mitotic (I_m) index after oestrogen treatment was mentioned. In her review of the effects of hormones on the cell cycle, Epifanova (208) has concluded that oestrogens are mitogenic hormones in both the target and non-target organs, and that the differences between the target and non-target organs are quantitative.

Contrary to these findings, one of the most actively renewing, non-target tissues in the body shows quite a different response to oestrogens. Several investigators (130, 188, 753) have documented that oestrogens inhibit erythropoiesis in bone marrow and cause anaemia from hypoplasia of bone marrow. It has also been reported that oestrogen treatment has retarded general body growth (513).

In view of these conflicting data, we have investigated systematically the effect of oestrogens on cell proliferation and differentiation using the descending colon of the mouse as an example of a non-target organ (328, 329), because particularly detailed morphological and kinetic studies of various types of epithelial cells have been performed at this site (95, 98).

4.5.2 EXPERIMENTS AND RESULTS

4.5.2.1 THE EFFECT OF THE OESTROUS CYCLE ON THE COLONIC CRYPT

For the study of the effect of the oestrous cycle on the colonic crypt, smears prepared from vaginal lavages were examined daily in young adult virgin female CF-1 mice 12 weeks old. Animals which had had two or more regular oestrous cycles were killed either at early dioestrus, late dioestrus, pro-oestrus, oestrus, early metoestrus or late metoestrus, employing smear staging criteria (13). All the mice were killed, under ether anesthaesia, between 0900 h and 1100 h to avoid the effect of diurnal variation on intestinal epithelial cell proliferation (93). Each mouse received 1 μCi ^{3}HTdR per g body weight one hour before death. A segment of descending colon was excised and processed for Epon-embedding and autoradiography as described previously (95). The methods of analysis of autoradiographs have also been detailed (95, 98, 329).

In the distal colon of the mouse the crypt size, expressed as the average number of epithelial cells lining one side of the longitudinally sectioned crypt, was 35 cells, and showed a minimal fluctuation during the oestrous cycle. Maxima were reached during early dioestrus and oestrus, whereas minima were exhibited during late dioestrus and late metoestrus (Table 4.5.1).

There are three epithelial cell lines in the crypt of murine descending colon: vacuolated-columnar, mucous (goblet), and enteroendocrine (argentaffin) (95). Since enteroendocrine cells constitute only about 1 to 2 percent of the total epithelial cell population and rarely divide, studies were carried out only on the vacuolated-columnar and mucous cell lines.

In the vacuolated-columnar cell line, vacuolated cells are located in the lower two-thirds of the crypt where they proliferate; on migration to the upper part of

Table 4.5.1 Changes in the numbers and labelling indices of different types of cells per crypt column in the colon of mice at various phases of the oestrus cycle

	Early dioestrus		Late dioestrus		Pro-oestrus		Oestrus		Early metoestrus		Late metoestrus	
	Number	% of total	Number	% of total	Number	% of total	Number	% of total	Number	% of total	Number	% of total
Total	35.7		34.2		34.9		36.1		35.3		34.5	
Columnar	8.7	24	5.4	16	6.1	17	9.8	27	10.4	29	8.6	25
Vacuolated	19.5	55	22.9	67	21.9	64	19.6	55	20.3	58	18.7	54
Mucous	7.5	21	5.9	17	6.9	19	6.7	18	4.6	13	7.3	21
Labelled Total	3.0	8.3	2.8	8.2	3.2	9.2	3.6	9.6	2.8	7.6	3.2	9.1
vacuolated	2.6	7.3	2.5	7.2	2.8	8.3	3.1	8.3	2.6	7.1	2.7	7.7
mucous	0.4	1.0	0.3	1.0	0.3	1.0	0.5	1.3	0.2	0.6	0.5	1.4
I_s (vacuolated and columnar) (%)	9.1		8.8		10.2		10.2		8.0		9.6	
I_s (mucous) (%)	4.7		5.0		5.5		7.2		4.3		7.2	

the crypt they lose their vacuoles and become non-proliferating columnar cells (95). During the course of the oestrous cycle, the number of proliferating vacuolated cells and non-proliferating columnar cells per crypt column was found to fluctuate (Table 4.5.1). The size of the vacuolated cell population increased during dioestrus, reaching its maximum during late dioestrus when it comprised 67 percent of the epithelial cell population per crypt column; from there it decreased to reach its minimum during late metoestrus when it occupied 54 percent of the cell population in the crypt column. On the other hand, a minimum in the size of the columnar cell population was observed during late dioestrus, when it occupied 16 percent of the crypt cell population, while the maximum was during early metoestrus when it represented 29 percent of the total.

The number of mucous cells decreased during dioestrus and then stayed fairly constant from late dioestrus through oestrus. It was smallest during early metoestrus, occupying 13 percent of the crypt cell population, and was largest during late metoestrus and early dioestrus when it comprised about 21 percent.

The proliferative activity of epithelial cells expressed as the labelling index also showed some slight variations during the phases of the oestrus cycle, increasing from late dioestrus to oestrus, declining from oestrus to early metoestrus, and being high again during late metoestrus.

The labelling index of vacuolated cells essentially followed a similar pattern to the overall I_s of epithelial cells in the crypt: a maximum during proestrus and oestrus and two minima during late dioestrus and early metoestrus. The labelling index of mucous cells fluctuated much less than that of vacuolated cells, but showed two peaks during oestrus and late metoestrus and two troughs during early metoestrus and late dioestrus.

4.5.2.2 THE COLONIC CRYPT IN OVARIECTOMISED MICE

In order to assess the effect of ovarian hormones on the colonic crypt, the populations of different cell types in ovariectomised and intact animals were compared. As shown in Table 4.5.2, the mean crypt size in mice three weeks after bilateral ovariectomy was significantly decreased to 27.4 cells per column from 35.1 cells in intact mice. This decrease was due to a 40 percent decrease in the numbers of columnar cells, 34 percent decrease in mucous cells and 11 percent decrease in vacuolated cells. Hence, each of the colonic epithelial cell populations seemed to depend on ovarian hormones for the maintenance of population size, but the mature cells were more dependent on these hormones than the immature cells. Consequently, the colonic crypts in ovariectomised mice had relatively more proliferating vacuolated cells than those of control animals.

In spite of the reduced numbers of cells, the crypt in ovariectomised mice had

Table 4.5.2 Changes in the numbers and labelling indices of different types of cells per crypt column in the colon of intact female, ovariectomised, and oestrogen-treated ovariectomised mice

	Intact		Ovariectomised Untreated		Ovariectomised, single oestrogen injection		Ovariectomised, multiple oestrogen injection	
	Number	% of total	Number	% of total	Number	% of total	Number	% of total
Total	35.1		27.4		25.7		24.1	
Columnar	8.2	22	4.9	18	4.1	16	3.3	14
Vacuolated	20.5	59	18.2	66	17.8	69	16.6	69
Mucous	6.5	18	4.3	16	3.8	15	4.2	18
Labelled								
Total	3.1	8.7	3.4	12.1	1.0	3.9	1.4	5.7
vacuolated	2.7	7.6	3.2	11.3	0.9	3.6	1.3	5.3
mucous	0.4	1.1	0.2	0.8	0.1	0.3	0.1	0.4
I_s (vacuolated (%) and columnar)	9.3		13.4		4.2		6.4	
I_s (mucous) (%)	5.7		4.9		1.6		2.6	

as many labelled cells, and consequently a higher I_s than normal animals. This was attributable to an increase in the number of vacuolated cells labelled.

These data indicate that three weeks after bilateral ovariectomy the colonic crypt appeared to have reached a new steady state, which was characterised by a small decrease in the number of differentiated cells, and an increase in the relative number of proliferating cells, when compared to the crypt of intact animals.

4.5.2.3 THE COLONIC CRYPT IN OVARIECTOMISED, OESTROGEN-TREATED MICE

For assessment of the effects of oestrogen alone on the colonic crypts, ovariectomised mice were given single or multiple injections of 10 ng per g body weight of 17β-oestrodiol (17β-E$_2$) and killed one hour after ^{3}HTdR injection. Oestrogen treatments decreased ^{3}HTdR incorporation into the DNA

Table 4.5.3 Incorporation of ^{3}HTdR in colonic mucosa of ovariectomised mice at various times after a single injection or the last of multiple injections of 17β-oestradiol. Results are expressed as percentages of the control value and significant differences from this are indicated by *($p < 0.05$), **($p < 0.01$), ***($p < 0.001$)

	Hours after end of treatment			
	4	8	16	24
Single injection	25**	68	36*	43**
Multiple injections	59*	63*	127	81

of the colonic mucosa most prominently 4 h after the single injection or the last of multiple injections (Table 4.5.3). The inhibitory effect of oestrogen on ^{3}HTdR incorporation was greater, and lasted longer, after a single injection than after multiple ones. With continuous exposure to oestrogen, effected by implantation of 17β-E$_2$-packed silastic capsules into the subcutaneous tissue, ^{3}HTdR incorporation into the colonic mucosa was 112 percent of the control value after 1 day, 106 percent after 2 days and 104 percent after 4 days; none of these values differed significantly from the control. In each of these experiments, the efficacy of oestrogen treatment was verified by an increase in both the wet and dry weights of the uterine horns of ovariectomised mice (328).

Such an oestrogenic effect was also observed in the colonic mucosa of intact male mice, and the size of the change was comparable to that in ovariectomised females. As shown in Table 4.5.4, intact males and ovariectomised females

Table 4.5.4 Thymidine incorporation in the colonic mucosa of intact male and ovariectomised female mice after two different treatment regimes. Results are expressed as percentages of the respective control values, and those significantly different from control values are indicated as in Table 4.5.3

	Male	Female
Multiple low dose	66*	76*
Implant	85	106

given four daily injections of 1 ng 17β-E$_2$ per body weight and killed 16 h after the last injection incorporated significantly less ^{3}HTdR than their respective controls. Two days of oestrogen implantation in male mice caused a 15 percent decrease in ^{3}HTdR incorporation into the colonic mucosa as compared to the control but the decrease was not statistically significant.

Moreover, induced cell proliferation in the colonic crypt was also inhibited by oestrogen. Incorporation of ^{3}HTdR into the colonic mucosa of ovariectomised mice fasted for 48 h was 20 percent of that in normally fed ovariectomised mice. Sixteen hours after refeeding, ^{3}HTdR incorporation increased significantly to 285 percent of the control value. In the refed mice given a single injection of 10 ng 17β-E$_2$ per g body weight, the specific activity was 240 percent of the control value, significantly lower ($p < 0.05$) than for the refed group not given oestrogen.

Autoradiographic studies were carried out to determine the sizes of different cell populations in the colonic crypt in two groups of ovariectomised mice 4 h after single and multiple injections of oestrogen, and these were compared to cell populations in untreated ovariectomised mice (Table 4.5.2). The effect of treatment was investigated at 4 h because ^{3}HTdR incorporation was inhibited most markedly at this time.

The number of epithelial cells per crypt column seemed to be somewhat reduced after single (6.3 percent) and multiple (12.2 percent) injections of 17β-E$_2$ as compared to the untreated ovariectomised mice. When the constituent cell types were analysed, the percentage decrease in the number of columnar cells was greater than that of other types of cells. Therefore, the colonic crypts of the oestrogen-treated mice had proportionally slightly more vacuolated cells and slightly fewer columnar cells than the colonic crypts of the untreated mice. The decrease in columnar cells was greater with multiple injections than with a single injection.

The labelling index decreased significantly in the colonic crypt after both of the oestrogen treatments, the reduction being greater after a single injection than after multiple injections, in accordance with the biochemical data presented previously. The decrease in the proliferative activity of vacuolated cells after oestrogen treatments was greater than that of mucous cells.

In short, oestrogen inhibited proliferation of epithelial cells in the colonic crypt for a short time, not only under physiological conditions in ovariectomised female and intact male mice, but also when the proliferative activity was enhanced by refeeding after 48 h of fasting. In ovariectomised mice, however, repeated administration of oestrogen diminished, and oestrogen implants abolished this inhibitory effect, indicating a tachyphylactic effect of oestrogen. At the same time, the total number of cells as well as of differentiated cells per crypt column failed to return to normal after oestrogen treatment. It appears, therefore, that oestrogen did not promote differentiation of epithelial cells in the colonic crypt.

4.5.3 DISCUSSION

Both biochemical and autoradiographic studies have shown that oestrogen has a short-lived inhibitory effect on cell proliferation in the colonic crypt, and this was not associated with any significant change in the DNA content, nor in the ratios of RNA or protein to DNA (328). Furthermore, in spite of a decrease in I_s after oestrogen administration, our observations show that the number of silver grains per labelled nucleus did not seem to differ between the oestrogen-treated and untreated animals. It is unlikely, therefore, that oestrogen reduces DNA synthesis in proliferating cells.

The duration of the S-phase in the duodenum, jejunum, ileum and colon of ovariectomised mice has been found to be substantially shorter after oestrogen treatment (244). On the other hand, repeated injections of oestrogen resulted in a decrease in ^{3}HTdR incorporation following growth response in the endometrium (677) and in the vagina (408). The oestrogen-induced growth response in target organs is generally believed to be due to the genome-mediated recruitment of cells from a dormant (G_0) cell population (208), resulting in the many-fold increase in labelled and mitotic cells. When most of the cells have been triggered to enter the proliferative cycle, additional injections of oestrogen inhibit [3]HTdR incorporation in target organs, a feature which has been called a 'refractory' phenomenon (677). The refractoriness is found to be independent of the availability of oestrogen cytosol receptor and is suggested to be secondary to a block in the G_1 phase (677). Another steroid, hydrocortisone, causes a G_1 to S block in the epithelium of the mouse forestomach (237). Although additional experimental evidence is needed to establish the existence of a G_1 to S block by oestrogen, such a block, in conjunction with the shortening of the S-phase, could explain the inhibitory effect of oestrogen on cell proliferation in colonic crypts. If this is the case, it appears that oestrogen only modulates the cell cycle in the non-target organ. In contrast, the action of oestrogen in the target organ not only involves the classical growth responses, but also modulates the cell cycle following the growth responses.

The existence of such a G_1 to S block and subsequent release can also explain other findings. Following a single injection of 17β-E_2, the inhibition of [3]HTdR incorporation was sustained for at least 24 h. However, recovery from the inhibition occurred by 16 h in the multiple injection treatment. Such an early recovery from the inhibition after multiple injections can best be explained by blockage and subsequent release of cells at the transition from G_1 to S. It is probable that the G_1 to S block by oestrogen is progressively weakened in the colon by repeated injections of oestrogen, which is reminiscent of a tachyphylactic effect. The latter is also evident in the relationship between the dosage schedule of oestrogen and the degree of inhibition of [3]HTdR incorporation. Moreover, the finding that the inhibitory effect of oestrogen is abolished by continuous exposure, by oestrogen implants, also supports the hypothesis that there is a tachyphylactic effect of oestrogen on the colonic mucosa.

The present data also reveal that oestrogen treatments could not restore the colonic crypt of ovariectomised animals to normal. It is most likely, therefore, that oestrogen does not promote differentiation of epithelial cells in the colonic crypt, and that progesterone is required for the maintenance of crypt size and the maturation of epithelial cells in the crypt. Since the effect of progesterone on cell proliferation in the colonic crypt has not been explored, any attempt to correlate changes in the blood levels of oestrogen and progesterone with changes in the various cell populations in the colonic crypt during the oestrus cycle would be premature. Figure 4.5.1, however, suggests that the number of mucous cells per crypt column fluctuates more or less is a similar pattern to the blood level of progesterone. There is a cyclic change in the number of

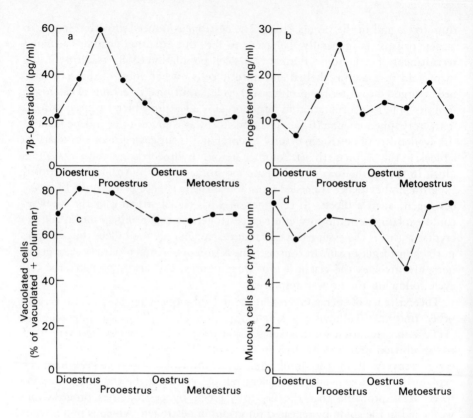

Figure 4.5.1 The changes in (a) 17 β-oestradiol and (b) progesterone blood concentrations during the oestrus cycle of the mouse (336, 475), together with those in (c) vacuolated and (d) mucous cell populations in the colonic crypt

proliferating vacuolated cells and differentiated columnar cells during the oestrus cycle: the number of vacuolated cells per crypt column increases in the preovulatory phase, while that of columnar cells increases in the post-ovulatory phase. A significant change in their population size occurs in the transition from prooestrus to oestrus, which is associated with successive peaks in the blood levels of oestrogen and progesterone. Because oestrogen appears to accelerate the proliferating cells through the S-phase and the cell cycle, and then to keep them from reentering the S-phase, it may be more than coincidence that those vacuolated cells which have been pushed through their terminal division under oestrogen and linger in their 'critical' phase (557) would have an extended opportunity to be affected by progesterone and induced to undergo differentiation. This hypothesis, however, needs to be tested by further experiments.

SECTION 5

EXPERIMENTAL CARCINOGENESIS AND CANCER

5.1 Experimental Carcinogenesis and Cancer in the Rodent Gut

J P Sunter

5.1.1 INTRODUCTION

Carcinoma of the large bowel is one of the commonest malignant diseases in westernised societies; in 1977, for example, it was estimated that 17 000 deaths occurred from this cause in England and Wales (505). Small-intestinal cancer is comparatively rare and the reasons for this difference between two such similar organs remain conjectural. A great deal of useful information on the way intestinal tumours arise has been gathered by the study of the cytokinetic events which accompany neoplastic development, and the study of cell proliferation in established tumours will yield important information on the nature of tumour growth and perhaps lead to improvements in treatment. Since an understanding of human disease processes is the ultimate goal in cancer research it would seem logical for the experimentalist to focus his attention on human material. However, in studies of intestinal cancer, as is so frequently the case in other situations, the practical and ethical constraints imposed by this approach are often too restrictive and resort is had to experimental animals.

5.1.2 SPONTANEOUS INTESTINAL TUMOURS IN RODENTS

It is the general experience that intestinal tumours which arise apparently spontaneously are rare in laboratory rodents. Several early studies involving huge numbers of rats failed to demonstrate the presence of any intestinal tumours at all (67, 465), but over the years reports of occasional small-intestinal and colonic tumours have appeared, and have been reviewed (547, 596, 780). The majority of these tumours 'are of epithelial origin: adenocarcinomas outnumber benign adenomatous lesions, colonic tumours are of more frequent occurrence than small bowel tumours, and the proximal part of the colon appears to be particularly involved. In the mouse the prevalence of spontaneous tumours is of a similar order to that seen in the rat, as is their distribution (596). An interesting phenomenon is the clustering of apparently spontaneous tumours (318, 474). This is in itself suggestive of intermittent exposure to some sort of unidentified environmental carcinogen; alternatively, changes in the thoroughness of pathological examination might be responsible for such an effect since in order to detect all intestinal tumours, particularly early ones, pathological examination has to be meticulous (596).

This very low incidence of spontaneous intestinal tumours, and the way in which most examples have presented (either as very advanced disease or as an unexpected finding at post-mortem examination) have precluded the development of inbred strains of animals manifesting a high incidence of spontaneous tumours. It has, however, proved possible to induce neoplasms in the rodent gut, both by the administration of chemical carcinogens and by exposure to ionising irradiation. The models employing chemical carcinogens have been most widely used and only these will be considered further.

5.1.3 EXPERIMENTAL CHEMICAL CARCINOGENESIS

The list of chemical substances shown to have a carcinogenic action on rodent intestinal mucosa is surprisingly long when one considers the rarity of spontaneous neoplasia. There have been a number of reviews (386, 547, 596, 777), and only an outline of the more important developments will be given here.

One of the first classes of chemicals shown to have a carcinogenic effect on the intestinal mucosa was the *polycyclic hydrocarbons*. In the early 1940s, Lorentz and Stewart demonstrated the occurrence of carcinomas of the small bowel in mice exposed to methylcholanthrene and to dibenzanthracene administered orally in an olive-oil emulsion (437). Occasional benign looking colonic neoplasms were also described (673). In rats, the topical application of methylcholanthrene (by means of an implanted chemically impregnated string) resulted in a high incidence of adenocarcinoma of the caecum (335), but local application of this chemical to the rectal mucosa of mice resulted not in the development of epithelial neoplasms, but in soft tissue tumour formation (41). More recently the intragastric administration of methylcholanthrene has resulted in the development of epithelial tumours of both small and large bowel in hamsters (147, 331). While the polycyclic hydrocarbons appear to be effective as intestinal carcinogens, their use has never been very great; more predictable models are available. Their role in natural human disease, however, may be considerable, given the epidemiological evidence for the implication of faecal bile salts and steroids in the genesis of human colonic cancer (322, 323, 565) and the possible production of carcinogens from these substances (323).

The second major group of intestinal carcinogens is the *aromatic amines*, and once again the early steps were taken in the 1940s. Bielschowsky demonstrated the production of small-intestinal neoplasms in up to 50 percent of rats given 2-acetyl-aminofluorene orally, with a much lower incidence of colonic neoplasms; strain differences in susceptibility were conspicuous (44, 45). Other workers confirmed the preponderance of small-intestinal tumours in treated rats (129), and demonstrated the occurrence of small-intestinal tumours in mice (236). The effects of parenteral administration of 4-aminodiphenyl and 3,2'-dimethyl-4-aminodiphenyl were described; this latter chemical proved to be a very potent colonic carcinogen, a majority of rats showing benign or malignant epithelial tumours of the colon after its subcutaneous administration (575). Strain differences in susceptibility exist (758), and these may in part account for the differences in reported tumour yield. Nevertheless this experimental model has been used quite widely (121, 364, 495, 662).

A third group of potent carcinogenic substances with effects in the intestinal tract is the *nitroso compounds*. Druckrey and his coworkers (186) observed the development of carcinomas of the colon in a minority of rats given a single intravenous injection of N-methyl-N-nitrosourea. Subsequent work has shown that intestinal tumours occur also after intraperitoneal or oral administration of the nitroso compounds (399, 633, 634), and that topical application (ie, intrarectal instillation) is associated with a particularly high incidence of neoplastic development in the colonic mucosa (562).

The most widely used intestinal carcinogens belong to a fourth group of substances which are all related to *cycasin*, a substance found in plants of the family *Cycadaceae*. These plants belong to a group which had its heyday in the late Jurassic and early Triassic periods. They resemble tree ferns and are perhaps the most primitive living seed-bearing plants. Occasionally, various products of these plants are used as food, and it was because suspicion had arisen that ingestion of cycad meal was associated with the development of the neurological disease amyotrophic lateral sclerosis that Laqueur and his coworkers performed experiments involving feeding crude cycad meal to laboratory rats. In this original work it was observed that two out of several hundred test animals developed large bowel neoplasms (396). This observation was followed up and it was confirmed that cycasin (the β-glycoside of methylazoxymethanol) was the chemical carcinogen concerned (392, 393). In these experiments the proportions of animals which developed colonic tumours were small, and a sex difference was apparent, males being much more vulnerable than females. Following observations on the metabolism of cycasin and its aglycone (375) further experiments involved the parenteral administration of methylazoxymethanol (MAM) (392, 394). In addition to benign and malignant colonic neoplasms, there was a high incidence of small-intestinal carcinomas, which occurred predominantly in the duodenum. Using weekly subcutaneous injections of 1,2-dimethylhydrazine (DMH), a chemical allied to cycasin and assumed to be metabolised to yield similar alkylating intermediate products to those of the dialkylnitrosamines, Druckrey and his coworkers (185) described very high incidences of small and large bowel carcinoma in rats. Not only was the tumour incidence high, but carcinogenicity appeared to be specific for the gut. These two properties combined to make DMH potentially a useful experimental carcinogen. Further experience has shown that DMH is not entirely gut-specific in its carcinogenic effects, but the incidence of tumours in other organs is acceptably low (184). Many groups of workers have amply confirmed the effectiveness of the DMH model of intestinal carcinogenesis in rats (455, 549, 760, 786) in mice (269, 519, 721, 787) and in hamsters (804), and it is at present the most widely used.

Subsequent sections will deal principally with the changes resulting from the experimental use of the cycasin group of chemicals.

5.1.4 THE EFFECTS OF THE CYCASIN-RELATED COMPOUNDS

5.1.4.1 METABOLISM AND BIOCHEMISTRY

The pioneer studies of Laqueur showed that cycasin itself was a relatively inert substance. Oral administration to germ-free animals failed to produce the usual acute toxic effects seen in conventional rats (392), and later studies showed that carcinogenicity was not manifest in cycasin-fed germ-free animals (395, 397). Cycasin administered by parenteral injection was not subjected to metabolic breakdown and was excreted unchanged, largely in the urine (375). The toxic nature of MAM, the aglycone of cycasin, was well established (393, 394) and it was considered that hydrolysis of cycasin by bacterial glycosidase in the intestine led to the formation of MAM which was then absorbed and metabolised with subsequent toxic and carcinogenic effects.

The metabolism of DMH suggested by Druckrey (184) (Figure 5.1.1), with successive production of azomethane, azoxymethane and MAM, is strongly supported by detailed chromatographic analysis (229, 230). MAM is an unstable compound in aqueous solution, and alkylating properties were observed both in vitro (464) and in vivo (641). The evidence suggests that methyldiazonium is indeed the highly reactive intermediary product (493), and that it is through the alkylating properties of this substance that the carcinogenic effects of the cycasin derivatives occur.

Clearly the distribution of these chemicals and their metabolites in the different tissues and body fluids is important in determining their conspicuous organotropism. Following parenteral administration of ^{14}C-labelled DMH, autoradiography has shown that activity is first concentrated in the liver, and then in the colonic epithelium (643). Pozharisski and his coworkers (550) found

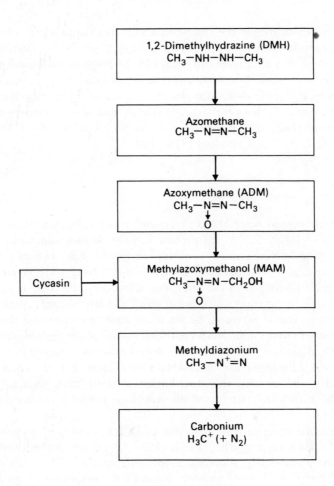

Figure 5.1.1 Steps involved in the metabolism of the cycasin-related compounds (184)

maximum levels of radioactivity in rat blood, bile and urine within 3 to 6 h of administration of ^{3}H-labelled DMH, and commented that while there was biliary secretion of DMH metabolites (777) this alone could not account for the very rapid alkylation of colonic DNA, RNA and protein. Others (305) have found no evidence of biliary secretion of DMH metabolites in the rat, and regard transport via the bloodstream as the major means of distribution. This would account for the undiminished toxic effects of MAM on the intestinal mucosa of animals having a diverted biliary flow (833).

The extent to which different organs appear to concentrate DMH or its metabolites, and the degree to which alkylation of nucleic acids is effected, consistently fail to mirror the extent to which those organs are vulnerable to neoplastic transformation (305, 550, 590, 643). Clearly other factors must be operative; these may simply be differences in the inherent biological properties of the different tissues, but within the bowel mucosa there are many factors acting at a local level to determine the ultimate nature of the response to these alkylating agents. Such factors include dietary and other constituents of the bowel contents (140, 323, 463, 565, 766), the proliferative status of the mucosa (36, 250, 687, 797) and heredity (170, 210).

5.1.4.2 ACUTE TOXIC EFFECTS

Parenteral administration of MAM to rats and mice results in marked reduction in synthesis of DNA, RNA and protein in liver, kidney and small intestine (835). These effects are most conspicuous in the first twenty-four hours following treatment, and begin in the first hour. Changes are greatest in the liver, but most prolonged in the intestine. Microscopically there is evidence of necrosis of cells in the mucosal crypts of small and large bowel, particularly in the duodenum; this is extensive by six hours after treatment and shows some improvement at twenty-four hours, with restoration of the normal pattern after several days. A similar sequence of microscopic changes occurs in rats and mice following the administration of DMH (304) (Figure 5.1.2). There is good evidence that the severity and distribution of acute toxic mucosal changes parallels the distribution patterns of the neoplasms arising in chronically treated animals (833).

In mice, subcutaneous administration of DMH is followed within 24 h by necrosis of colonic crypt epithelial cells (150). Crypts are markedly reduced in size and morphologically abnormal crypt cells appear with occasional multinucleate forms or bizarre mitotic figures. A compensatory proliferative response evidenced by increased ^{3}HTdR-labelling index (I_s) results in a state of crypt hyperplasia by the fourth day following treatment. During this phase labelled cells are transiently present in the upper third of the crypt. By seven days after treatment normality appears to have been restored (150). As well as having these notable effects when administered parenterally, DMH produces rapid changes when administered topically. Following intrarectal instillation of solutions of the chemical, crypt cell loss, as evidenced by loss of prelabelled cells, occurs within 30 min in the descending colon. Labelling indices in crypt epithelium show an increase which is first apparent at 24 h, and is sustained for up to 2 weeks (92). In none of these experiments on rectal instillation did the ascending colon show any evidence of toxic effects, and this implies a strictly local action of DMH in this situation, with an insignificant degree of absorption and systemic distribution.

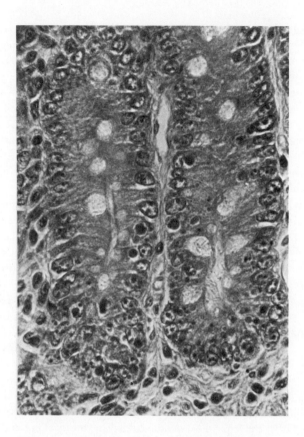

Figure 5.1.2 Crypt cell damage in the jejunum occurring 8 h after administration of 60 mg/kg DMH in the rat (haematoxylin and eosin (H & E) × 1000)

5.1.4.3 HYPERPLASTIC CHANGES IN MUCOSAL CRYPTS

Occurring quite separately from the acute toxic changes described above there are a variety of hyperplastic changes in the intestinal crypts of animals treated chronically with chemicals of the cycasin group, and most workers agree that it is in the setting of such a generalised mucosal abnormality that there arise the dysplastic and in-situ neoplastic changes which are thought to precede the development of the grossly recognisable tumours.

Inflammatory changes occurring in the intestinal mucosa of chronically treated animals have occasionally been commented on (549, 710, 804). It seems that such changes are an effect of acute toxicity and are not of primary importance in the development of hyperplasia or neoplasia.

The elevation of crypt I_s seen two weeks following intrarectal instillation of DMH solutions in mice (92) may represent either a late phase in the recovery from acute toxic effects, or the earliest part of some chronic hyperplastic response; the absence of any associated morphological change makes it difficult to be sure which. In the colon of mice given repeated subcutaneous injections of DMH, most workers have found that the chronic hyperplastic changes begin several weeks later than this. In one detailed study (710) focal colonic crypt hyperplasia had appeared by 38 days after the start of weekly injections, and became more severe and generalised by 109 days, with dysplastic and neoplastic changes occurring at some time after this. In the abnormal colonic crypts I_s increased, and DNA-synthesising cells were found to have an abnormal distribution within the crypt, spreading into the upper third and even as far as the crypt mouth. In the jejunum, which remained morphologically normal, I_s and the distribution of labelled cells also remained normal. The changes in crypt size in descending colon of mice have been observed by other workers (94, 574), as have the changes in I_s and in the distribution of the proliferating cells within the crypt (94, 149, 150, 574). In one of these studies (574) there were no detectable differences in the major parameters of the cell cycle (calculated from fraction of labelled mitoses (FLM) data) between the cells in the abnormal hyperplastic crypts and in colonic crypts of control animals. Recent observations, however, have shown prolongations of the cell cycle times (T_c) and the duration of G_1 in treated animals (97).

In the rat colon there appears to be less agreement about the sequence of events during what may be termed preneoplastic hyperplasia. Wiebecke and his coworkers (786) described 'more or less localised mucosal hyperplasias' often occurring towards the tips of mucosal folds; in these elongated crypts the distribution of proliferating cells remained normal despite increased values for I_s. It was in these hyperplastic areas that the earliest features of neoplasia were found. Other workers (549, 736) have described increases in the size of the proliferation compartment without elongation of the crypts, although a larger cell population was observed in one of these studies, due to an increased crypt circumference (736). In these latter crypts cell birth rates were similar to control values, but the basal zone of slowly cycling cells appeared to have become extended. Recently a progressive crypt hyperplasia, with increasing size of proliferation compartment not associated with elevated labelling indices, has been described in the descending colon of DMH-treated rats (456). Abnormalities worsened progressively with duration of DMH treatment, but the distribution of proliferating cells within the enlarged crypts remained essentially normal. In addition to this picture of progressive hyperplasia other workers have described irregular areas of mucosal atrophy (499).

Observations on the small bowel during this preneoplastic phase of carcinogenesis are relatively few. In mice no obvious abnormalities have been reported (710). In rats mucosal hyperplasias have been described in animals treated with DMH (499, 786), while the considerably elevated levels of DNA and RNA seen in rat jejunal mucosa following chronic administration of azoxymethane are evidence of a similar hyperplastic response (797). We have studied development of this hyperplastic state, and have attempted to define it in kinetic terms (686).

Our results show that soon after the start of DMH injections the mean crypt length in the upper jejunum becomes significantly greater than normal (Figure 5.1.3). This state of modest hyperplasia presumably represents some compen-

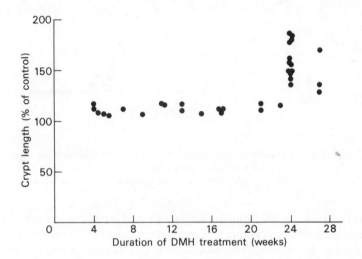

Figure 5.1.3 Mean length of jejunal crypts as a percentage of the control value (33.7) versus weeks of DMH treatment. Each point represents a separate animal

satory response to the toxic effects of DMH, and is sustained during the succeeding treatment until at about 24 weeks a sudden further lengthening of the crypts occurs, with mean values of up to twice normal. At about this time approximately one third of the animals are affected by neoplasms of the upper small bowel, but the hyperplastic response is seen in all treated animals, and not only where there are adjacent tumours. Over the period of observation the circumference of the crypts remains constant.

Whole-crypt labelling indices remain steady during the experimental period, perhaps only slightly greater than control values. The distribution of ^{3}HTdR-labelled cells within the crypt retains the usual form (Figure 5.1.4), but there is

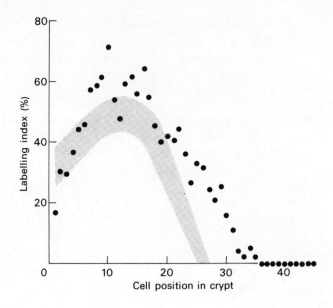

Figure 5.1.4 Distribution of labelled cells within the jejunal crypt of an animal treated with DMH for 27 weeks: the 95% confidence limits of the control group are superimposed

an increase in maximum I_s and a displacement of proliferating cells to higher cell positions within the crypt. Thus the size of the proliferation compartment, as judged by the position of half-maximum I_s, increases in absolute terms but relative to the total size of the crypt actually decreases. The major cell cycle parameters calculated from FLM studies show little change (Table 5.1.1) save for a slight reduction in T_c at the base of the crypt. But the estimates of growth fraction (I_p) for the crypt as a whole, derived from I_s and FLM data, show that the abnormal crypts have significantly lower values (Table 5.1.1). This reduction in growth fraction appears to have arisen as a result of a fall in I_p within the expanded proliferation compartment; this suggestion is confirmed by a generalised reduction in the birth rate calculated from stathmokinetic data (Table 5.1.2).

These results show a great deal in common with the changes which occur in the colon. Clearly they represent a preneoplastic state, but hyperplasias can occur in many situations which are not obviously associated with the later development of neoplasms (82, 432, 691). Whether or not there are any characteristics distinguishing those states of intestinal mucosal hyperplasia which have a neoplastic potential, from those which do not, is at present unknown.

Table 5.1.1 Estimates of T_c and t_s at various positions in the jejunal crypts of DMH-treated rats and of normal animals (6), with estimates of the growth fraction for the whole crypt

Cell positions	DMH treated		Normal	
	T_c(h)	t_s(h)	T_c(h)	t_s(h)
1–4	12.1	7.4	15.5	8.6
5–8	13.4	7.7	12.3	7.1
9–12	12.7	7.9	11.2	6.4
13–16	10.6	6.7	10.8	5.9
17–20	10.9	6.6	11.0	5.9
21–24	10.3	6.5	10.7	6.0
25 +	10.7	6.0	—	—
Whole crypt	10.9	6.9	11.3	6.5
Whole crypt growth fraction	0.49		0.62	

Table 5.1.2 Comparison of birth rates (cells/1000 cells/h) in the jejunal crypts of normal and DMH treated rats

Cell position	Normal	DMH treated
1–4	46	17
5–8	77	37
9–12	86	46
13–16	86	55
17–20	63	58
21–24	30	63
25–28	10	47
29–32	—	49
33–36	—	48
37–40	—	29
Whole crypt	62	46

5.1.4.4 DYSPLASIA AND NEOPLASIA

While there is clear evidence that tumours can arise directly from the epithelium of normal looking crypts (549), most workers agree that it is in the setting of some generalised hyperplastic abnormality of the mucosa that there arise the foci of dysplasia and of atypia which are the source of established neoplasms.

The morphology of these dyplastic and early neoplastic lesions has been described in some detail (786). In the small bowel of the rat they appear as zones of abrupt loss of cellular differentiation of the crypt epithelium. The enterocytes assume an abnormal form, with basophilic cytoplasm and densely staining nuclei; occasionally the appearance is that of a syncytium. In the rat

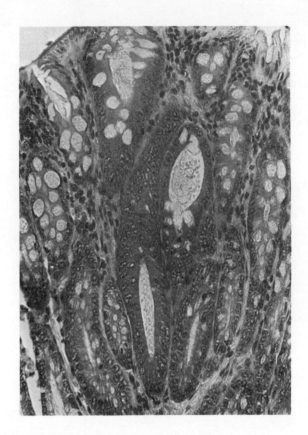

Figure 5.1.5 Dysplastic lesion within a crypt of the descending colon of a rat
treated for 24 weeks with DMH (H & E × 300)

colon similar changes occur (Figure 5.1.5). A striking feature on autoradiography is the abnormal labelling activity of these lesions situated, as they so
frequently are, in the upper part of the crypt (549, 760, 786). The severity of
cell change varies a great deal, and, dependent on this, the lesions may be
classed as degrees of dysplasia or as in-situ carcinoma. It is considered that
from these fairly well differentiated lesions arise adenomas and well differentiated
carcinomas which tend to grow first into the lumen of the bowel (549, 760).
On the other hand, poorly differentiated carcinomas originate as highly invasive
mucosal lesions without any recognisable in-situ precursor stage, and often arise
in relation to lymphoid aggregates; even minor degrees of dysplastic change
have recently been noted to occur preferentially at the base of crypts overlying
lymphoid aggregates (499). The histogenesis of the tumours induced in the

colon of mice will be dealt with later (Section 5.2), and hereafter only lesions occurring in the rat will be considered.

There are many factors of importance in determining the ultimate yield of tumours in any experimental situation, including hereditary susceptibility and a variety of influences presumably operating via co-carcinogens of various sorts. One factor of major importance is the precise manner in which the carcinogen is given: the route of administration, dosage and frequency of dosage all influence the outcome of treatment.

Most workers have administered DMH by weekly subcutaneous injection, usually at a dosage of between 10 and 20 mg of DMH base per kg body weight. At the lower dosage the incidence of colonic neoplasms is almost 100 percent but that of small-intestinal neoplasms is much lower. The larger dose results in a higher incidence of upper small-intestinal tumours, and a shortening of the induction period from around eight months to less than six months (89, 184, 786). The subcutaneous administration of a single large dose of DMH is associated with the development of colonic neoplasms in a minority of animals after a prolonged induction period (184). Oral (184) and intraperitoneal administration (421) are similarly associated with development of small-intestinal and colonic tumours in a substantial proportion of treated animals. The subcutaneous administration of azoxymethane on a weekly basis results in the development of a high incidence of both small and large-intestinal tumours and there are similar dose-dependent effects to those of DMH (763). Azoxymethane too is active following a single subcutaneous injection (834).

Many workers have produced histopathological classifications of the different types of tumour seen in these cycasin-related drug models. In general, despite variations in numbers of tumours observed and in the relative frequencies in small and large bowel, there appears to be a fairly predictable distribution pattern for the different histological types of tumour.

In the small intestine there is a predominance of lesions in the duodenum and upper jejunum, and histologically nearly all of them are well differentiated tubular or tubulovillous adenocarcinomas (455, 686, 760, 763, 786). Often these upper small-intestinal neoplasms are relatively large and show extensive local spread (Figure 5.1.6) or systemic metastasis (686, 760, 763). Lesions arising lower down the small bowel, although of rather infrequent occurrence, are often poorly differentiated by comparison (760, 786).

We have recently published our findings on the pathological features of the colonic tumours, and have described a classification which is a useful compromise between descriptive complexity and oversimplification (687). The animals used were female Wistar Porton rats, and they were given weekly subcutaneous injections of DMH, the dose being 15 mg (base) per kg body weight. The first colonic tumours were noted at 19 weeks of treatment and groups of animals were killed until 30 weeks after the start of injections. A total

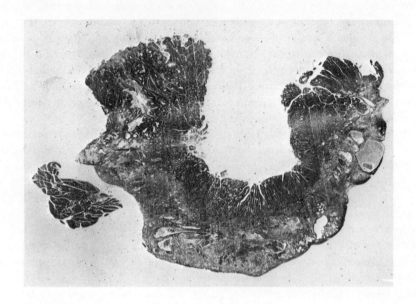

Figure 5.1.6 An ulcerated small intestinal carcinoma which has spread
through the full thickness of the jejunal wall (H & E × 5)

of 142 animals was observed over this 11 week period, and the 378 separate
colonic neoplasms found were studied. After 24 weeks over 90 percent of
treated animals showed colonic tumours, and the mean prevalence of tumours
was 2.7 per animal. The distribution of all tumours along the length of the
colon is shown in Figure 5.1.7. The proximal tenth of the colon was invariably

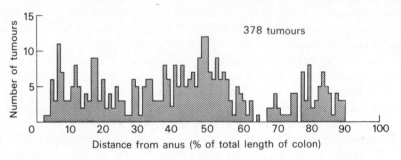

Figure 5.1.7 Distribution of all colonic tumours along the length of the
bowel. Zero represents the anus, and 100% the colocaecal junction

free of tumours, and there were fewer than average lesions at the junction of its proximal and middle thirds, around the site where the character of the mucosa changes (688). This relatively uniform distribution is similar to that noted by some others using a similar dosage (421, 549, 760, 786), but different from that described elsewhere, where a clear and rather striking predominance of lesions was seen around the middle third (89, 456).

The tumours were classified into four groups according to their microscopic appearances. The benign *adenomas* manifest a tubular or a tubulovillous structure (Figure 5.1.8), and are uniformly well differentiated with no evidence of cellular atypia nor of invasive growth through the muscularis

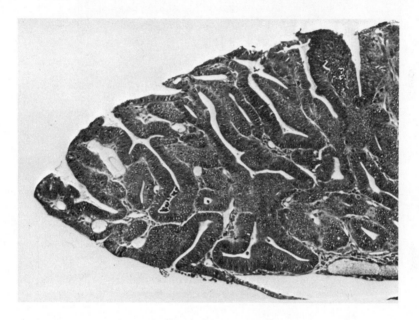

Figure 5.1.8 Benign tubular adenoma. Note the lack of malignant cellular atypia (H & E × 300)

mucosae. Macroscopically these lesions appeared as sessile or pedunculated mucosal polyps, and they accounted for 26 percent of observed lesions. *Group 1 carcinomas* showed similar gross appearances to the benign adenomas, and histologically are indistinguishable save for the presence of localised invasion through the muscularis mucosae (Figure 5.1.9); some 16 percent of all tumours fall into this group. The largest group of tumours, comprising about 40 percent of the total were the *group 2 carcinomas*. These have the appearance of moderately

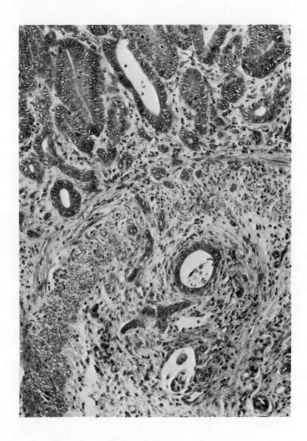

Figure 5.1.9 Group 1 carcinoma; the earliest evidence of neoplastic glandular acini penetrating the muscularis mucosae (H & E × 300)

well differentiated invasive adenocarcinomas often extensively infiltrating the bowel wall. Macroscopically they appear as mucosal polyps or plaques, often with surface ulceration as a conspicuous feature. At the periphery there is often a shoulder of residual 'adenomatous' tissue suggesting an origin in an antecedent benign neoplasm (Figure 5.1.10). The *group 3 carcinomas* are a heterogeneous group of adenocarcinomas which show a variety of histological appearances (Figures 5.1.11 and 5.1.12), but which have in common that they are poorly differentiated. Ulceration is usually a conspicuous feature, and macroscopically they present as ill defined mucosal thickenings often resembling a plaited loaf. This is the only form of colonic tumour from which distant metastases arise with any frequency.

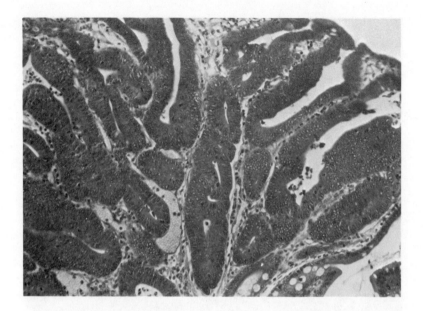

Figure 5.1.10 The periphery of a group 2 carcinoma showing residual adenomatous tissue lacking malignant cellular atypia (H & E × 300)

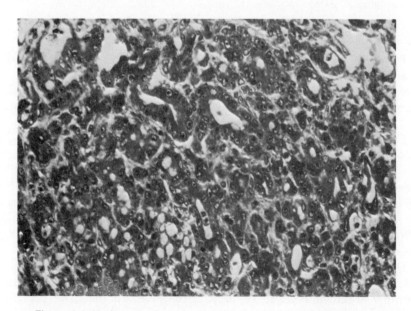

Figure 5.1.11 A group 3 carcinoma, showing its poorly differentiated appearance (H & E × 600)

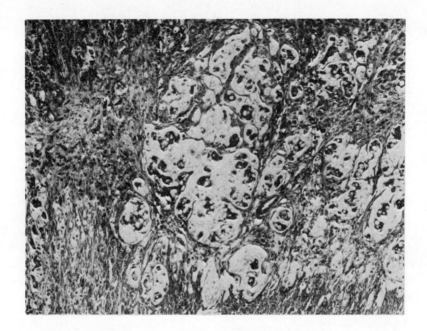

Figure 5.1.12 A group 3 carcinoma—so called colloid carcinoma
(H & E × 300)

The range of colonic tumours we have observed is similar to that observed by most other workers, although in one report it was emphatically stated that no benign tumours were convincingly demonstrated (456). With the possible exception of purely villous adenoma virtually every type of epithelial neoplasm seen in the human colon is duplicated in the rat model.

The distributions of the different tumour types along the length of the bowel show some interesting variations (Figure 5.1.13). The poorly differentiated group 3 carcinomas are concentrated in the proximal part of the colon, while adenomas and group 1 carcinomas are virtually confined to the distal half. Group 2 carcinomas have a more widespread distribution. These observations are in keeping with those of others (561, 760), and the tumour distributions reflect the changes in morphology (760) and cytokinetic organisation (688) of the colonic crypts from one site to another along the length of the bowel.

The changes in the incidences of the different tumour types at different times after the start of DMH treatment are given in Table 5.1.3. The frequencies of the different tumour types are similar, and the increase in the overall prevalence of tumours is brought about almost exclusively by the increase in the frequency of the group 2 carcinomas.

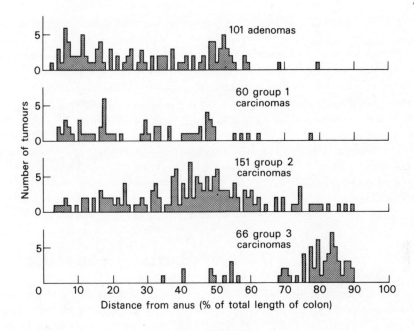

Figure 5.1.13 Distribution of the different tumour types along the length of the bowel. Zero represents the anus and 100% the colocaecal junction

Table 5.1.3 The mean number of different types of tumour per rat at different times after the start of DMH treatment

	Duration of treatment (weeks)	
	24	27 to 30
Adenomas	0.7	0.8
Group 1 carcinomas	0.4	0.5
Group 2 carcinomas	0.9	1.7
Group 3 carcinomas	0.5	0.4
Total	2.5	3.3

5.1.5 THE POLYP-CANCER SEQUENCE

As far as human beings are concerned there is a strong case to be made that, if one excludes patients with ulcerative colitis, the majority of colonic carcinomas will have resulted from malignant change occurring in benign adenomatous polyps. The evidence has recently been reviewed (487). Most workers feel that there is little to support the suggestion that a polyp-cancer sequence exists in the DMH-treated rat (455, 456, 549, 760). While there is good evidence that a substantial proportion of these experimental carcinomas do arise de novo, we agree with Wiebecke and his colleagues (786) that there is histological evidence in favour of a polyp-cancer sequence in some lesions, particularly those situated in the distal half of the colon. The common anatomical distribution of adenomas and group 1 carcinomas provides additional support, and the increase in frequency of group 2 lesions with duration of DMH treatment suggests a continuous process of formation of benign polyps which rapidly progress to group 2 carcinoma. As many as half the carcinomas observed in DMH-treated rats might have their origin in polypoid adenomas, lesions whose malignant propensity parallels but greatly exceeds that of colonic adenomas in man, very rapidly developing the property of tissue invasion.

5.1.6 CYTOKINETIC STUDIES OF INDUCED COLONIC TUMOURS

There have been relatively few studies of cell proliferation in chemically induced colonic tumours either in rats or in mice. The findings in the mouse are discussed in detail later (see Section 5.2), and only the situation in the rat will be dealt with here.

A number of years ago a study was published which gave ^{3}HTdR-labelling indices for neoplastic and non-neoplastic colonic epithelium and also the results of an FLM study (626). In adenocarcinomas mean I_s was 38 percent, considerably greater than the value of 24 percent calculated for the proliferation compartment of normal-looking crypts. From the FLM study, values for the duration of DNA synthesis (t_s) were 7.9 h and 8.0 h for tumours and normal colon respectively, and from the ratio of t_s to I_s values for T_c were obtained of 21 h and 32 h. Other workers (551), using the colchicine-thymidine technique, found much variation in the cell cycle parameters from one tumour to the next. Both t_s and T_c were longer than in non-neoplastic colonic crypts. The mean labelling indices in adenomatous polyps have also been calculated at around twice the value found in normal mucosa (786).

Tutton and Barkla have used the stathmokinetic technique to measure cell proliferation in large bowel mucosa and tumours. In the adenocarcinomas, cell birth rates are slightly less than the values seen in the region of fastest proliferation in the normal crypt, but they are comparable with the rates seen at the crypt base (736). Various factors have been shown to influence significantly cell birth rates in normal and neoplastic colonic epithelium, and often a differential effect is observable (737, 738, 740). Stathmokinetic results must, however, be interpreted with caution in view of the possible effects of undiscernable alterations in growth fraction or cell loss.

We have performed ^{3}HTdR labelling studies on our rat colonic tumours, and have analysed the data by tumour type. As far as possible we have drawn comparisons with the cell cycle parameters derived from the normal mucosa at the site of maximum prevalence of particular types of tumours, to compare cell proliferation in tumours with that of their antecedent epithelia.

It is well known that within tumours there is considerable variability in the uptake of thymidine from one site to another, dependent on vascular and other local factors (703). Therefore counts of I_s were made only in specified zones. In benign adenomas, for example, I_s was calculated for the surface 0.05 mm and for a 0.1 mm thick strip of tissue 0.1 mm below the surface. Table 5.1.4 shows

Table 5.1.4 Labelling indices (%) at two sites within six benign adenomas studied at various times after the start of DMH treatment

| | \multicolumn{6}{c}{Duration of treatment (weeks)} | |
	23	24	24	27	27	28	Mean
Surface I_s(%)	2.0	3.4	3.1	7.5	4.4	6.4	4.5
Subsurface I_s(%)	23.3	22.3	20.7	22.1	28.8	24.5	23.6

I_s values in six benign adenomas encountered at various times after the start of DMH injections. Corresponding results are consistent, but the mean I_s of the surface zone is only 4.5 percent and the mean value for the subsurface region is 23.6 percent, which illustrates the size of variation within tumours that may be expected. The fact that mitotic index parallels I_s in these results suggests that what is observed is not simply an artefact due to inadequate penetration of labelled thymidine to the surface.

Table 5.1.5 summarises mean labelling indices in the different tumour types, indices calculated for specific sites within tumours, and for regions of a particular histological appearance. These values are compared with the maxi-

Table 5.1.5 Mean labelling indices (%) of tumours and the corresponding values in normal mucosa

Tumour	Site	I_s(%)	Mucosal I_s(%)
Adenoma	Surface zone	5	
	Subsurface zone	24	
Group 1 Carcinoma	Subsurface zone	20	21
	Invasive glands	22	
Group 2 Carcinoma	Raised margin	21	
	Deep central zone	26	16
	Deeply invasive glands	19	
Group 3 Carcinoma	Small acini	16	16

mum I_s values occurring in the proliferation compartment of the normal colonic crypts in sites corresponding to maximum tumour prevalences. Thus adenomas and group 1 carcinomas are compared with descending colon, group 2 carcinomas with transverse colon and group 3 carcinomas with ascending colon (688). The mean labelling indices for the tumours are seen to be very similar to the peak values obtained in the normal colon, save for group 2 carcinomas which show greater labelling indices than are observed in the antecedent epithelium.

Results of analysis (251) of FLM studies for the different tumour types are presented in Table 5.1.6, along with the corresponding parameters calculated

Table 5.1.6 Estimates of T_c and t_s(h) derived from FLM data for various types of tumours, and the corresponding values in normal mucosa

Tumour type	T_c	t_s	Site	T_c	t_s
Adenoma	23	7.0 ⎱	Descending colon	58	9.0
Group 1 carcinoma	21	7.3 ⎰			
Group 2 carcinoma	17	7.1	Transverse colon	42	9.1
Group 3 carcinoma	22	7.2	Ascending colon	35	8.8

for the crypts in the normal mucosa at the different sites along the length of the bowel (688); the mean values represent the whole of the proliferating epithelium in the crypt, not any specific part of it. It is evident that cell cycle times in the tumours are very similar to one another with similar values for t_s also. Both these parameters are substantially shorter than the values for normal mucosa.

Our results are clearly at variance with some of the results described above, and in particular the discrepancies in labelling index are difficult to explain.

5.1.7 SUMMARY AND CONCLUSIONS

There are a number of effective experimental models of intestinal cancer available, the most popular of which relies on the fairly specific carcinogenicity for the gut of the cycasin group of compounds. On histological grounds this would appear to be a model that closely mimics human intestinal neoplasia.

Its use has led to an awareness of the hyperplastic and other changes which occur in mucosae which are undergoing neoplastic transformation, and further work is necessary to establish whether there are any particular features which will characterise the state of 'preneoplastic hyperplasia' prior to the development of dysplasia or in situ neoplasia which herald frank malignancy.

At present there is perhaps more scepticism shown about the 'polyp-cancer sequence' in the experimental animal than in the human being.

The available labelling studies on established colonic tumours in rats show some conspicuous differences between tumour cell proliferation and the proliferative status of normal intestinal mucosa, and stathmokinetic results show differential responsiveness to a wide variety of drugs and other stimuli. These differences, if they reflect accurately the situation in human beings, may be of great value as far as therapy is concerned.

ACKNOWLEDGEMENTS

I would like to thank the North of England Council of the Cancer Research Campaign for generous financial support. Mrs E Wallace and Mrs M Hughes provided invaluable technical assistance.

5.2 Pathogenesis and Biological Behaviour of 1,2-Dimethylhydrazine-Induced Colonic Neoplasms in the Mouse

William W L Chang

5.2.1 INTRODUCTION

The understanding of the detailed mode of formation and evolution of experimental colonic neoplasms is a basic problem in tumour biology which may lead us to better methods of preventing and treating colonic cancers. An experimental model for colonic neoplasia has been provided by the pioneer works of Laqueur (393) and Druckrey and his colleagues (185). Since then it has been repeatedly shown that symmetrical 1,2-dimethylhydrazine (DMH) and related compounds (184) induce neoplasms specifically in the colon of the rat (455, 456, 549, 551, 627, 667, 687, 736, 760, 763, 786, 834) and the mouse (94, 149, 211, 269, 710, 720, 721, 786, 787).

Although tumours are produced mainly in the descending colon and rectum in rodents after administration of DMH, the mode of tumour formation appears to be species-specific: the neoplasms are isolated in the rat and broader-based and widespread in the mouse (786). Thus the mouse seems to be the better experimental model with which to analyse the pathogenesis of multiple adenomas (adenomatosis) with subsequent development of adenocarcinomas. We have taken advantage of the high reproducibility and multiplicity of neoplasms in the descending colon in CF-1 mice after DMH treatment (710) to study the mode of formation and evolution of colonic neoplasms in relation to the changes in proliferation, differentiation, and migration of epithelial cell populations in the crypt (94, 97).

5.2.2 MATERIALS AND METHODS

Young adult female CF-1 mice were given subcutaneous injections of DMH.2HCl in a dose of 20 mg per kg body weight weekly for 3 to 26 weeks and killed at various times after the start of treatment; the details of these experiments have been published (94, 97). Animals also received 1 μCi tritiated thymidine (³HTdR) per g body weight 45 to 60 minutes before being killed. Autoradiographs were prepared from sections of Epon-embedded descending colon (with tumours if present), which were prestained by the periodic acid-Schiff (PAS) reaction and by iron-hematoxylin (95). The details of analytical methods have also been published previously (95, 97, 98).

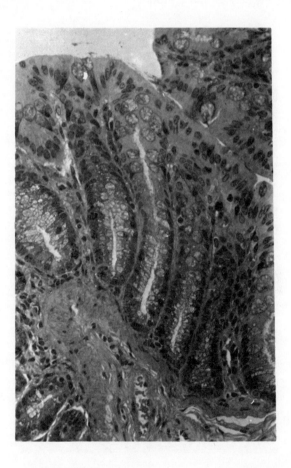

Figure 5.2.1 Autoradiograph of normal colonic crypts. Proliferating vacuolated cells with occasional ³HTdR labelling are located in the lower half of the crypt, whereas absorptive columnar cells are in the upper half. Mucous cells are scattered throughout the crypt (×350)

5.2.3 RESULTS AND INTERPRETATION

5.2.3.1 HYPERPLASTIC RESPONSE OF COLONIC CRYPTS TO DMH

Following weekly injections of DMH, the distal half of the colon (the descending colon including the rectum) became progressively enlarged, the mucosa thickened, and the crypts elongated and hyperplastic (Figures 5.2.1 and 5.2.2). These changes were noted by 9 weeks after the start of DMH administration and became more pronounced after further treatment with the

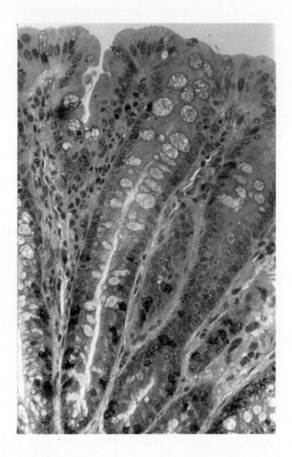

Figure 5.2.2 Autoradiograph of hyperplastic crypts in a DMH-treated mouse. Proliferating cells in the lower half of the crypt show a varying degree of vacuolation, and many of them are devoid of vacuoles (×350)

carcinogen. The degree of these responses, however, varied from animal to animal and also from crypt to crypt even in the same animal.

The crypt length, defined as the mean number of epithelial cells lining one side of a longitudinally sectioned crypt, was significantly increased 62 and 125 days after commencement of DMH injections (Table 5.2.1). Further elongation

Table 5.2.1 Length and labelling index of colonic crypt in control and DMH-treated mice 62 and 125 days after the start of treatment

Time after start of treatment	Treatment	Crypt length (cells)	Labelling index ($\%$)
62 days	Control	37	10.2
	DMH	49	11.4
125 days	Control	33	9.9
	DMH	53	14.1

and hyperplasia of the crypts were observed in some mice with further DMH treatment, sometimes accompanied by an increase in the girth. However, quantitative analysis using the crypt as a unit became very difficult due to progressive elongation, distortion, tortuosity and branching.

In the descending colon of normal mice there are three populations of epithelial cells: 83 percent vacuolated-columnar, 16 percent mucous (goblet) and 1 percent enteroendocrine (argentaffin) (95). Since a majority of epithelial cells in the crypt belong to the vacuolated-columnar cell line, the crypts have a distinctive appearance due to the presence of proliferating vacuolated cells in the lower two-thirds of the crypt and of non-proliferating columnar (absorptive) cells in the upper one-third. In DMH-treated mice, however, the hyperplastic crypts showed various cytological alterations. In many of them, proliferating epithelial cells of the vacuolated-columnar cell line contained few or no vacuoles (Figures 5.2.1 and 5.2.2), whereas in some, vacuolated cells were unusually numerous and present up to the mouth of the crypt (94). However, the relative frequency of the three populations of epithelial cells was not altered. These findings suggest that, after treatment with DMH, the epithelial cells in the main vacuolated-columnar cell line show various degrees of derangement in differentiation, but differentiation of stem cells into the three cell populations appears not to be disturbed (94).

The rate of proliferation of epithelial cells per crypt column as expressed by the labelling index (I_s) was also increased in the hyperplastic crypts. This increase was significant 125 days after the start of DMH administration (Table 5.2.1). In order to investigate the distribution of proliferating cells in the crypt, the crypts were divided into ten equal segments (95), and I_s was estimated for each segment. As the crypt length and I_s increased, the proliferation zone of the crypt progressively expanded with DMH treatment.

However, the general pattern of distribution of labelled cells in the hyperplastic crypts was similar to that in the normal crypts (Figure 5.2.3) and followed what has been described as the slow cut-off model (84). This indicates that the cessation of proliferation takes place in the hyperplastic crypts as it does normally (98).

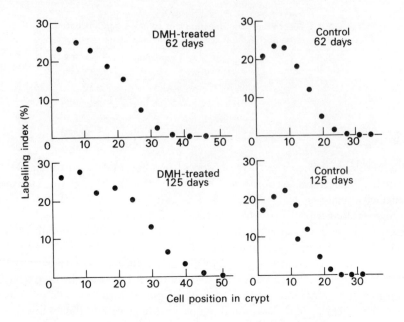

Figure 5.2.3 Labelling index distribution along the length of colonic crypts of DMH-treated and control mice.

In our murine model, hyperplastic (metaplastic) polyps (359, 389, 486) as described in man were not observed, but hyperplasia of crypts occurred diffusely in the mucosa of the descending colon. In the hyperplastic polyps the crypts are elongated, with an increased number of epithelial cells per crypt column, and appear serrated due to focal flattening of the lining epithelial cells; cellular differentiation occurs normally and no epithelial atypia is found (486). Hyperplastic polyps are, therefore, distinctly different from adenomatous polyps and do not give rise either to adenomas or to adenocarcinomas (359, 389). Whether or not hyperplastic polyps in man and diffuse hyperplasia of crypts in the murine model are related needs further investigation. Both conditions are quite similar in terms of such important properties as the distribution of proliferating cells and the maintenance of the three epithelial cell lines in the crypt.

Our current belief is that the diffuse crypt hyperplasia following DMH treatment represents a reaction to the injury caused by the carcinogen. According to several investigators' (92, 433) as well as our own observations, some epithelial cells in the crypts degenerate and die following a single administration of DMH; the surviving cells usually regenerate and repopulate the crypts to such an extent that there is an increase in the proliferative activity and in the epithelial cell population. With repeated administration of DMH, therefore, hyperplasia of crypts may or may not occur depending upon the degree of overcompensation. Such crypt hyperplasia after DMH treatment has been noted in all the experiments using mice (94, 149, 710, 786). In the rat, it has been observed by some investigators (456), but not by others (549, 736). Such a discrepancy may be attributable to differences in species and strains of experimental animals, but may also indicate that hyperplasia of crypts does not necessarily occur during colonic tumorigenesis.

5.2.3.2 FORMATION OF EARLY NEOPLASTIC LESIONS IN THE COLON

By 9 or more weeks after the start of DMH treatment, early neoplastic lesions were observed sporadically in the upper part of the thickened mucosa (Figure

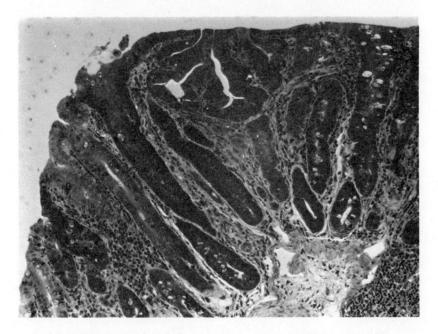

Figure 5.2.4 An early neoplastic lesion in the upper part of the colonic mucosa in a DMH-treated mouse (×160)

5.2.4). Such lesions were identified as adenomatous structures lined with pseudostratified or stratified columnar epithelium without mucous cells. The constituent neoplastic cells were basophilic, had a high nuclear to cytoplasmic ratio and prominent nucleoli, and were capable of proliferation as indicated by mitotic and labelled cells. The number and size of such neoplastic lesions increased with treatment and with time.

Searching for a precursor of the early neoplastic lesion, we observed among the hyperplastic crypts abnormal crypts of various widths (Figures 5.2.5 to 5.2.7).

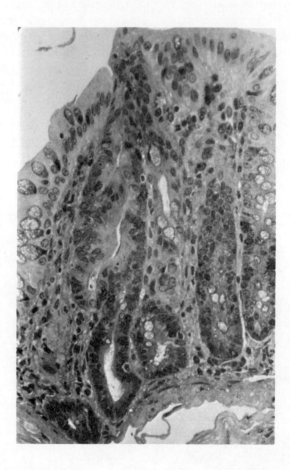

Figure 5.2.5 Abnormal crypt composed of a homogeneous population of basophilic cells with a high nuclear-cytoplasmic ratio. The crypt has increased frequency of labelled cells and becomes tortuous and branched in the upper half (×350)

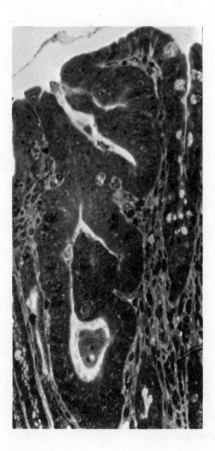

Fig. 5.2.6 Autoradiograph of the upper half of an abnormal crypt showing
tortuosity, irregular foldings of epithelial lining, and labelled cells (×350)

These were isolated and infrequent, possibly due to their transient and
metastable nature. The lining epithelium was mainly simple, but focally
pseudostratified or stratified, especially in the upper part of the crypts. It
consisted of a homogeneous population of cuboidal or columnar basophilic
epithelial cells with a high nuclear to cytoplasmic ratio, but without vacuoles or
mucous droplets. Mucous cells were usually absent, but in a few instances a
single cell or a group of them was seen being extruded into the lumen in the
lower part of the crypt (94), suggesting that transformation from stem cell to
mucous cell might take place there, but that most of these mucous cells were
extruded or died prematurely. The abnormal crypts had an increased number of
labelled cells, distributed not only in the lower part but also in the upper part of

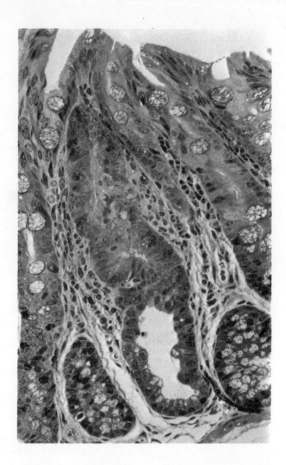

Figure 5.2.7 Autoradiograph of an abnormal crypt with labelled cells
scattered throughout the crypt. Note the tortuosity of the crypt in the upper
half and the dilatation in the lower half ($\times 350$)

the crypt (Figures 5.2.6 and 5.2.7). Most of the abnormal crypts showed
evidence of accumulation of these proliferating, basophilic cells in the upper
part of the crypt, where tortuosity, budding and branching occurred.

Our morphological studies revealed early neoplastic lesions being formed in
the upper part of abnormal crypts. However, the lower half of the corresponding crypts could hardly be identified in most instances, even by serial sectioning
(Figures 5.2.4 and 5.2.8). Ultrastructurally, the constituent cells of the early
neoplastic lesions contained numerous free ribosomes and polysomes, poorly
developed rough endoplasmic reticulum, a rudimentary Golgi complex, and
scattered lysosomes and mitochondria in addition to prominent nucleoli in a

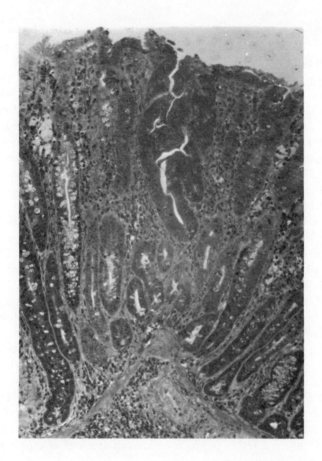

Figure 5.2.8 An early neoplastic lesion in the upper half of the mucosa
following DMH treatment (×160)

relatively large nucleus. Neither vacuoles nor mucous droplets were evident.
These cytological features characterise the undifferentiated stem cells located at
the base of the crypt in normal colon.

On the basis of these findings, we have postulated a hypothesis of two-stage
colonic tumorigenesis (94). In the first stage, a given crypt is repopulated,
following damage by a carcinogen, by a homogeneous population of basophilic
epithelial cells that resemble the undifferentiated stem cells located at the base
of the crypt. These cells are apparently transformed stem cells incapable, or only
partially capable, of phenotypic expression or differentiation. Hence, typical
vacuolated cells, columnar cells, mucous cells and enteroendocrine cells
normally present in the crypt are usually absent from this abnormal crypt. The

transformed stem cells are capable of proliferation as attested by their ability to incorporate ^{3}HTdR. Their descendants migrate normally in the proliferation compartment of the crypt, and repopulate not only the lower part of the crypt but also the upper part. In these aspects, the abnormal crypts differ from the hyperplastic crypts in the colonic mucosa of DMH-treated mice and also from the crypts in the hyperplastic polyps in man. Our morphological observations suggest that the abnormal crypts are probably of transient and metastable nature. Most of them seem to progress to form neoplastic lesions, but the possibility exists that some such crypts revert to normal by differentiation of transformed stem cells or their descendants under certain environmental conditions. If this does occur it is likely to happen before the formation of an aberrant proliferative focus in the upper part of the abnormal crypt.

The second stage begins with the accumulation of the descendants of transformed stem cells in the upper part of the abnormal crypt to form an aberrant proliferative focus from which a neoplasm develops. The detailed mechanism by which the descendants of transformed stem cells form the earliest identifiable neoplastic lesion only in the upper part of the abnormal crypt is not entirely clear. As discussed previously (98) the migration of epithelial cells in the crypt is due mainly to the population pressure created by mitoses in the lower half of the crypt, and the cells stop dividing before migrating out of the crypt onto the surface. In the abnormal crypt, the transformed stem cells and their descendants migrate upwards normally in the lower part of the crypt, but appear to have difficulty in migrating out of the crypt, possibly because of their proliferative activity. Consequently, continued cell division leads to an accumulation of abnormal cells in the upper part of the crypt, forming the earliest identifiable neoplastic lesion. A somewhat similar view has been expressed (390) as a result of studies on serial sections of early adenomatous lesions in familial polyposis.

After such an aberrant proliferative lesion is formed, the descendants of transformed stem cells seem to be unresponsive to the normal negative feedback control and so gain autonomy. Thus the process of neoplastic transformation becomes seemingly irreversible. As more transformed cells are produced in the aberrant lesion in the upper part of the crypt, the cells in the lower part of the crypt become stagnant in their migratory and proliferative activities and undergo degeneration. Hence, the lower part of the crypt in which the neoplastic lesion arises often undergoes cystic degeneration and eventually disappears (94).

Since all the epithelial cells in a crypt are progeny of a stem cell or stem cells located at the base of the crypt (90, 95, 103) the finding that a neoplasm originates in a single crypt is in accord with the view that the newly formed neoplasm is of monoclonal origin. Evidence also indicates that separate neoplasms may be formed in separate crypts concomitantly or sequentially. As neoplasms grow larger, they may form conglomerates and therefore become multiclonal (94).

5.2.3.3 BIOLOGICAL BEHAVIOUR OF COLONIC NEOPLASMS

Sequential examinations of colonic mucosa following initiation of DMH treatment showed that the earliest identifiable neoplastic lesions were first formed in the upper part of the mucosa (Figures 5.2.4 and 5.2.8), and then expanded in various directions (Figure 5.2.9) to produce sessile polypoid lesions (Figure 5.2.10) or discoid ones (Figure 5.2.11), depending upon the local environmental factors. These include the response to the neoplasm of the connective tissue and wandering cells in the lamina propria, the proliferative activity of the neoplastic lesion, and the interaction between the neoplastic lesion and the adjacent non-neoplastic crypts. Presumably due to these factors,

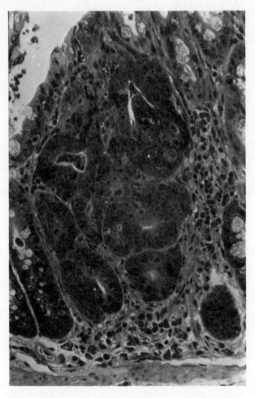

Figure 5.2.9 An expanding neoplastic lesion occupying four-fifths of the mucosa. Note the increased complexity of adenoid structures (×350)

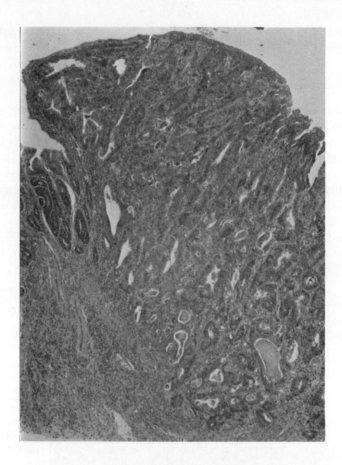

Figure 5.2.10 A sessile polypoid neoplasm occupying the entire thickness of the mucosa, with early invasion through the muscularis mucosae (×56)

individual neoplasms grew at different rates, and the neoplastic lesions were not homogeneous in size, appearance, or progression, even in the same animal. Also, neoplasms possibly arose at different times.

The progression and biological behaviour of neoplasms appeared to be determined by the extent of the local invasion of the subjacent bowel wall. This was associated with cystic degeneration and loss of underlying non-neoplastic crypts (94). The location of the downward leading edge of the most advanced neoplastic lesions was analysed in all the tumour-bearing mice killed at various times after the start of DMH treatment in various experiments (Table 5.2.2). At 9 weeks after initial DMH injection the most advanced lesions were localised in the upper part of the mucosa; at 11 weeks some had extended to the middle

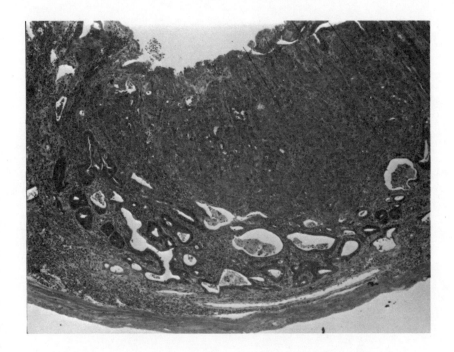

Figure 5.2.11 A discoid neoplasm with cystic changes in the lower portion
of the mucosa (×56)

third of the mucosa; at 18 weeks half of the animals analysed had lesions
extending down to the muscularis mucosae. Penetration of the leading edge of
neoplastic lesions through the muscularis mucosae, an indication of invasion,
was observed in more than two-thirds of treated animals by 25 to 26 weeks
(Figure 5.2.12). In mice killed 28 weeks after initiation of DMH administration 97 percent had colonic neoplasms, and invasive adenocarcinomas were
found in 81 percent of the tumour-bearing animals.

The progression of colonic neoplasms could hardly be correlated with their
histology, because there was a continuous spectrum in the histology of early and
invasive neoplasms. In addition, the progression of early neoplastic lesions to
invasive adenocarcinomas occurred in a short time in the animal model.
Therefore, as several investigators have suggested (456, 549), DMH-induced
colonic neoplasms could be interpreted as being malignant from the outset.

However, the early neoplastic lesions in the upper part of the mucosa grew by
addition of cells through mitosis, and they usually lacked morphological
evidence of invasiveness. Metastasis did not take place when the lesions were
limited to the upper part of the mucosa (488). Only when the neoplasms

Table 5.2.2 Numbers of mice with one or more tumours, and the location of the leading edge of the most advanced tumour per animal, in groups of mice subjected to different periods of DMH administration and killed at different times after the start of treatment

Number of weekly DMH injections	Weeks from start of treatment to examination	Number of mice	Number of tumour-bearing mice	Leading edge of most advanced neoplasm in each tumour-bearing mouse				
				Upper 2/3 of mucosa	Whole mucosa	Submucosa	Muscularis externa	Serosa
9	9	4	4	4	2			
18	18	4	4	2	2			
26	26	4	4		2	2		
26	32	4	4			4		
3	25–26	16	3	1	1	1		
12	25–26	16	16		6	7	2	1
22	25–26	14	14		4	8	2	
11	11–12	32	26	26				
15	28	32	31	1	5	15	3	7

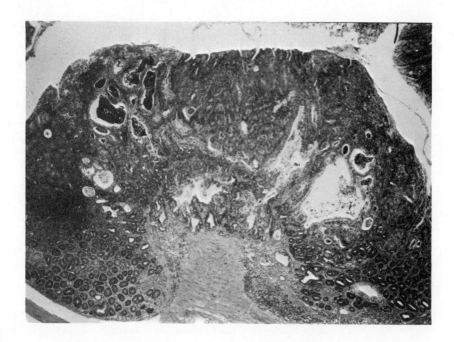

Figure 5.2.12 An adenocarcinoma invading the submucosa. Note the areas
of cystic changes (×35)

reached the deeper part of the mucosa and involved the muscularis mucosae,
were invasiveness and metastasis characteristic of malignant tumours observed
(219, 488). This phenomenon is explicable in that lymphatics are present only
in these areas of the colonic mucosa (219). Some authorities (219, 488) favour
the view that the best criterion of malignancy in the colon is invasion through
the muscularis mucosae, and that neoplastic lesions in the upper part of the
mucosa are benign in their biological behaviour. Such a definition may be too
restrictive, because it excludes carcinoma-in-situ and superficial carcinoma.
However, the latter two disease entities are ill-defined, since the criteria for
their diagnosis are purely morphological and their biological behaviour has not
been clarified.

Even in this animal model for colonic neoplasms, the long-standing problem
of the relations between adenomas (adenomatous polyps) and carcinomas (90,
206, 490, 665) can not yet be settled. Animal experiments have shown,
however, that both adenomatous polyps and adenocarcinomas can be produced
by the same carcinogens (549, 663, 710, 786). This may suggest that they
share the same aetiological factors, but their development appears to be
determined by their local environment. How the local environment influences

the development of benign and malignant neoplasms needs further investigation.

5.2.3.4 CELL PROLIFERATION IN INDUCED COLONIC NEOPLASMS

In DMH-induced colonic neoplasms and their adjacent colonic mucosa, we have analysed the parameters of cell population kinetics using a computer program (439, 440) for the fraction of labelled mitoses (FLM) method (557). The cell cycle parameters were compared with those of three groups of epithelial cells in the crypts of the descending colon of normal mice (97, 98). In this way we sought to relate the cell kinetic behaviour of the normal and neoplastic colonic cells to differentiation of epithelial cells in the crypt, and also to determine if colonic neoplastic cells had any proliferative advantage over non-neoplastic epithelial cells.

For investigation of the relationship between cell kinetic parameters and cell differentiation, epithelial cells in the colonic crypt were divided into three groups (98). *Group I* included vacuolated cells at the base of the crypt, cell positions 1 to 3, which presumably represented the first generation of cells in the vacuolated-columnar cell line, and which were also the presumptive stem cells giving rise to group II and group III cells as well as enteroendocrine cells. *Group II* comprised vacuolated and columnar cells in cell positions 4 and above to the mouth of the crypt, and presumably represented the second and third generations as well as part of the fourth generation of cells in the vacuolated-columnar cell line. *Group III* consisted of all the cells in the crypt identifiable as mucous cells by the presence of intracytoplasmic PAS-positive materials.

According to the computer analysis (Table 5.2.3), these three groups of epithelial cells showed similar cell cycle times (T_c) and also G_1 and S-phase

Table 5.2.3 Cell kinetic parameters of epithelial cells in normal colonic crypts, colonic neoplasms a colonic crypts adjacent to neoplasms

	Vacuolated cells positions 1–3	Vacuolated and columnar cells positions 4+	Mucous cells	Neoplastic cells	Epithelial cells in crypts adjacen to neoplasms
t_G(h)	10.1	10.4	10.1	14.5	18.0
t_s(h)	10.0	9.9	9.8	6.1	7.8
t_{G_2}(h)	1.6	1.1	1.0	1.3	0.9
t_m(h)	1.5	1.8	2.4	1.2	4.8
T_c(h)	23.2	23.2	23.2	23.2	31.5
CV of T_c(%)	23	22	22	48	(35)
I_s(%)	22.4	8.8	5.1	18.2	8.9
I_m(%)	3.0	1.4	1.1	3.0	4.9
I_p(%)	48	19	11	60	33

durations. The G_2-phase was longest in the presumptive stem cells (group I), and became shorter in the differentiating cells (groups II and III). The duration of mitosis appeared to be prolonged as the cells became more differentiated and specialised; it was longest in mucous cells. The proliferative activity, as shown by the labelling and mitotic indices, and the proliferative pool of cells, as shown by the growth fraction, decreased with differentiation of epithelial cells in the colonic crypt.

In DMH-induced colonic neoplasms T_c was similar to that of epithelial cells in normal colonic crypts (97). However, the duration of various phases of the cell cycle varied. Neoplastic cells had a longer G_1-phase (14.5 h versus 10.4 h), a shorter S-phase (6.1 h versus 9.9 h) and a shorter mitotic duration than epithelial cells in normal colon. Similar findings have been reported in other chemically induced tumours (571). The duration of the G_2-phase in neoplastic cells fell between the values of presumptive stem cells (group I) and differentiating cells (groups II and III). This lends support to the hypothesis that colonic neoplastic cells are derived from transformed stem cells defective in cellular differentiation.

Our analysis also revealed that neoplastic cells had a much greater variance for T_c and for t_{G_1} than epithelial cells in normal colon. This indicates a heterogeneity in the proliferative behaviour of neoplastic cells, particularly in the G_1-phase, which is not well understood.

Neoplastic cells had a growth fraction of 60 percent which is larger than for any group of epithelial cells in normal colon, but the proliferative activity of neoplastic cells (as shown by the labelling and mitotic indices) was comparable to that of presumptive stem cells (group I). In spite of this similarity, presumptive stem cells are situated only at the bottom of the crypt, whereas neoplastic cells may be anywhere in the mucosa, submucosa or even muscularis propria depending on the extent of the neoplasm. This may imply a change in the local environment in the development and progression of neoplasms.

Epithelial cells in non-neoplastic colonic crypts located immediately adjacent to neoplasms in tumour-bearing mice behaved differently from other groups (97). In the FLM curve the first wave of the fitted curve was low but peaked, but the second wave became damped and the position of its maximum was thus ill-defined. This implies high variability in cell cycle phase durations, with some cells having a longer cell cycle time. In addition it may be that some cells leave the cell cycle while others are lost by degeneration or exfoliation.

By assuming an arbitrary but reasonable value for the variance of T_c, we were able to estimate the mean T_c as well as other cell cycle parameters for those cells cycling normally. They had a significantly longer T_c than epithelial cells in normal colon or neoplastic cells in induced colonic tumours. This resulted from a longer G_1-phase and a longer mitotic duration. As for the duration of the S-phase, epithelial cells in adjacent mucosa had a value intermediate between that of epithelial cells in normal colon and that of neoplastic cells. The duration of the G_2-phase in these cells was not significantly different from the majority of epithelial cells in the colonic crypt of normal mice represented in group II, but it was significantly different from presumptive stem cells (group I) and neoplastic cells. In addition, they had an unusually high mitotic index (4.9 percent) in comparison to their labelling index (8.9 percent). The estimated duration of mitosis was prolonged to 4.8 h. These findings are, at present, best explained by some kind of mitotic arrest or blockage. Now, if intestinal crypt cells were arrested in metaphase by colchicine for more than 4 h, many of them would degenerate and die (332). Hence, the possibility of mitotic blockage with eventual loss of some of these labelled cells may explain the damped second wave in the FLM curve. The main cause of such mitotic blockage of these cells seems to be a mechanical pressure created by expansion of neoplasms, but a possible role of diffusible substances produced by neoplasms, such as tumour angiogenesis factor (233), collagenase (183), or dipeptidase (690), as well as other factors, cannot be ruled out. If mitotic blockage of cells in the colonic crypt adjacent to neoplasms does occur, this may be one of the mechanisms which facilitate the expansion of neoplasms.

5.2.4 SUMMARY

The pathogenesis and biological behaviour of colonic neoplasms and the associated changes have been investigated in mice given DMH. This animal model has proved very useful in elucidating the early changes of tumorigenesis in the colon.

Hyperplasia of colonic crypts, which occurs in mice following DMH treatment, seems to be a reaction to injuries caused by the carcinogen and does not appear to be directly related to colonic tumorigenesis.

Among hyperplastic crypts, we have observed a few isolated abnormal crypts of transient and metastable nature, which we believe are precursors of neoplastic lesions. Our morphological and cell kinetic data are in favour of the hypothesis that neoplastic cells are derived from transformed stem cells located at the base of the crypt. In contrast to the progeny of normal stem cells in the crypt, the descendants of transformed stem cells are capable of proliferation even though they migrate to the upper part of the crypt, but are incapable or only partially capable of differentiation. With accumulation of these transformed proliferating cells, an early adenomatous neoplastic lesion is first formed in the upper part of an abnormal crypt as an aberrant proliferative focus, and then expands in various directions. From the biological point of view, the downward growth of neoplasms through the muscularis mucosae seems to be a crucial determining factor in the development of malignant behaviour.

ACKNOWLEDGEMENT

Figures 5.2.1, 5.2.5 and 5.2.6 are reproduced from an article in the Journal of the National Cancer Institute (94).

5.3 A Final Common Pathway Promoting Cell Proliferation in Normal and in Neoplastic Intestinal Epithelia

P J M Tutton and D H Barkla

5.3.1 INTRODUCTION

A wide variety of systemic hormones, local hormones and neurotransmitter substances have now been shown to influence the rate of cell proliferation in the epithelium of the jejunal crypt and the colonic crypt and in dimethylhydrazine (DMH)-induced adenocarcinomas of rat colon. Some of the agents that have been shown to influence cell division in rat colonic tumours have now also been shown to have a similar influence on human colonic tumours propagated as xenografts in immune-deprived mice (746).

In the case of the jejunal crypts, where our studies have been most extensive, we have postulated that cell proliferation is controlled by the interaction of a highly localised neural system and a more diffuse endocrine system (734). The neural system, by virtue of its topographical localisation, could adjust crypt cell proliferation to match cell loss in a particular region of the small intestine; this system has been termed the *villous longistat* (735). By contrast, the endocrine regulating system, acting on the entire length of the small intestine, could modulate cell production and hence change villous length to meet the overall nutritional requirements of the organism.

It has been observed that the response to a particular hormone or neuro-transmitter varies markedly between each of the tissues examined. For example, alpha-adrenoceptor agonists promote cell division in jejunal crypts (745) and in colonic crypts, but not in colonic adenocarcinomas (738). Beta-adrenoceptor agonists, on the other hand, inhibit cell proliferation in jejunal crypts (209, 367, 745) and in colonic tumours, but not in colonic crypts (738). Both histamine and serotonin promote cell division in jejunal crypts (731, 732) and colonic tumours, but not in colonic crypts (741, 742). However, prostaglandin F_{2a} stimulates jejunal crypt-cell proliferation, appears not to influence colonic crypts, and inhibits both rat colonic tumours and human colonic tumour xenografts (743).

Cyclic nucleotides have been shown to be intracellular mediators for the action of many hormones and neurotransmitters, and it has been proposed that various cellular responses, including cell division, are regulated by the molar ratio of 3',5-cyclic adenosine monophosphate (cAMP) to 3',5-cyclic guanosine monophosphate (cGMP) within the cell: the *Yin Yang* hypothesis of Goldberg and his colleagues (256, 257). However, perusal of recent literature reveals that, whilst the *Yin Yang* hypothesis may be valid for some cellular responses, a review of the available data for cell proliferation (558) indicates that cAMP may either promote or inhibit this process. This present paper reports the influence of dibutyryl cGMP (db cGMP) on cell proliferation in the jejunal crypt epithelium, the colonic crypt epithelium, and DMH-induced adenocarcinomas of rat colon.

5.3.2 MATERIALS AND METHODS

Colonic adenocarcinomas were induced in rats by weekly injections of DMH for 26 weeks (185). Epithelial cell birth rates were measured using a stathmo-kinetic technique as previously described (736).

5.3.3 RESULTS

Cell proliferation was stimulated by db cGMP in each of the tissues examined. However, DMH-induced adenocarcinomas required a higher dose (2.0 mg per kg compared to 0.02 mg per kg) than did either jejunal or colonic crypts. The birth rates are shown in Table 5.3.1.

Table 5.3.1 Birth rates (cells/1000 cells/h) in three tissues after different doses of db cGMP

Tissue	Control	db cGMP		
		0.02 mg/kg	0.2 mg/kg	2 mg/kg
Jejunal crypts	35	49	89	53
Colonic crypts	24	57	63	35
Colonic adenocarcinoma	25	19	24	61

5.3.4 DISCUSSION

The present results indicate that db cGMP increases the birth rate in each of the tissues examined, but of course do not indicate the kinetic mechanism involved in this process. It is obviously important to establish which phases of the cell cycle, if any, are influenced by agents such as cyclic nucleotides, and whether these agents alter the growth fraction within a tissue. There appear to be no reports on the direct influence of cyclic nucleotides on the cell cycle or growth fraction in the intestinal epithelia. However, the effect on ileal crypt cell proliferation of isoprenaline, a beta-adrenergic agonist whose major pharmacological properties are mediated by cAMP, has been studied using the fraction of labelled mitoses technique (367). The results were analysed using both a graphical method (557) and a computerised technique (693). Using the graphical method of analysis, it was found that isoprenaline increased the duration of the G_1, S, and G_2 phases and was without significant effect on the growth fraction. Computerised analysis, on the other hand, suggested a substantially lower growth fraction in isoprenaline-treated animals and a prolonged cell cycle time caused predominantly by an increase in the duration of the S phase and of mitosis. Reinterpretation of these results (for 28-day-old rats) using another computer model (670) suggested that isoprenaline treatment extended the median cell cycle time from 11.2 h to 14.1 h and that this was attributable to increases in the mean duration of G_1 (by 0.7 h), S (by 1.0 h) and G_2 (by 1.4 h). Subtraction of the median phase durations of G_1, S and G_2 from the median cell cycle time suggests that the mitotic time was also extended (by 0.7 h) in isoprenaline-treated rats. The standard deviations of the durations of G_1 and S were also increased by isoprenaline treatment.

Injection of dibutyryl cyclic nucleotides into intact animals is obviously a very gross approach to the investigation of intracellular mechanisms controlling cell division and, because of the diversity of the effects of cyclic nucleotides on endocrine glands, many artefacts can be envisaged. However, cyclic nucleotides have been demonstrated in the intestinal epithelium using immunocytochemistry (506) and in homogenates of DMH-induced colonic tumours (672) using radioimmunoassay. We have also observed them in colonic mucosa by the latter method. In addition many agents, such as adrenaline, which are known to exert many of their cellular effects via alterations in cyclic nucleotide metabolism, have been shown to influence epithelial cell proliferation. The *Yin Yang* hypothesis of cellular regulation by opposing influences of cAMP and cGMP (in the case of cell division, cGMP activating and cAMP inhibiting) is in part supported by the present data. However, because of the possibility of indirect endocrine influences on cell proliferation, the current report must be interpreted with caution. Future investigations relating cellular cyclic nucleotide levels, under various conditions, to cell proliferation rates may well clarify the situation.

Notwithstanding these reservations, the present results are compatible with our earlier observation that alpha-adrenergic agonists, serotonin, and prostaglandin $F_{2\alpha}$ are able to promote cell proliferation in one or more of the tissues under consideration, since each of these agents has been shown to elevate cGMP levels in other tissues. Alpha-adrenergic agonists have been shown to elevate cGMP in smooth muscle cells (649) and in platelets (258); serotonin has been shown to increase cGMP in lymphocytes (615) and uterine smooth muscle cells (258); and prostaglandin F_{2a} elevates cGMP levels in vascular smooth muscle (189). In addition, beta-adrenergic agonists, known to inhibit cell proliferation in some tissues, have been shown to lower cGMP levels in lung (381) and in smooth muscle (189).

Two obstacles still confront the hypothesis that cGMP represents a common pathway mediating the effects of agents promoting cell division in the tissues examined. These obstacles are, firstly, the observation that histamine, apparently acting through a histamine H_2-receptor, promotes cell division in two of the tissues, and secondly, that prostaglandin F_{2a} inhibits, rather than promotes, cell division in colonic tumours. The effects of histamine H_2-receptor agonists are now generally believed to be mediated by an increase in intracellular cAMP without any change in cGMP levels (122) and hence the influence of histamine on cell proliferation would appear to be an exception to any generalisation regarding the role of cyclic nucleotides in the control of cell division. The evidence that histamine does influence cell proliferation via an H_2- rather than an H_1-receptor appears to be sound. In the case of jejunal crypt-cell proliferation the effect of histamine was blocked by the H_2-receptor antagonist metiamide at a dose of 0.5 mg per kg and was not influenced by the H_1-receptor antagonist mepyramine at a dose of 2.5 mg per kg (732). This dose of mepyramine is nearly 10^6 times the threshold dose for blockade of vascular H_1-receptors in the rat (60). In the case of DMH-induced adenocarcinomas the evidence that histamine acts via an H_2-receptor is even stronger, since the receptor was also activated by dimiprit, at a dose of 0.1 mg per kg. Dimaprit is over 10^6 times more potent for H_2-receptors than for H_1-receptors (191). The recent literature reveals that the relationship between histamine receptors and cyclic nucleotide metabolism is more variable than previously suspected. Whilst in most cases which have been investigated, H_1-receptors are linked to guanylate cyclase and H_2-receptors are linked to adenylate cyclase, a group of H_1-receptors linked to adenylate cyclase have now been described (38) and evidence for two subclasses of H_2-receptors termed H_{2A} and H_{2B} has been presented (213). Thus the possibility that histamine stimulates cell proliferation via an H_2-receptor-cGMP pathway cannot, at present, be totally rejected.

The relationship between prostaglandins and cyclic nucleotide metabolism has been investigated in numerous tissues, and most commonly prostaglandin E_2 stimulates adenylate cyclase, and prostaglandin F_{2a} can interact with the prostaglandin E_2-receptor and thus stimulate adenylate cyclase (379). This is unlikely to be the explanation of inhibition of DMH-induced adenocarcinomas by prostaglandin F_{2a} since prostaglandin E_2 itself was ineffective (743). Further analysis of this issue must await clearer definition of prostaglandin receptors.

If the same group of hormones (biogenic amines) activating the same intracellular 'second messenger' system (guanylate cyclase—cGMP) promote cell division in malignant cells and closely related non-malignant cells, what aspect of the control system is deranged in malignancy? Two possibilities seem particularly worthy of discussion in the present setting. Firstly, the enzyme cyclic nucleotide phosphodiesterase, which is responsible for the degradation of cGMP may be defective, and secondly, the location of guanylate cyclase may be different in malignant cells, allowing persistent inappropriate activation.

At present, there appear to be little data on cGMP-phosphodiesterase and its regulation in malignant cells, and further research in this field is clearly needed. Guanylate cyclase is known to exist in two distinct forms, a particulate membrane-bound form and a soluble cytoplasmic form (363). The colonic carcinogen N-methyl-N'-nitro-N-nitrosoguanidine (MNNG) has been shown to cause a change from particulate to soluble guanylate cyclase in rat colonic mucosa (148). If cytoplasmic rather than surface-membrane-bound guanylate cyclase is to be activated directly by biogenic amines, the cells would need to have an uptake mechanism by which the amines could enter their cytoplasm. It has been shown that inhibition of the enzyme monoamine oxidase, which is responsible for the degradation of intracellular amines such as serotonin, accelerates cell division in DMH-induced colonic tumours but not in jejunal or colonic crypts (737). In addition, the administration of 5,6-dihydroxy-tryptamine, a toxic congener of serotonin, causes rapid onset of cytoplasmic damage in DMH-induced adenocarcinomas but is without effect on the crypt epithelium (739). Thus, there is evidence that, in non-malignant intestinal epithelial cells, proliferation is promoted by hormonal signals acting transiently on surface membrane receptors, the hormones then being cleared in the usual manner. By contrast, in malignant cells, proliferation may be promoted by hormones taken into the cytoplasm where they may not be subject to the normal clearance process and hence may persist and lead to inappropriate cell division.

ACKNOWLEDGEMENT

This work was done during the tenure of a research grant awarded by the Anti-Cancer Council of Victoria.

5.4 Promotion of Intestinal Carcinogenesis by Adaptive Mucosal Hyperplasia

Robin C N Williamson and Ronald A Malt

5.4.1 INTRODUCTION

Several agents which alter intestinal cell kinetics affect the development of colorectal cancer. Bile acids, which have a direct co-carcinogenic action after intrarectal instillation in rats (494), may stimulate the growth of intestinal mucosa (796). Similarly, the microflora of the gut, which reflects dietary intake and may convert bile acids into potential carcinogens (321, 563), also affects intestinal cell turnover (793). The susceptibility of colonic mucosa to cancer in ulcerative colitis (214) may be associated with the increased cell proliferation that accompanies chronic mucosal damage (195).

Subtle kinetic changes leading to the accumulation of dividing cells on the luminal surface of the colon occur in 'premalignant' mucosa, both in patients with polyposis coli and in rats receiving the intestinal carcinogen 1,2-dimethylhydrazine (DMH) (423). A triphasic response can be identified in colon exposed to DMH or related derivatives of cycasin: an immediate toxic effect, followed by mucosal healing, is succeeded after several weeks by hyperplasia and later by the development of neoplasms (510, 736, 833). As in human cancer, benign polypoid adenomas may precede the development of carcinomas (760).

If hyperplasia preconditions the lining of the bowel to neoplastic transformation, intestinal adaptation to surgical stimuli such as partial resection might be expected to enhance the development of cancer in susceptible mucosa. This hypothesis, which could in part account for metachronous colorectal cancers, is supported by our recent finding of increased numbers of colonic tumours induced by DMH in rats having ileal resection (510). The present paper reviews data showing similar promotion of colonic neoplasia by proximal small-bowel resection in animals given the related carcinogen, azoxymethane. Partial enterectomy produces at least a transient hyperplasia of the colonic mucosa (501, 795). Since compensatory hyperplasia of the small bowel is proportional to the loss of functioning mucosa (792), subtotal enteric resection or bypass might cause maximal enhancement of colonic neoplasia. On these grounds, therefore, patients undergoing jejunoileal bypass for obesity might be expected to have an increased risk of developing colonic cancer. In the rat, however, enteric bypass was found to have a protective effect against chemical colonic carcinogenesis.

The distribution of tumours induced by cycasin derivatives might reflect their metabolic pathways. It has been suggested that the proximate carcinogen, methylazoxymethanol, is secreted in the bile following hepatic conjugation and passes in an inactive form through the small bowel to the colon, where bacterial enzymes split the conjugate and release the active agent into the lumen (184, 777). Overloading of the conjugation mechanism might liberate active carcinogen directly into the bile and thus explain the appearance of tumours in the proximal small bowel at higher doses. We have found, however, that distal diversion of papillary secretions before the administration of azoxymethane does not prevent the formation of duodenal tumours, although it does predispose to colonic neoplasia. This shows that the biliary secretion of carcinogenic metabolites is not of overriding importance in the development of upper-small-bowel tumours.

5.4.2 MATERIALS AND METHODS

5.4.2.1 EXPERIMENTAL TECHNIQUES

Male Fischer rats were received into the animal quarters 7 to 10 days before the start of the experiments and weighed between 100 and 170 g at the time of operation. Quarters were lighted in 12 h cycles and animals were housed in groups of 5 in cages with open wiremesh bottoms. Rats were allowed Purina rat chow and water ad lib, apart from the first 24 h after operation, when food was withdrawn.

Operations were performed under light ether anaesthesia. The small bowel was delivered and measured between the ligament of Treitz and the caecum. All intestinal anastomoses were performed with a single layer of continuous 6/0 silk sutures.

Azoxymethane was diluted in sterile water and solutions were stored at $-20\,°C$ until required. Groups of rats received a course of subcutaneous injections of either azoxymethane or vehicle. Animals were weighed weekly and were observed for evidence of intestinal tumours: namely, weight loss, listlessness, abdominal distension or frank rectal bleeding. These features seldom developed within 20 weeks of the first injection of carcinogen.

Rats were killed when moribund or after 30 to 36 weeks. At autopsy the entire intestinal tract was delivered, flushed clean and scrutinised for macroscopic tumours. The remainder of the body, including the ear canals, was also examined for possible tumours. All tumours were charted, measured and stored in 10 percent formalin for histological examination. One paraffin block was prepared from each tumour, and histological sections were cut at 2 or 3 different levels to determine the level of invasion. In certain animals mucosal scrapings were obtained from relevant segments of small bowel and colon and were immediately frozen in liquid nitrogen for subsequent estimation of RNA and DNA, as previously described (see Section 4.4.2.1). In addition, other specimens of intestine not involved by tumour were stored in formalin for histological measurement of villus height and crypt depth (small bowel) or crypt depth alone (large bowel). The internal circumference of the small bowel was measured with a ruler.

Tumours were classified as early neoplastic lesions or adenocarcinomas, depending on invasion of the muscularis mucosae. Early neoplastic lesions included adenomas, foci of mucosal atypia and severe dysplasia or carcinoma-in-situ. Carcinomas were classified according to their dominant histological pattern, whether papillary, tubular or mucinous (colloid). Ear-canal tumours were common at higher doses of azoxymethane, often attaining considerable size and invading the adjacent tissues of the face. These tumours exhibited various histological patterns, including sebaceous adenoma, squamous cell carcinoma and malignant fibrohistiocytoma. Tumours were frequently bilateral and caused bleeding or interfered with feeding.

Statistical analyses comprised Student's t-test for unpaired data, unless otherwise indicated. The χ^2 test, Fisher's exact probability test and the Mann-Whitney U test were also used, as appropriate.

5.4.2.2 PROXIMAL ENTERECTOMY

Seventy-six rats were allocated to one of 4 groups: azoxymethane and resection, azoxymethane alone, vehicle and resection, vehicle alone. Azoxymethane was administered in 16 weekly injections of 10 mg per kg per week. Resection involved removal of the proximal 50 percent of the small bowel 8 to 12 days after the last injection. Intestinal continuity was restored by end-to-end anastomosis immediately distal to the ligament of Treitz. Two contiguous 5-cm segments of bowel were cut from the centre of the resected jejunum for biochemical analysis.

Surviving rats were killed 30 weeks after the start of the experiment and mucosal scrapings were again obtained from 5-cm segments of the ileum and colon in healthy animals. Enteric segments were situated proximal to the ileocaecal valve by 39 to 44 cm (upper ileum) and 11 to 16 cm (lower ileum). Colonic segments were situated distal to the caecum by 3 to 8 cm (right colon) and 14 to 19 cm (left colon). Adjacent specimens were obtained for histological measurements.

5.4.2.3 PANCREATOBILIARY DIVERSION (PBD)

One hundred and fourteen rats were allocated to receive 16 weekly injections of azoxymethane (10 mg per kg per week) or vehicle. Animals from each group underwent PBD immediately before the first injection; controls had no operation. In a further group, PBD was delayed until 10 days after the last injection of azoxymethane. PBD was performed, as previously described (795), by transposition to mid small bowel of a duodenal segment containing the papilla, followed by restoration of duodenal continuity, as in Figure 4.4.1.

Surviving rats were killed at 30 weeks and mucosal scrapings were obtained for assay of RNA and DNA from 5-cm segments of upper and lower ileum and right and left colon as above. In addition, a jejunal specimen was obtained from 94 to 99 cm proximal to the ileocaecal valve. Adjacent specimens were used for histological measurements.

Eight rats from each group (weighing about 300 g) were isolated in individual hanging cages 23 to 26 weeks after the start of the experiment. Faeces were collected daily for 4 days, pooled, homogenised and frozen. Bile acids were later extracted from lyophilised homogenates treated with ethanol, after removal of neutral sterols. Methylated bile acids were subsequently separated from lipids, quantified with steroid dehydrogenase and individually identified by gas–liquid chromatography, as previously described (798).

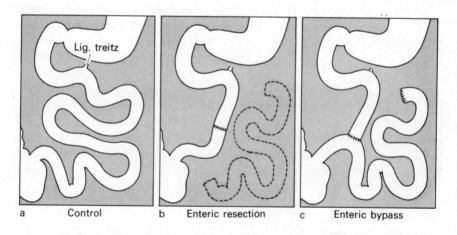

a   Control   b   Enteric resection   c   Enteric bypass

Figure 5.4.1 Schematic representation of the operations of enteric resection and enteric bypass. Subtotal enteric resection entailed removal of between 85 and 90% (75 to 80 cm) of the jejunoileum, leaving 5-cm stumps of jejunum and ileum that were directly anastomosed. In subtotal enteric bypass, between 85 and 90% of the jejuno-ileum was defunctioned as a self-emptying blind loop

5.4.2.4 JEJUNOILEAL BYPASS AND RESECTION

One hundred and forty rats were randomised to one of 3 groups (Figure 5.4.1). Controls had no operation. Subtotal enterectomy was carried out by resection of 85 to 90 percent of the combined jejunoileum, leaving short 5-cm stumps of jejunum and ileum that were united by end-to-end anastomosis. Subtotal enteric bypass was carried out by end-to-side jejunoileal bypass, leaving similar 5-cm segments of jejunum and ileum in circuit, with a long (75 to 80 cm) self-emptying blind loop.

One week after operation animals in each group received the first of 6 weekly injections of azoxymethane (15 mg per kg per week) or vehicle. Surviving rats were killed 36 weeks postoperatively. For morphometric estimations, segments 1 cm in length were cut from the small bowel, 3 cm (terminal ileum) and 35 cm (mid ileum) proximal to the ileocaecal valve; from the large bowel they were cut 3 cm (right colon) and 15 cm (left colon) distal to the caecum.

5.4.3 RESULTS

5.4.3.1 PROXIMAL ENTERECTOMY (797)

Azoxymethane did not affect body weight until the latter stages of the experiment, when tumours developed. Small-bowel resection caused a 10 to 15 percent fall in body weight, followed by a return towards control values. The operative mortality was 15 percent. In all, 14 rats dying before the 24th week were excluded from the statistical analysis, because post-resection hyperplasia seemed unlikely to have had a chance to promote neoplasia within this period (less than 6 weeks after operation). In fact colonic tumours were not encountered until 26 weeks.

Mean values from contiguous jejunal segments obtained at the time of resection (17 to 18 weeks) showed that azoxymethane increased RNA by 27 percent ($p < 0.05$) and DNA by 26 percent ($p < 0.01$) compared with values from rats receiving vehicle alone. No consistent differences between vehicle and carcinogen groups were found at 30 weeks, however. Whatever the nature of the preoperative injections, proximal enterectomy caused substantial elevations of RNA and DNA in ileal mucosa 3 months postoperatively (Table 5.4.1). Moreover, resection significantly increased villous height, crypt depth, and luminal circumference in the ileum at this time, and variable but limited increments in colonic RNA and DNA were seen.

Most rats had at least one small-bowel tumour (Table 5.4.2). This was most commonly an adenocarcinoma of the duodenum, exceeding 5 mm in diameter and arising within 10 mm of the pylorus. In unoperated controls a few jejunal

Table 5.4.1 Nucleic acid contents per 5 cm mucosa in ileum and colon 3 months after 50% proximal small bowel resection (PSBR). Results are mean values for between 8 and 10 rats per group. Values significantly different from controls are indicated by *(p <0.05), **(p <0.01) or ***(p <0.001)

Location	Operation	RNA (mg)		DNA (mg)	
		Vehicle	Carcinogen	Vehicle	Carcinogen
Upper	Control	1.69	1.97	1.54	1.40
Ileum	PSBR	2.98***	2.79***	2.58***	2.73***
Lower	Control	1.55	1.73	1.58	1.40
Ileum	PSBR	2.27***	2.90***	1.93	2.64***
Right	Control	1.50	1.76	1.55	1.47
Colon	PSBR	1.85*	1.88	1.63	1.81*
Left	Control	1.45	1.75	1.38	1.39
Colon	PSBR	1.42	2.09	1.30	2.06***

Table 5.4.2 Mean number of tumours per rat in small and large bowel after 50% proximal small bowel resection (PSBR). Significant differences from controls are indicated as in Table 5.4.1

	Treatment	
Site in bowel	Control (18 rats)	PSBR (16 rats)
Duodenum	1.05	0.56
Anastomosis	—	0.25
Jejunum	0.22	0.00
Ileum	0.11	0.00
Total small intestine	1.38	0.81
Right colon	0.50	1.12
Left colon	1.00	1.37
Recto-sigmoid	0.11	0.43
Total colon	1.61	2.92*
Total bowel	2.99	3.73

tumours were found, usually mucinous cancers, but only two tumours arose more distally in the ileum. Partial resection did not significantly alter the prevalence of enteric tumours, which were confined to the duodenum and to the site of the small-bowel anastomosis.

Proximal enterectomy increased the yield of colonic tumours by 82 percent but did not affect their distribution or size (Table 5.4.2). Papillary and tubular adenocarcinomas predominated in both groups. Mucinous cancers in particular were slightly commoner after enterectomy (p <0.05), and often arose in the ascending colon. About half the tumours occurred in the descending and pelvic colon and the caecum was never affected. Metastases were largely confined to regional lymph nodes and were commoner after resection (63 percent) than in controls (33 percent), but this difference was not statistically significant. Ear-canal tumours were equally common in control and operated groups.

5.4.3.2 PANCREATOBILIARY DIVERSION

After pancreatobiliary diversion (798), an immediate postoperative weight loss of 15 percent was recovered after about 10 weeks in rats given vehicle, but animals with azoxymethane as well as PBD remained 5 to 10 percent lighter than unoperated groups throughout the experiment. All groups receiving carcinogen lost weight slightly in the last 3 to 4 weeks of the experiment when tumours became manifest. The operative mortality rate of PBD varied from 22 to 36 percent, being higher in azoxymethane-treated groups.

Table 5.4.3 Nucleic acid contents per 5 cm mucosa in jejunum, ileum and colon 30 weeks after pancreatobiliary diversion (PBD) to mid small bowel. Results are mean values for between 8 and 10 rats per group. Values significantly different from controls are indicated as in Table 5.4.1

Location	Operation	RNA (mg) Vehicle	RNA (mg) Carcinogen	DNA (mg) Vehicle	DNA (mg) Carcinogen
Jejunum	Control	1.76	2.31	1.57	1.65
	PBD	1.94	1.84	1.46	1.81
Upper Ileum	Control	1.69	1.97	1.54	1.40
	PBD	2.80***	2.70***	2.20**	2.83***
Lower Ileum	Control	1.55	1.73	1.58	1.40
	PBD	2.16***	2.32***	1.76	2.34***
Right Colon	Control	1.50	1.76	1.55	1.47
	PBD	1.94*	1.70	1.75	1.92*
Left Colon	Control	1.45	1.75	1.38	1.39
	PBD	1.63	1.97	1.36	1.81*

Data concerning intestinal adaptation to PBD are summarised in Table 5.4.3. No alterations in RNA and DNA content were detected in jejunal mucosa deprived of pancreatobiliary secretions for 30 weeks. By contrast, ileal contents of nucleic acids were much higher in rats with PBD. Like proximal enterectomy, PBD caused only modest and patchy elevations of these values in the colon. Amounts of RNA and DNA tended to be higher in groups receiving azoxymethane than in the equivalent group receiving vehicle, but only a few of these differences reached statistical significance (798).

Rats showed marked individual variation in the amount and type of bile acids excreted in the faeces, but no quantitative or qualitative differences from unoperated controls could be detected either between 6 and 8 weeks or between 23 and 26 weeks after PBD, nor did azoxymethane have an obvious effect as opposed to vehicle. Deoxycholic acid was the commonest single bile acid in all groups.

Although PBD did not affect the prevalence of tumours in the normal duodenum and jejunum (Table 5.4.4), it did alter their site of predilection

Table 5.4.4 Mean number of tumours per rat in small and large bowel in animals with pancreatobiliary diversion (PBD) performed before or after azoxymethane (AOM). Significant differences from controls are indicated as in Table 5.4.1

| | | Treatment | |
Site in bowel	Control (23 rats)	PBD + AOM (25 rats)	AOM + PBD (10 rats)
Duodenum	0.86	1.08	0.90
Duodenal stump	—	0.92	0.10
Jejunum	0.39	0.12	0.30
Ileum	0.08	0.04	0.10
Total small intestine	1.33	2.16*	1.40
Caecum	0.00	0.36	0.20
Ascending colon	0.26	0.64	0.70
Transverse colon	0.39	0.60	1.10
Descending colon	0.52	1.04	0.50
Recto-sigmoid colon	0.08	0.52	0.20
Total colon	1.25	3.16***	2.70*
Total bowel	2.58	5.32***	4.10*

from the normal juxtapyloric segment to the point of duodenal reanastomosis about 2.5 cm distal to the pylorus. Anastomotic cancers appeared sometimes to be closely related to residual suture material or local diverticula. The total number of small-bowel tumours was increased in rats receiving PBD before the course of azoxymethane, because of a large crop of tumours in the transposed duodenal stump. As in the orthotopic duodenum, tumours in the short papillary segment were mostly congregated at one or other end, in close apposition to suture lines. Ileal tumours were very uncommon in all groups.

PBD increased colonic tumour yields from 1.3 to 3.1 per rat when operation preceded carcinogen and to 2.7 when carcinogen preceded operation (Table 5.4.4). The increased number of tumours was distributed throughout the large bowel, although the caecum was involved only in rats with PBD.

The distribution of different histological types was similar to that in the first experiment and was not specifically affected by PDB, although a modest increase in the number of metastases was observed (798). The prevalence of auditory canal tumours was not affected by operation.

5.4.3.3 JEJUNOILEAL BYPASS AND RESECTION (799)

Operative mortality rates were 16 percent for subtotal enteric bypass and 20 percent for enterectomy; initial weight loss was also slightly greater after resection (20 percent versus 12 percent). Thereafter, rats with resection gained weight more rapidly and appeared healthier than those with bypass. At 36 weeks, rats with bypass weighed 62 percent of unoperated control animals, and rats with resection 79 percent. Azoxymethane did not affect weight gain. During the early postoperative weeks when diarrhoea was profuse, operated animals were voracious and extremely thirsty. The yields of rats surviving 30 weeks were 85 percent (controls), 69 percent (bypass) and 63 percent (resection).

Dilatation and hypertrophy of the functioning stumps of jejunum and ileum contrasted with macroscopic atrophy of the defunctioned loop after jejunoileal bypass. Resection increased villous height in the terminal ileum by 32 percent (p < 0.01). Bypass resulted in more conspicuous changes: an 84 percent increase in villous height (p < 0.001) and a 22 percent increase in crypt depth (p < 0.05). Bypass did not alter significantly these measurements in the defunctioned mid-ileum. Neither operation altered colonic crypt depth at 36 weeks.

The smaller total dose of azoxymethane used in this experiment (90 mg per kg), as compared with the first two experiments (160 mg per kg), resulted in a lower incidence of tumours of the small bowel (Table 5.4.5) and auditory canal in control animals. Tumours were distributed through the small and large bowel as before. Fewer rats developed intestinal tumours after enteric bypass

Table 5.4.5 Mean number of tumours per rat after jejunoileal resection or bypass. Significant differences from controls are indicated as in Table 5.4.1

Site in bowel	Control (22 rats)	Treatment Resection (20 rats)	Bypass (22 rats)
Duodenum	0.13	0.40	0.00
Jejunum	0.09	0.45	0.00
Anastomosis	—	0.50	0.13
Ileum	0.13	0.05	0.05
Total small intestine	0.35	1.40***	0.18
Right colon	0.60	0.46	0.17
Left colon	0.54	0.36	0.09
Rectum	0.22	0.13	0.05
Total colon	1.36	0.95	0.31***
Total bowel	1.71	2.35	0.49***

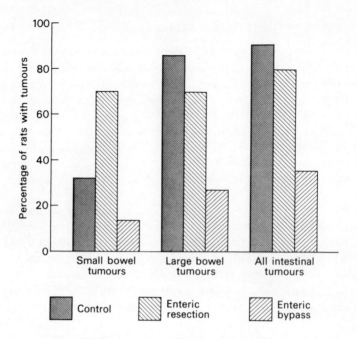

Figure 5.4.2 Percentage of rats with tumours after different operations: There were 22 control rats, 20 rats with jejunoileal resection, and 22 rats with jejuno-ileal bypass. For large bowel and total intestine, frequency of tumours after enteric bypass is significantly lower than after enteric resection (p < 0.01) or than in controls (p < 0.001). For small bowel, frequency of tumours after enteric resection is significantly higher than after enteric bypass (p < 0.001) or than in controls (p < 0.05)

than after either resection or no operation (Figure 5.4.2). Only 4 small-bowel tumours were seen in rats with bypass: 3 at the anastomosis and 1 in the adjacent terminal ileum. Twenty-two control rats had a total of 30 large-bowel tumours. The same number of rats with bypass had 7 tumours.

After enteric resection the number of rats with tumours of either small or large bowel was substantially greater than in those animals in which a similar segment of bowel had merely been defunctioned (Figure 5.4.2). Compared with controls, resection did not affect colorectal tumour yield, but in the small bowel there was an eightfold increase (Table 5.4.5). This increase resulted partly from more duodenojejunal tumours and partly from a large number of tumours arising at the jejunoileal anastomosis. A smaller proportion of tumours was invasive, however. Neither operation altered the number of metastases.

In all three experiments no neoplasms occurred in any of the rats receiving vehicle, although occasional ulcers and suture granulomas were encountered at intestinal anastomoses.

5.4.4 DISCUSSION

Adaptive hyperplasia seems the most plausible explanation for the surgical promotion of intestinal carcinogenesis shown both in these three experiments and in a previous study using ileal resection (510). The compensatory response to partial enterectomy involves the stomach and colon as well as the remaining small bowel, though changes seem to be greatest in adjacent segments (792). Increased cell proliferation has been demonstrated in colonic mucosa during the first month after removal of either proximal, mid or distal small bowel (501, 713, 795). The shortest and least intense response would logically be expected when resection was confined to the jejunum, leaving the ileum to undergo progressive adaptation. Despite one report of increased cell renewal in the colon three months after jejunectomy (838), our present results show only patchy increments in colonic RNA and DNA either three months after proximal small-bowel resection or seven months after pancreatobiliary diversion.

An alternative explanation for the promotion of colonic carcinogenesis by proximal or distal enterectomy, or PBD, could lie in the fact that all three operations bring the large-bowel epithelium closer to the duodenal papilla. With or without bacterial degradation, bile acids might act as carcinogens or co-carcinogens to the colon (321, 494). Increased amounts of bile acids in faeces have been implicated in the promotion of colonic cancer in rats by either cholestyramine, transposition of the bile duct, or high-fat diets (30, 106, 563). Bile-acid excretion is also reported to be higher in patients with colorectal cancer (324, 566). Nonetheless, we have been unable to show any gross alteration in the nature or amount of bile acids excreted in the faeces either six weeks or six months after PBD, though excretion studies admittedly reveal only one aspect of bile-acid metabolism. Presumably larger amounts of bile do enter the colon immediately after operation, but ileal adaptation to jejunectomy (and by inference to PBD) will increase the absorption of bile acids by the distal small bowel (521).

Relatively transient changes in either luminal contents or post-operative growth rates could therefore explain the observed enhancement of colonic carcinogenesis. Yet only adaptive hyperplasia can readily account for the increased tumour yields found in the upper small bowel, proximal to the site of jejunoileal resection. Azoxymethane itself causes hyperplasia before the development of intestinal neoplasia. Compensatory growth may act simply by expanding the population of cells susceptible to malignant transformation. Similar mechanisms could explain increased carcinogenesis in mouse colon rendered hyperplastic by infection with *Citrobacter freundii* (36) and in rat liver after partial hepatectomy (546). Moreover, hypoplasia following faecal diversion inhibits colorectal carcinogenesis, whereas hyperplasia after restoration of colonic continuity promotes the development of tumours (87, 706).

The absence of any enhancement of colorectal carcinogenesis following subtotal loss of functioning small bowel appears at first sight to contradict the theory that adaptive growth promotes bowel cancer. Indeed, jejunoileal bypass actually protects against tumour development throughout the intestinal tract. Although there is some evidence of differential colonic adaptation to enteric resection and bypass (795), changes in body weight seem more likely to explain the discrepancy in tumour yields. Moderate (20 percent) reductions in body weight might prevent the anticipated increase in distal tumours after jejunoileal resection; extreme (40 percent) reductions could explain the substantial decrease in tumours after jejunoileal bypass. Obesity, which increases bile-acid excretion (308), may be commoner in patients with colorectal cancer (825), and starvation profoundly affects epithelial-cell turnover in the large bowel as well as the small bowel (281). Alternatively, bacterial products elaborated in the long blind loop of rats with bypass might conceivably protect the colon by interfering with the local metabolism of carcinogens.

The ileum remains relatively resistent to the induction of tumours in this experimental model, despite surgical stimulation of marked and persistent hyperplasia. Even interposition of ileal segments within the colon fails to render them susceptible to cancer (250). This resistance accords with the peculiar rarity of clinical carcinoma of the ileum and could result from local absence of enzymes capable of catalysing the production of the ultimate carcinogen or from protective immunological mechanisms, since the ileum is a major source of IgA (438). Intestinal tumours induced by a single intraperitoneal injection of N-nitroso-N-butylurea are also confined to the duodenum and jejunum (762), but ileal cancers do develop in large numbers after direct irradiation or intraperitoneal administration of methyl(acetoxymethyl)nitrosamine (509, 761). Carcinoma may also complicate Crohn's disease of the ileum, even after defunctioning ileotransverse anastomosis (214, 265).

Anastomotic suture lines appear to excite adjacent tumour formation whether they are duodenal, duodenoileal or jejunoileal. We have lately shown a similar phenomenon around anastomoses in the transverse colon (706), and chronic irritation from non-absorbable sutures in the caecum also predisposes to local cancer (548). These findings may relate to suture-line 'recurrences' in human colorectal cancer, since desquamated tumour cells are of doubtful viability (591).

Since transposition of the papilla before giving azoxymethane does not reduce the total number of duodenal tumours, the carcinogen must be delivered to the bowel at least in part by the bloodstream. In support, tumours still arise in colonic segments defunctioned by proximal colostomy (87). In fact, rather fewer tumours occur in the juxtapyloric segment after PBD, and the adjacent anastomosis seems to contribute to the overall yields in the duodenum. This observation is consistent with the finding of small amounts of methylazoxymethanol in bile (778) and with the development of gall-bladder cancers in hamsters after administration of cycasin derivatives (659).

5.4.5 SUMMARY

Adaptive growth of the bowel in response to various surgical stimuli has been investigated as a possible promoter of chemical carcinogenesis in rat intestine. Like dimethylhydrazine, azoxymethane causes intestinal hyperplasia before the appearance of macroscopic tumours. Both resection of the proximal half of the small bowel and pancreatobiliary diversion (PBD) to the ileum produce prolonged ileal hyperplasia, but only patchy colonic hyperplasia, 3 to 7 months postoperatively. Despite this adaptive response, neither operation makes the ileum susceptible to azoxymethane carcinogenesis. Proximal enterectomy increases the prevalence of colonic tumours, however, and PBD causes a similar effect, whether operation precedes or follows the course of azoxymethane. In the absence of any qualitative or quantitative change in faecal bile acids after PBD, enhanced colonic carcinogenesis is attributed to transient postoperative hyperplasia. Adaptive growth probably also explains increased numbers of tumours in the residual proximal small bowel after 85 to 90 percent mid-enterectomy. By contrast, end-to-side jejunoileal bypass strongly inhibits the development of intestinal cancers, perhaps because of the profound weight loss associated with this operation. All intestinal anastomoses appear to be favoured sites for tumour formation.

ACKNOWLEDGEMENTS

The original work reviewed in this paper was supported by a grant (CA-17324) from the National Cancer Institute through the National Large Bowel Cancer Project and by the Shriners Burns Institute, Boston Unit. We are grateful to Dr F L R Bauer, Dr J E A Oscarson, Dr J S Ross, Dr O T Terpstra, Dr J B Watkins and Mrs Rebecca Adjoyan for assistance. Original illustrations were kindly supplied by Mr G James, Medical Artist, and Miss Elizabeth Hurst, Superintendent Photographer, of the Department of Medical Illustration, Bristol Royal Infirmary.

5.5 Some Observations on the Effect of Prolonged Asbestos Ingestion on Cell Proliferation in the Intestine of Aged Rats

R E Bolton and D R Appleton

5.5.1 INTRODUCTION

Prolonged exposure to asbestos fibre has been shown to be associated with the development of pulmonary fibrosis and the occurrence of certain forms of cancer. The links between exposure, asbestosis and lung cancer are particularly strong, with cigarette smoking having a synergistic effect on the incidence of tumours (638), and there is also good epidemiological evidence for an association between the development of mesothelioma and a history of asbestos exposure (754). Some studies have reported an increased incidence of gastrointestinal cancers in individuals occupationally exposed to asbestos (448, 639) and, although the risks appear to be less than those associated with the pulmonary and pleural tumours, there is evidence for a threefold increase in incidence among heavily exposed individuals (202). The discovery that water from Lake Superior was polluted with an asbestos-like mineral led to speculation that the ingestion of these fibres might be associated with an increased risk of gastrointestinal cancer in the general population; the realisation that many beverages and drugs contained asbestos fibres (22, 142), and that asbestos cement piping was widely used for water supplies, provided additional impetus for research into the potential hazards of asbestos ingestion. The present study was undertaken as part of that research.

A preliminary report (51) has shown that continuous exposure of rats to ingested asbestos for periods up to one year was not associated with any significant widespread damage or evidence of fibres penetrating the gastrointestinal mucosal tissues, despite the rats being given about 50 000 times the calculated likely human maximum (630); a continuation of the study to 130 weeks has confirmed these findings. However, it is possible that the ingestion of asbestos is associated with subtle changes in cell proliferation of the gastrointestinal mucosa, since force feeding of large amounts of asbestos has been shown to cause a temporary increase in mucosal proliferation as measured by the uptake of tritiated thymidine (22, 23). We shall describe experiments in which we examined mucosa from selected gastrointestinal sites in rats exposed to a more realistic dose regimen of continual asbestos ingestion, which was nevertheless many thousands of times higher than the calculated human maximum ingestion.

5.5.2 MATERIALS AND METHODS

Male Wistar rats, of the AF/HAN strain, ten weeks old at the start of the study, were used throughout. They were housed two per cage and maintained on standard pelleted laboratory diet. Eight treated animals were given free access to a dietary supplement of margarine containing 5 mg amosite asbestos per g. Amosite was chosen because it is most similar to the contaminating fibres in Canadian drinking water, and the UICC standard reference sample was used (572, 716); the asbestos was administered in margarine to prevent the generation of airborne fibres. Five positive control rats received the margarine supplement without amosite, and eight negative controls received only the normal diet. The animals given margarine consumed 50 to 60 g per week, corresponding to between 250 and 300 mg of asbestos fibre for those animals given the margarine-amosite formulation.

The cytokinetic analyses were performed when the animals were 120 weeks old. Two approaches were used; the first procedure involved estimating the amount of tritiated thymidine (^{3}HTdR) incorporated by the gastrointestinal tissues, using liquid scintillation counting (22); the second employed auto-radiography to obtain the pattern of intestinal crypt cell proliferation, and a stathmokinetic determination of the cell birth rate. Animals were injected with either 0.5 μCi ^{3}HTdR per g body weight (three amosite-treated and three negative control), or 1 μg vincristine sulphate per g body weight (five from each treatment group), all injections being performed at 0900 h to try to avoid the effects of diurnal variability in proliferative activity (652). Animals were killed by cervical dislocation 60 minutes after ^{3}HTdR, and 30, 60, 90, 120 and 150 minutes after vincristine.

The upper, mid, and lower small-intestinal tissue samples were taken from the first 10 cm, the region between 35 and 45 cm, and the distal 10 cm respectively, of the excised small intestine. Similarly, the ascending and descending colon samples were taken from the first 5 cm and the region between 15 and 20 cm of the excised colon.

5.5.2.1 DNA EXTRACTION AND ASSAY

Immediately after death the rats given ³HTdR were exsanguinated and samples of glandular stomach, upper, middle and lower small intestine, caecum, ascending and descending colon, liver and spleen were immersed in liquid nitrogen and then stored at −70°C. Subsamples of 100 mg wet weight were used for the assays, care being taken to avoid the Peyer's patches in the samples of small-intestinal tissues, and these subsamples were homogenised in cold 10 percent trichloroacetic acid (TCA) using a motor-driven teflon pestle and glass tubes. After the homogenate had stood over ice for 20 minutes, the precipitate was collected, washed twice with cold 95 percent ethanol and twice with one part ethanol to three parts ether; then it was centrifuged, collected again, resuspended in cold 6 percent TCA, and divided into two equal parts. One half was used for the radioactivity estimations by liquid scintillation counting: the precipitate was recovered from the TCA, and dissolved in 1 N NaOH at 90 °C; then the solution was neutralised with 6 N HCl and bleached with hydrogen peroxide. Duplicate samples of the preparation were mixed with NE260 scintillant and counted at 4 °C after overnight equilibration. Full quench calibrations were prepared, and the activity of the tissue samples expressed as mean disintegrations per minute (dpm). The other half of the precipitate was used for total DNA estimations: it was hydrolysed in 6 percent perchloric acid at 100 °C and triplicate samples of the hydrolysate were analysed using Burton's modification of the diphenylamine assay for DNA (76) with calf thymus DNA standard.

Three 100 mg samples of each tissue were processed for each rat and the mean activities (in dpm per μg DNA) in treated and control groups were compared using analysis of variance.

5.5.2.2 CYTOKINETIC ESTIMATIONS

Tissues from the three small-intestinal sites and from the descending colon were fixed in cold Carnoy's fluid for six hours and embedded in paraffin wax. Histological sections 3 μm thick were stained with Harris's haematoxylin and eosin. For those rats given ³HTdR, autoradiographs were prepared by a dipping technique and exposed for two weeks. From each sample of tissue 100 axially-sectioned crypts were analysed (82, 818) and from transversely sectioned crypts the column count and Tannock's factor (702) were estimated. The product of the mean crypt length and column count was taken to be an estimate of the total number of cells per crypt, and the slope of the line of best fit to the data relating corrected mitotic index to time after vincristine administration (from 30 minutes onward) was multiplied by this total to give an estimate of the crypt cell production rate (CCPR). The cut-off position, at which the average cell begins its final cycle, was also calculated (28, 84).

5.5.3 RESULTS

The animals used for these investigations were 120 weeks old at the time of assay, and as such displayed some of the usual age-associated pathology (72). The renal hypertensive tubular damage frequently described in aged rats was present to some degree in all animals, and those given access to margarine were obese, having a mean body weight of 720 g compared to 510 g for the negative controls, and showed widespread hepatic periportal fatty change. None of the animals had any specific pathological lesion which could be considered to have had a major effect on gastrointestinal cell proliferation.

5.5.3.1 DNA ESTIMATIONS

Table 5.5.1 summarises the results of the DNA estimations for the amosite-

Table 5.5.1 A measure of DNA-synthetic activity in various tissues in amosite-treated and negative control rats. Units are dpm/μg of DNA, and numbers given are the means of triplicate estimates on each of three rats

Tissue	Control	Amosite
Glandular stomach	80	59
Upper small intestine	370	370
Mid small intestine	590	670
Lower small intestine	190	200
Caecum	510	610
Ascending colon	180	180
Descending colon	220	150
Liver	23	37
Spleen	150	180

treated rats and the negative controls. Only in the descending colon are the two counts significantly different ($F_{1,4} = 35.48$; p <0.01), where the treated animals incorporated less labelled thymidine than the controls, suggesting a depression in proliferative activity associated with the ingestion of asbestos and margarine.

5.5.3.2 MORPHOMETRIC AND CYTOKINETIC ESTIMATIONS

Table 5.5.2 summarises the dimensions of the crypts at different sites in those animals used for stathmokinetic experiments; there was one anomaly in that the crypts of the descending colon in the five rats used for labelling index estimation were on average some 10 cells longer than in those which took part

Table 5.5.2 Values of morphometric and cytokinetic variables in the crypts at different sites in the gut of amosite-treated and negative-control 120-week-old rats

	Treatment	Upper small intestine	Mid small intestine	Lower small intestine	Descending colon
Crypt length (cells)	Control	36.0	32.1	31.8	41.8
	Amosite	35.7	32.6	31.4	41.1
Column count	Control	22.0	20.1	21.1	20.8
	Amosite	20.0	20.8	20.4	20.2
Total cells per crypt	Control	790	650	670	870
	Amosite	710	680	640	830
Corrected mitotic index (%)	Control	1.95	2.02	2.06	2.13
	Amosite	2.50	2.21	1.92	1.10
Labelling index (%)	Control	26.9	25.0	27.2	12.5
	Amosite	28.3	26.8	25.2	8.7
CCPR (cells/crypt/h)	Control	39	26	28	24
	Amosite	40	45	22	13

in the stathmokinetic experiment. There were no significant differences in crypt size at any site between control and treated rats. The table also shows the mitotic and labelling indices for the whole crypt, and the cell birth rate; the only consistent difference is the apparently decreased proliferative activity in the descending colon of the treated rats. Figure 5.5.1 illustrates the labelling index at each cell position at that site in the two groups.

Table 5.5.3 gives further data for the descending colon, and includes results for the margarine-fed controls; also presented are comparative results for 12 week old rats (688). Because of the small numbers of animals available, the birth rate estimates have rather large standard errors, being some 25 percent of

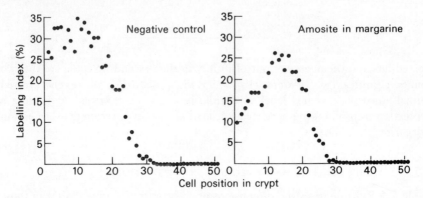

Figure 5.5.1 Labelling index distributions in the descending colon of (a) control rats and (b) rats given amosite in margarine supplement

Table 5.5.3 A comparison of variables in the descending colon of differently treated 120-week-old rats and 12-week controls (688). Cell cycle times are based on a constant growth fraction estimate of 0.34 (688)

Treatment	Crypt length (cells)	Cut-off position	Birth rate (cells/crypt/h)	Cell cycle time (h)
Amosite in margarine	41	11	13	23
Margarine-fed controls	39	10	9	29
Negative controls	42	8	24	12
12-week controls	42	11	7	34

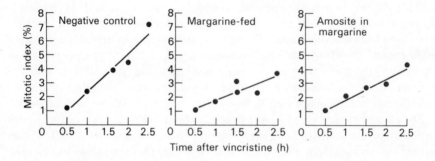

Figure 5.5.2 Mitotic accumulation data after vincristine administration in the descending colon of (a) rats given a normal diet, (b) rats given margarine supplement, and (c) rats given amosite in margarine supplement

the estimates themselves; Figure 5.5.2 shows the metaphase accumulation data which gave rise to them.

5.5.4 DISCUSSION

There was no clear-cut effect of prolonged ingestion of asbestos on cell proliferation in the rat intestine. The findings of the DNA extractions and the cytokinetic analyses were similar, confirming that bulk estimation of the extent of DNA synthesis can provide useful information on proliferative activity. It is interesting that both techniques showed a depression in activity in the descending colon of amosite-treated animals compared to negative controls, but further comparison with margarine-fed controls suggests that this is more likely to be associated with the high intake of margarine than with asbestos fibre ingestion; indeed it is the high cell birth rate in the negative-control rats which is difficult to explain, as it is considerably in excess of that found in younger animals (see Table 5.5.3). It is not clear whether a depressive effect of a high fat diet should be attributed to reduction in cell attrition arising from changes in food transit time, to the composition of either the luminal contents or the intestinal flora, or alternatively to some direct regulatory influence as yet unknown.

Although ingestion of asbestos has been shown to be associated with an increase in gastrointestinal DNA synthesis (22, 23, 347, 348), these findings were concerned with the effects of a challenge with massive doses of the more toxic chrysotile form of asbestos, and may be attributable to a combination of cytotoxicity and the sort of alteration to regulatory mechanisms of proliferation which is known to occur in response to such non-specific stimuli as changes in intestinal flora (2) or secretions (7), starvation and refeeding (18, 110), parasitic infection (431) and diet (409). If one may draw such conclusions from animal experiments, the absence of any adverse effect of amosite ingestion previously reported (51), taken with our current findings, suggests that low levels of asbestos fibre contamination in food, beverages, and drinking water are unlikely to have any major significance for the health of the general population.

The present studies are of a more general interest for their observations on the proliferative characteristics of gastrointestinal tissues of aged rats as such. Under normal circumstances the male SPF Wistar rat of the HAN strain may live for up to three years, with 80 percent mortality occurring by about 130 weeks. The animals used in this study were 120 weeks old and therefore represent a survivor population of aged animals. A detailed description of the morbidity and mortality of the animals exposed to chronic asbestos ingestion will be the subject of a future paper.

It has been suggested that intestinal proliferative homeostasis is less effective in aged mice and that proliferative activity is reduced as a result of a decrease in the size of the proliferation compartment in the crypt (241, 414). A study of rats at several ages up to a year old (116) demonstrated an increase with age in the ratio of crypts to villi, but little change within the crypts themselves. A comparison of our results in the descending colon shows that there is probably little change in the size of the crypt, and leaves us uncertain about how age affects crypt cell production rate. In the small intestine the picture is clearer: we may compare our results (Table 5.5.2) with those previously published (6, 814, 818) for rat jejunum. Our crypt length and column count are not far from the 32.9 and 22.3 cells respectively given in these reports, and our corrected mitotic index, labelling index and crypt cell production rate are all rather less than the respective values of 3.1 percent and 57 cells per crypt per hour for three-month-old animals. This is consistent with a decrease in the size of the proliferation compartment in the aged rats: in fact the cell position at which the labelling index is half of its maximum is some three or four positions lower in the crypt than for younger rats, implying a cut-off position a cell or two lower. However, assuming a cell cycle time of 10.9 h over the relevant part of the crypt (6) we can estimate the cut-off to occur at cell position 12 from data on all three small-intestinal sites in the aged amosite-treated and control rats, and at position 11 in three-month-old animals. It therefore remains a possibility that the cell cycle time in the older rats is longer; but if this is not to result in an upward movement of the position of half-maximum labelling index it must be brought about by an increase in the duration of G_2.

We do not consider that we have enough data to assert that G_2 is indeed increased, but comparison of the phase duration in the same strain of rats of different ages by a single worker would be of interest.

ACKNOWLEDGEMENTS

We would like to thank Professor Sir Alastair Currie and Dr D Lamb for the use of the facilities of the Pathology Department of the University of Edinburgh. Thanks are also due to Dr N A Wright for his helpful suggestions in the earlier phase of this work.

SECTION 6

NORMAL AND DISEASED STATES IN MAN

6.1 Measurements of Cell Proliferation and Associated Risk Factors in the Identification of Population Groups with Increased Susceptibility to Colonic Cancer

Martin Lipkin

6.1.1 INTRODUCTION

In recent years several new approaches to the control of large-bowel neoplasia have been proposed. These include attempts to improve the early identification of population groups at increased risk for colorectal cancer, and associated studies of environmental and physiological elements believed to contribute to its pathogenesis. In parallel studies, methods of intervention in high risk groups have been started, and attempts to halt the progression of colorectal neoplasms have been initiated.

Early studies of cell proliferation in the gastrointestinal tract of man have made these new approaches possible, because of their delineation of the normal cell cycle parameters and the boundaries of the proliferation and maturation compartments of cells within the gastrointestinal mucosa. An example of tritiated thymidine (^{3}HTdR)-labelling of epithelial cells in the colonic crypts of man is shown in Figure 6.1.1; Figure 6.1.2 illustrates distributions of labelled cells in human colonic crypts which give indications of the boundaries of the proliferation and maturation compartments; and Figure 6.1.3 shows a fraction of labelled mitoses (FLM) curve from which the cell cycle parameters were estimated. We have recently reviewed these findings (156) and the relevant data are summarised in Table 6.1.1.

These techniques have now been applied to the study of high risk groups, and have led to the identification of predisposing factors before the appearance of clinically detectable lesions, or during early growth of benign and malignant neoplasms. Known high risk groups are enumerated in Table 6.1.2 and our recent approaches attempting to identify useful determinants in some of these groups are summarised in Table 6.1.3.

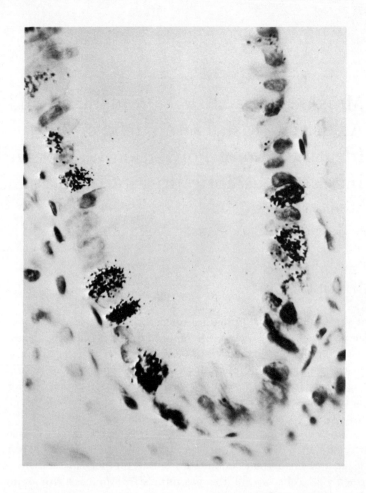

Figure 6.1.1(a) Autoradiograph showing labelled DNA in the human colonic crypt 2 h after injection of ³HTdR (Haematoxylin & eosin × 400)

6.1.2 DISEASES WITH AN HEREDITARY PREDISPOSITION TO COLORECTAL CANCER

6.1.2.1 FAMILIAL POLYPOSIS (INHERITED ADENOMATOSIS OF THE COLON AND RECTUM)

Cases of intestinal polyposis have been recorded for 250 years, and more recently several subgroups have been delineated. There are several recent reviews (14, 77, 488, 751).

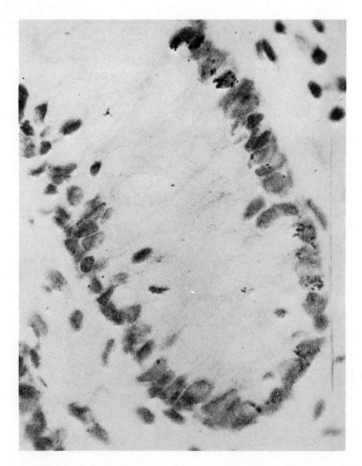

Figure 6.1.1(b) Autoradiograph showing labelled DNA in the human
colonic crypt 8 days after injection of ³HTdR (H & E × 400)

It is now clear that the disease is inherited as an autosomal dominant genetic
defect, expressed phenotypically about 80 percent of the time. While there
appears to be general agreement that classical familial polyposis is due to a
single dominant gene, the genetics of sporadic cases and the various associated
syndromes is more controversial. Some believe that sporadic cases can be
explained by new mutations, but others argue that this is true of only a small
proportion. It has also been suggested that environmental modification would
render the inheritance and expression of the disease virtually polygenic.

Analysis of age at onset of disease has proved important in the identification
of familial polyposis and other diseases where familial predisposition increases
the risk of colorectal cancer. In Figure 6.1.4 the cumulative distributions of age

Table 6.1.1 Summary of proliferative parameters in the gastrointestinal tract of man (156)

a. Gastric mucosa

Type of tissue	$I_s(\%)$	$I_m(\%)$	$t_{G_1}(h)$	$t_s(h)$	$t_{G_2}(h)$	$T_c(h)$
Normal cardia	13.1	1.3				
Normal fundus	4.2–14.0	0.8–1.0	62	7–10	1–4	48.72
Normal antrum	12.8–15.2	1.4		16	1–6	>30
Fundus in atrophic gastritis	14–19					
Antrum in atrophic gastritis	12.9	2.9				
Cardia in gastric cancer	20.1	2.1				
Fundus in gastric cancer	13.4					
Antrum in gastric cancer	16.2					
Zollinger-Ellison Syndrome	15.7	0.8	36	6	1	45

b. Small intestine

Type of tissue	$I_m(\%)$	$t_{G_1}(h)$	$t_s(h)$	$t_{G_2}(h)$	$t_m(h)$	$T_c(h)$	$I_p(\%)$
Normal duodenum	2.36				1.1	48–54	83
Normal jejunum				1.5	1.1	42–48	
Ileal conduit		22	11	1–2	1	24–36	
Duodenum-jejunum with ileal conduit	5.1				1.3–1.5	21–22	61
Small intestine in sprue	5.2						55

c. Large intestine

Type of tissue	$I_s(\%)$	$I_m(\%)$	$t_{G_1}(h)$	$t_s(h)$	$t_{G_2}(h)$	$t_m(h)$	$T_c(h)$	Turnover time (h)
Normal colon (in vivo)	12–18		14	11–20	1–6	1	40	72–96
Normal rectum (in vivo)	18–25			9–14	2		24–48	96–192
Normal rectum (in vivo)	1–17			7–11			77–90	58–87
Colon in active ulcerative colitis	26			9.2				34
Colon in remitted ulcerative colitis	7							
Adenoma { rectum (in vitro)	23			7.4–12.0				32
rectum (in vivo)	2			15				>40
Carcinoma (in vivo)	13–23	1.1–2.9		14				26–244
Carcinoma (in vitro)	4–32	0.3–2.8		19				30–177

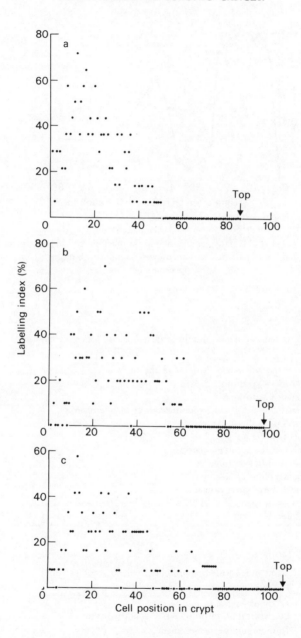

Figure 6.1.2 Labelling index distributions in human colorectal crypts after injection of 20–200 μCi/kg ^{3}HTdR; (a, b) colon after 30 min, (c) rectum after 1 h

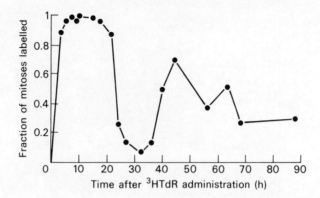

Figure 6.1.3 FLM data for histologically normal colonic tissue of a 50-year-old male patient. Specimens were obtained through a colostomy opening site

Table 6.1.2 Population groups at increased risk for colorectal cancer

Familial polyposis syndromes:
   Inherited adenomatosis of colon and rectum
   Gardner's syndrome
   Turcot's syndrome
Previous colonic, breast, endometrial, or bladder cancer
Site-specific colonic cancer
Woolf syndrome
Hereditary adenocarcinomatosis
Cancer family syndrome
Sporadic colorectal adenomas
Inflammatory bowel disease
Residence in geographical areas having high frequencies of
   colorectal cancer

Table 6.1.3 Recent approaches to identification of high risk groups

Study of environmental factors
Quantification of proliferative abnormalities
Immunological measurements
Study of cutaneous cells
Study of nuclear protein and enzyme alterations
Examination of faecal contents
Haemoccult, radiological and endoscopic studies

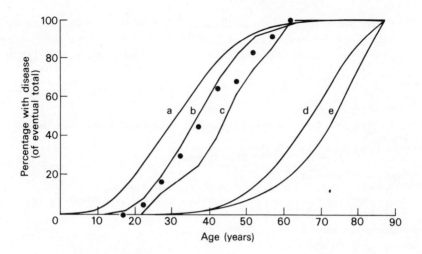

Figure 6.1.4 Distributions of age of onset as cumulative percentages of all those contracting (a) nonmalignant polyposis; or (b) colonic cancer in individuals with familial polyposis; and (c) colon-cancer-prone individuals without polyposis. Curves (d) and (e) show the corresponding data for colorectal cancer in the general population of the USA and Japan respectively. The points are also for colonic cancer in familial polyposis. More details on these cases are available (429)

at onset of familial polyposis and subsequent colonic cancer are shown, and comparisons made with other population groups. From these data the magnitude of increased risk at every age can be estimated.

6.1.2.2 GARDNER'S SYNDROME

This disease is a variant of familial polyposis, an autosomal dominant disorder showing a high degree of penetrance. Adenomatous polyps are formed in the colon, and occasionally in the small intestine, and have a propensity for development of adenocarcinoma. The syndrome is now recognised on the basis of characteristic clinical findings, and has an estimated incidence of 1 in 14 000 births, a lower incidence than that of familial polyposis.

Adenomatosis of the large intestine, multiple osteomas of the skull and mandible, multiple epidermoid cysts and soft tissue tumours of the skin were the features reported by Gardner in 1951 (248). Other possible associated lesions include carcinoma of the thyroid, the adrenal glands, the ampulla of Vater, and the duodenum; adenomas and carcinoid tumours of the small intestine; in-situ carcinoma of the gall bladder; tumours of the central nervous system; and lymphoid polyps of the ileum.

Gene expression is variable, with some individuals having the various manifestations of the major triad of Gardner's syndrome, while others have intestinal neoplasms alone. Periampullary carcinomas have been reported in the recent literature.

Table 6.1.4 Phenotypic characteristics recently reported in population groups at increased risk for colorectal cancer

Phenotypic characteristic

1. Colonic epithelial cells—
    (a) Adenomatous morphology leading to adenoma-cancer sequence
    (b) Abnormal proliferation of cells in individuals with familial polyposis and Gardner's syndrome
2. Extraintestinal neoplasms
3. Immunological abnormality—
    Inappropriate suppression of normal lymphocyte response to allogeneic stimulus in non-polyposis familial aggregates and in individuals with Gardner's syndrome
4. Cutaneous cells—
    (a) Heteroploidy of cutaneous epithelial cells in individuals with Gardner's syndrome
    (b) Modifications in the growth of cutaneous fibroblasts in familial polyposis and Gardner's syndrome
5. Faecal contents—
    (a) Decreased faecal degradation of cholesterol in familial polyposis and in some individuals in the general population
    (b) Conversion of bile acids and cholesterol by faecal microflora, and modifications of faecal bacterial enzyme activities
    (c) Mutagen activity in faeces of human subjects in the general population
    (d) Conversion of nitrogenous compounds to nitrosamines with carcinogenic activity

6.1.2.3 TURCOT'S SYNDROME

This disease has been described as polyposis coli associated with malignant tumours of the central nervous system (727). Two family members, a boy and a girl with polyposis, died with medulloblastoma of the spinal cord and a cerebral tumour respectively. Several other similar instances have been reported, and may be examples of tumour association as found in Gardner's syndrome.

6.1.3 APPROACHES TO EARLY IDENTIFICATION OF HIGH-RISK GROUPS

Recent approaches to the early identification of high risk groups have been carried out mainly on familial aggregates with an hereditary predisposition to cancer, and on individuals in the general population residing in regions having high and low incidences of colorectal neoplasia. Phenotypic characteristics recently reported in population groups at increased risk for colorectal cancer are summarised in Table 6.1.4, and are discussed in the following sections.

6.1.3.1 PROLIFERATIVE ABNORMALITIES IN COLONIC EPITHELIAL CELLS OF INDIVIDUALS WITH FAMILIAL POLYPOSIS

Studies of cell proliferation have aided our understanding of events that occur during neoplastic transformation of colonic cells, both in the hereditary diseases leading to large bowel cancer and in the sporadic large bowel cancers believed to be caused mainly by environmental or endogenously produced carcinogens. In familial polyposis, colonic epithelial cells predestined to develop neoplasia show characteristic proliferative changes. During progressive stages of abnormal development, epithelial cell phenotypes appear which have gained an increased ability to proliferate and to accumulate in the mucosa (49, 126, 153, 154, 345, 424, 747).

In the normal colon of man, the major proliferative activity occurs in the lower and mid-regions of the crypts, occupying about three-quarters of the crypt columns. Approximately 15 to 20 percent of the proliferating cells are engaged in DNA synthesis at any given time. The number of cells in the proliferative cycle diminishes as they advance to the luminal region of the crypts; within hours these cells undergo further differentiation and proliferative activity ceases as they approach the mucosal surface.

In individuals with familial polyposis, patches of flat (apparently normal) mucosa can be detected having colonic epithelial cells that fail to repress DNA synthesis during migration up the crypt, a finding which has been observed in normal-appearing colonic epithelial cells before as well as after the development of adenomatous lesions. This feature has been noted in 80 percent of random biopsy specimens from such patients (424), occuring with a higher frequency than in the general population.

Current observations in our laboratory also indicate a significantly higher frequency of abnormal proliferative activity of this type in colon-cancer-prone families without familial polyposis; these and other data are summarised in Table 6.1.5 (see Section 6.5). We are continuing to quantify several proliferative abnormalities as they are observed in colonic mucosae of high and low risk population groups, to determine better their discriminatory value in population groups in different geographical regions.

Failure of colonic epithelial cells to repress DNA synthesis in the normal manner also occurs in other diseases, including ulcerative colitis (195). Likewise, in atrophic gastritis, a condition associated with the development of gastric malignancy, epithelial cells fail to repress DNA synthesis and undergo

Table 6.1.5 Labelling distribution—percentage of labelled cells in the upper third of colonic crypts in normal appearing mucosa

Population group	Number of individuals	Ratio of mean labelling index in the upper third of the crypt to that found in a control group
Control group	13	1.0
Cancer free family	26	1.9
Primary colonic cancer	13	1.8
Familial polyposis		
Symptomatic	18	3.2
Asymptomatic	8	4.0
Colon-cancer-prone individuals		
Symptomatic	8	4.1
50 percent risk	23	4.1

abnormal maturation as they migrate (162, 803). A similar phenomenon occurs in precancerous disease of the cervix uteri in human beings (789), and in the cervix of rodents after exposure to a chemical carcinogen (302). Thus, during the development of neoplasms in other organs as well as in the colon, persistent DNA synthesis occurs in cells that normally would be terminal or end cells. Associated pathological changes accompany this development leading to atypias, dysplasias and malignancies, as also occurs in familial polyposis.

In familial polyposis, as colonic epithelial cells which do not repress proliferative activity undergo abnormal maturation and accumulate in the mucosa, they develop the morphological changes characteristic of adenomas; these further develop tubular or villous structures. In terms of cell proliferation we have estimated that most epithelial cells in these adenomas are extruded, while only a minor fraction are retained (420). The distribution of labelled cells in adenomas of man is shown in Figure 6.1.5. Carcinomas develop with increasing frequency as these adenomas enlarge (390).

The sequence of events believed to lead to malignancy can be summarised as follows. Cells having the germinal mutation fail to repress DNA synthesis (phase 1 proliferative lesion) (423). Additional events then occur, giving rise to new clones from the original cell population. An early event leads to the development of the adenomatous cells that proliferate and accumulate near the surface of the mucosa (phase 2 proliferative lesion) (423). In familial polyposis, according to this concept, a further event then occurs in the cells, giving rise to invasive malignancy. This concept of a sequence of events allows for a contribution of endogenous or exogenous carcinogenic or promotor elements to interact with the cells having an hereditary predisposition to neoplasia. It also provides a theoretical basis for the introduction of preventive measures to block the steps leading to malignant transformation of cells.

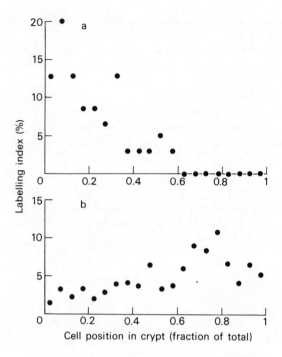

Figure 6.1.5 Labelling index distributions in (a) normal colonic mucosa and (b) adenomas from an individual with inherited adenomatosis of colon and rectum

6.1.3.2 CARCINO-EMBRYONIC ANTIGEN IN COLONIC LAVAGE OF INDIVIDUALS FROM HIGH-RISK GROUPS

Although plasma carcino-embryonic antigen (CEA) has been disappointing as an indicator of early lesions, increased CEA has been noted in colonic lavage specimens obtained from members of polyposis family aggregates. The CEA concentrations in individuals with large adenomas and cancer are elevated compared to those in individuals without evidence of colonic disease. We have measured CEA concentrations in colonic lavage specimens from hereditary polyposis families, nonpolyposis colon-cancer-prone families, and individuals without evidence of colonic disease or familial predispositions to colonic cancer. Our findings indicate an elevation of CEA in many individuals in familial polyposis aggregates who do not have visible adenomas (528), as summarised in Table 6.1.7. The reasons for this elevation are unknown at present, but it may be associated with early hyperplasia or inflammation.

Table 6.1.6 Similarities between characteristics of colorectal neoplasms induced in rodents by chemical carcinogens, and those found in man

1. Production of atypias, hyperplasias, adenomatous polyps, metaplasias and carcinomas
2. Expansion of the proliferation compartment in colonic crypts, with proliferating epithelial cells reaching the crypt surface
3. Proliferation of neoplastic epithelial cells near the surfaces of expanding colonic neoplasms
4. Modifications of the cell cycle of epithelial cells
5. More rapid growth of small nodules than of larger tumours
6. Ability to induce colonic neoplasms with dominant pattern of inheritance

Table 6.1.7 Carcino-embryonic antigen (CEA) in colonic lavage of individuals in familial polyposis and familial colonic cancer aggregates. ***indicates $p < 0.001$ compared to controls

Group	Number of individuals	Mean CEA (pg/mgp)
Familial polyposis		
affected	8	1.6
potential	14	2.0***
Familial colonic cancer		
affected	5	0.3
50% risk	19	1.2
Controls	17	0.4

6.1.3.3 STUDIES OF CUTANEOUS CELLS OF INDIVIDUALS WITH FAMILIAL POLYPOSIS

Recent studies have indicated that phenotypic expressions of the genetic defect leading to familial polyposis can be detected in cutaneous cells. Increased heteroploidy in cutaneous epithelial cells derived from individuals with Gardner's syndrome has been reported (144). It was also noted that cutaneous fibroblasts derived from individuals previously diagnosed as having familial polyposis or Gardner's syndrome have abnormal growth characteristics (522). Recent studies have shown differences from normal in the distribution of the cytoskeletal protein actin within cultured cells from individuals with familial polyposis (377). In order to determine the specificity of these observations additional measurements are presently being carried out on cutaneous cells from larger groups of individuals known to have a low risk of colorectal cancer, and from families with various patterns of inherited polyposis and large bowel cancer.

6.1.3.4 IMMUNOLOGICAL STUDIES

An immunological abnormality has recently been reported in individuals from colon-cancer-prone families without polyposis (42). When cell-mediated immunity in cancer-free individuals was studied, 44 percent demonstrated an apparent perturbation of adherent-cell function which manifested itself as an inappropriate suppression of the normal lymphocyte response to an allogeneic stimulus. This in-vitro defect in recognitive immunity was the same as that demonstrated in individuals with established malignancies; several patients with Gardner's syndrome showed the same defect (42). These studies are being extended to asymptomatic individuals in additional familial aggregates having the various disorders leading to large bowel cancer, and offer the possibility of a new, immunological approach to the early detection of susceptible population groups.

6.1.3.5 EXAMINATION OF FAECAL CONTENTS

In familial polyposis and related disorders, studies are in progress to identify those constituents of faecal contents that may be abnormal, and to examine their potential carcinogenic activity on colonic cells. The bile acids and their bacterial conversion products are a group of compounds currently under examination. Several recent reports have analysed and compared the faecal neutral steroids and bile acids in patients with familial polyposis and in controls other than relatives (182, 560, 767, 791). Individuals with familial polyposis excreted more cholesterol and less of its degradation products, coprostanol and coprostanone. The results of one of these studies is shown in Table 6.1.7. Non-degradation of cholesterol has also been found in a few individuals in the general population, whose background and related characteristics have not been defined (791).

Table 6.1.8 Faecal neutral sterols in patients with familial polyposis, relatives of patients, and controls consuming a mixed western diet

	Patients with familial polyposis (8)	Relatives of patients (controls) (10)	Controls (10)
Neutral sterols (mg/g dry weight of faeces)			
Cholesterol	11.9	1.5	1.2
Coprostanol	2.2	13.4	14.7
Coprostanone	0.5	2.5	2.1
Total	14.6 ± 1.4	17.4 ± 2.8	18.0 ± 1.8

Current results have suggested differences in metabolic activity of faecal microflora in members of familial polyposis aggregates, compared to controls matched for age and sex, who consumed similar western-style diets. These differences have previously been shown in population groups at increased risk for large bowel neoplasia. Further studies are in progress to extend these findings to individuals in the familial colon-cancer-prone groups in order to assess the utility of these variations in the metabolic activity of faecal microflora and in the excretion of cholesterol and its metabolites. Findings of this type may contribute to the screening of siblings in polyposis families, and could point to mechanisms of initiation or promotion of large bowel carcinogenesis.

An additional and potentially important lead to the identification of factors involved in the development of colonic cancer was provided by detection of mutagenic activity in the faeces of human beings (388, 748). It was suspected that a nitroso-group exchange reaction occurred by transfer from nitrosamine to an amide moiety, resulting in the generation of highly reactive nitrosamide compounds in faeces (449), and that endogenous nitrites might lead to formation of carcinogens (701). Patients in the familial polyposis and hereditary colon-cancer-prone (non-polyposis) aggregates are under study; this topic remains an interesting one for further development. We now have a variety of approaches to the analysis of faecal contents of individuals in high and low risk categories.

6.1.3.6 INDUCTION BY CARCINOGEN OF PROLIFERATIVE AND PATHOLOGICAL CHANGES IN COLONIC MUCOSA

Comprehensive analyses of proliferative and pathological changes induced in the colonic epithelial cells by chemical carcinogens have been carried out, revealing similar abnormalities to those observed in man. Rodent strains have different susceptibilities to the induction of colonic cancer, as occurs among human beings. In rodents the cell transformations can be induced by 1,2-dimethylhydrazine (DMH), methylazoxymethanol (MAM), N-methyl-N'-nitro-N-nitrosoguanidine (MNNG), and N-methyl-N-nitrosourea (MNU) (94, 157, 159, 362, 710). A main site of activity is the distal colon, as in man. In mice multifocal tumours, ranging from adenomatous polyps to metaplasias and carcinomas, grow from the mucosa and then protrude into the sigmoid colon and rectum. Early focal atypias and hyperplasias located mainly on the mucosal folds, adenomatous polyps, and carcinomas appear to be part of the progressive pathological changes which develop in mice and rats following DMH administration. These changes are accompanied by an increased proliferative activity in the cells. DMH and MNNG both induce an extension of the proliferation zone of the flat mucosa toward the surface (Figure 6.1.6).

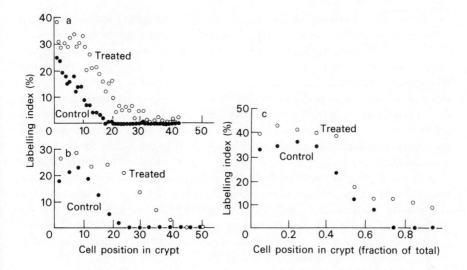

Figure 6.1.6 Labelling index distributions in (a) mice treated for 87 days with weekly injections of DMH, (b) mice 125 days after the start of weekly injections of DMH (94), and (c) rats given intrarectal installation of MNNG (362)

Thus, some of the colonic epithelial cells of rodents exposed to repeated injections of DMH continue to synthesise DNA throughout most of their life-span. Labelled cells show an increase both in their distance from the crypt base and their total number; these cells also show a shift into expanding adenomas and carcinomas. The tumours that develop manifest a proliferation of neoplastic epithelial cells near their surface with a continued expansion into the colonic lumen. Table 6.1.6 summarises similar characteristics of carcinogen-induced colorectal neoplasms and those observed in man.

6.1.4 APPROACHES TO THE PREVENTION OF COLORECTAL CANCER

In view of the numerous observations made on the pathogenesis and early detection of colorectal neoplasms, can rational approaches to the prevention of onset and progression of these lesions be developed? In support of this possibility are observations on modifications of lesion development and growth in a variety of experimental model systems and in man. Current experimental approaches proposed for the prevention of large bowel neoplasms comprise a new and expanding field of research (46, 146, 346, 664, 770–773, 824). They involve the deletion from, or addition to, the human diet of naturally occurring substances, or addition of a variety of compounds to experimental models.

Thus, in addition to studies on mechanisms leading to carcinogenesis, a variety of experimental approaches to active intervention and chemoprevention of colorectal neoplasia have been initiated. Experimental programmes are in progress in various laboratories to elucidate mechanisms of carcinogenesis and cell transformation in man, in animals, and in cell lines, which can lead to active intervention by deletion or addition of natural and synthetic substances. As efforts of this type become directed to human populations, the presence of early preclinical phenotypic characteristics can be recorded and quantified for experimental programmes, as described above. Degrees of abnormal cellular change, and other related phenotypic abnormalities, can be quantified to characterise current risk, and then to predict the probability of natural evolution of disease in individuals who are at specified ages in well defined population groups (425, 429). Risk profiles for this purpose are being developed and are reported elsewhere (429).

Based on available information on the expected age of development of disease in individuals in these well defined high risk groups, and on the observed evolution of disease when individuals are entered into specified treatment regimens, it will be possible to study the utility of experimental treatment programmes on the prevention of, as well as on the early detection of phenotypic abnormalities associated with, human colorectal cancer development.

6.2 Functional Maturity of Villus Enterocytes in States of Accelerated Cell Turnover without Villus Atrophy

Anne Ferguson, Frances Allan, and Dawood M Al-Thamery

6.2.1 INTRODUCTION AND HYPOTHESIS

The cell populations of the small-intestinal mucosa include not only those of the epithelium and the lamina propria, but also immunologically functioning cells of the lymphoid series. It may be that immune reactions within the mucosa directly affect epithelial cell proliferation, for in several gastrointestinal diseases associated with local small-intestinal immune reactions, such as infections, food hypersensitivities, and Crohn's disease, mucosal architecture is abnormal with crypt hyperplasia and short villi. We have conducted a series of experiments to investigate the role of cell-mediated immune reactions in the pathogenesis of this type of mucosal lesion. Experimental models included heterotransplanted grafts of rodent small intestine (226), graft-versus-host disease (442) and helminth parasite infection of T-cell-depleted animals (224). The results of conventional histological assessment (441), measurements of epithelial cell proliferation (442), and scanning electron microscopy (223) have shown that in the cell-mediated reaction of allograft rejection, destruction of the mucosa is preceded by considerable changes in epithelial cell proliferation. The reaction evolves in two stages: *phase 1* with virtually normal histology, including villi of normal length, but with an accelerated crypt cell production rate (CCPR) precedes *phase 2* in which CCPR remains high but villi are short or absent (222, 225, 442). Some of the features of these two phases are summarised in Table 6.2.1. The existence of the proposed enteropathic lymphokines has found some support (203).

Although cell-mediated immune reactions may be an important component of mucosal immunity, phase 2 is likely to have the disadvantage of causing malabsorption. In this paper we shall consider a possible disadvantage of phase 1, namely that the acceleration of epithelial cell proliferation may result in the villi being clothed by immature cells, deficient in absorptive and other

Table 6.2.1 Two stages of change in small-intestinal architecture and cell proliferation in experimental cell-mediated immune reactions

Feature	Phase 1	Phase 2
Villus and crypt measurements	Villi normal; crypts normal or lengthened	Villi shortened or absent; crypts lengthened
Crypt cell production rate	Elevated	Elevated
Postulated locally produced, 'enteropathic' lymphokines from T cells	'Crypt mitogenic factor'	'Crypt mitogenic factor'; 'enteropathic factor' causing collapse of villus core
Possible advantages	More rapid exfoliation of adherent bacteria, intracellular parasites	Loosening of attachment site of burrowing worms; reduced surface area possibly causing impairment of anti-peristaltic movement of parasites
Possible disadvantages	Possible immaturity of enterocytes covering villi	Reduction in number of enterocytes as a consequence of villus shortening; malabsorption

enzymes. It has been established that many enzymes are synthesised as cells move up the sides of the crypts towards the villi (56, 500). Clinically, perhaps the most relevant of these enzymes is the brush-border disaccharidase, lactase, which is necessary for hydrolysis and absorption of the milk sugar lactose. Lactase deficiency, with clinical lactose intolerance, may be seen in children recovering from infections and in other enteropathies (756), ie, in situations where there is an increased production and migration of enterocytes.

It would seem a reasonable hypothesis that when there is an increased rate of cell migration towards the tips of the villi, as a consequence of immunological or other stimuli, synthesis of lactase is reduced (573). We have collated results from several clinical and experimental studies to investigate the validity of this hypothesis.

6.2.2 MATERIALS AND METHODS

For measurements of the rates of crypt cell production we have used stathmokinetic techniques based on the work of Clarke (109). In mice, colchicine was used to block cells in metaphase, and vincristine has been used for studies in gnotobiotic lambs.

Villi and crypts of human small-intestinal biopsies were also examined and measured by a microdissection technique. In order to obtain some information on crypt mitotic activity in human disease, mitoses were also counted in single, microdissected, squashed crypts using Feulgen-stained biopsies (228). We have

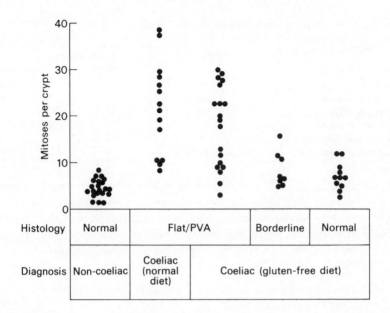

Figure 6.2.1 Mean numbers of mitoses per microdissected crypt in jejunal
biopsies from 52 patients with coeliac disease and 21 normal subjects
(PVA: partial villous atrophy)

found in our work on coeliac disease that this crypt mitotic count correlates well
with the clinical state of the patient and also with intestinal architecture as
assessed by conventional histology (Figure 6.2.1).

Tissue disaccharidases were assayed by the method of Dahlqvist (143). The
results are expressed as units of activity per g wet weight of tissue, one unit of
activity being the number of micromoles of glucose hydrolysed per minute at
37 °C.

6.2.3 EXPERIMENTS AND RESULTS

6.2.3.1 EFFECTS OF GLUTEN CHALLENGE ON SMALL-INTESTINAL
ARCHITECTURE AND DISACCHARIDASES IN DERMATITIS
HERPETIFORMIS

Parallel changes in mucosal architecture and enzymes are illustrated by a
recently completed clinical study of patients with dermatitis herpetiformis (48).
As shown in Table 6.2.2 comparison of jejunal biopsies from each of the five
dermatitis herpetiformis patients, taken first when the patient was on a

Table 6.2.2 Effects of gluten challenge on small-intestine biopsies from 5 patients with dermatitis herpetiformis (48). Morphometric variables estimated by microdissection

Feature	Before gluten (mean)	After 2 weeks gluten (mean)	Normal range
Villus length (μm)	485	397	500–1100
Crypt length (μm)	239	309	150–300
Mitoses per crypt	9.7	14.4	1–12
Tissue lactase (units/g)	1.32	0.14	1.0–7.0
Tissue sucrase (units/g)	4.06	1.29	2.5–9.3
Tissue maltase (units/g)	10.99	4.30	8.5–30.6

gluten-free diet, and then after two weeks of 20 g wheat gluten administration per day, showed that after gluten challenge villi were shorter, crypts were longer, and there was an increase in the crypt mitotic count in all five patients studied. Moreover, in every patient there was a considerable drop in brush-border disaccharidase activity, affecting lactase, sucrase, and maltase.

6.2.3.2 SMALL-INTESTINAL ARCHITECTURE AND DISACCHARIDASES IN GIARDIA-INFECTED MICE

It is for this model that we have the most complete documentation that a phase 1 type of alteration in intestinal architecture is present. The effects of chronic protozoal infection on intestinal architecture of mice are virtually undetectable by conventional histological assessment, apart from an increase in the number of intra-epithelial lymphocytes. Measurements showed that chronic infection did not influence villus length or crypt length. However, the CCPR doubled in giardia-infected animals (443). We confirmed by using autoradiography that there was accelerated transit of enterocytes up the villi (443). Results of

Table 6.2.3 Effects of chronic *Giardia muris* infections on the small intestine of 6 mice. Values significantly different from those of 6 uninfected controls are indicated by *(p < 0.05), **(p < 0.01), or ***(p < 0.001)

Feature	Uninfected mice (CBA strain) mean	Infected mice (Sha sha strain) mean
Villus length	760	775
Crypt length	119	152**
Crypt cell production rate (cells/h)	7.6	13.6**
Tissue lactase (units/g)	0.7	0.3
Tissue sucrase (units/g)	1.6	3.1**
Tissue isomaltase (units/g)	2.4	1.4
Tissue trehalase (units/g)	3.6	2.5*
Tissue maltase (units/g)	17.5	13.9

disaccharidase assays in six infected and six uninfected animals are shown in Table 6.2.3. Mean values for four of the five disaccharidases studied were lower in the infected group, trehalase significantly so, while sucrase was significantly increased. This subject has been further investigated by sequential examination of groups of CBA mice, at weekly intervals after infection with 1000 cysts of *Gardia muris*. Villus height remained normal after infection but CCPR increased to a maximum at four weeks. Assay of lactase and sucrase in the jejunum has shown these to be much reduced with the lowest values at two weeks (16). By comparing cell kinetic results, disaccharidase assays, and the parasite load as measured by trophozoite count, we have found that the lowest enzyme levels correlate with the peak of infection and not with the CCPR. We have therefore concluded that the lactase deficiency which is seen in giardiasis is likely to be due to damage directly produced by the parasites, rather than being the result of the altered cell proliferation.

6.2.3.3 SMALL-INTESTINAL ARCHITECTURE AND LACTASE MEASUREMENT IN ROTAVIRUS AND ASTROVIRUS INFECTION OF LAMBS

Small intestinal infection with viruses known to cause gastroenteritis, such as rotavirus and astrovirus, results in severe intestinal damage, with the villi and crypts being most affected in the mid-intestine and ileum (2, 89, 656, 657). We have examined cell proliferation and lactase levels in these infections (227). The results, summarised in Tables 6.2.4 and 6.2.5, illustrate that there is an

Table 6.2.4 Effects of rotavirus infection on the mid-small intestine of gnotobiotic lambs (227, 657). Villus and crypt lengths were measured in histological sections; there were 6 controls and 2 infected animals

Feature	Uninfected Controls (extreme range of 6 animals)	Day 2 post-infection (height of clinical illness) (single animal)	Day 8 post-infection (4 days after clinical recovery) (single animal)
Villus length (μm)	840–1250	590	850
Crypt length (μm)	120–210	229	220
Crypt cell production rate (cells/h)	3.2–9.0	13.6	17.5
Tissue lactase (units/g)	2.9–7.3	0.8	5.8

increase in CCPR when the illness is worst, with shortening of the villi and low levels of tissue lactase. However, after the animal has clinically recovered and the villus length has been restored, although CCPR remains high, lactase levels are normal. We have therefore concluded, particularly from the findings in rotavirus infections, that the capacity for maturation of brush border lactase can

Table 6.2.5 Effects of astrovirus infection on the proximal and mid-small intestine of gnotobiotic lambs (656). Villus and crypt lengths were measured in histological sections; there were 6 controls and 2 infected animals

Feature	Proximal small intestine				Mid small intestine			
	Controls		Day 2 post-infection	Day 5 post-infection	Controls		Day 2 post-infection	Day 5 post-infection
	Mean	SD			Mean	SE		
Villus length (μm)	690	34	732	713	613	17	306	804
Crypt length (μm)	124	10	167	225	115	3	161	178
Tissue lactase (units/g)	(range) 2.9–6.1		2.8	7.6	(range) 2.9–7.3		1.3	2.3

be maintained despite a considerable increase in CCPR above its base line. Altered cell proliferation may contribute to the enzyme deficiencies at the height of infection, but at this stage there is also marked villus shortening with reduction in the number of absorptive cells, and this too must contribute significantly.

6.2.3.4 TISSUE LACTASE IN JEJUNAL BIOPSIES WITH NORMAL VILLI AND HIGH MITOTIC COUNTS

A lack of correlation between crypt mitotic activity (and hence presumably CCPR) and tissue lactase is also occasionally seen in clinical studies. Although in the majority of our patients with abnormal jejunal biopsies due to coeliac disease, disaccharidase deficiency parallels changes in tissue architecture, we have in the last two years seen 10 instances where this correlation did not exist. Diagnoses included treated coeliac disease, idiopathic diarrhoea, malabsorption after radiotherapy, and hypogammaglobulinaemia. As illustrated in Figure 6.2.2, in the 10 jejunal biopsies studied, villi were normal, mitotic activity in the crypts was high, but enterocyte enzymes including lactase were normal.

6.2.4 CONCLUSIONS

There are many disease states in man and in animals, in which alterations in small-intestinal epithelial cell proliferation are accompanied by disaccharidase deficiency, as may be shown by the contrasting effects of gluten-including and gluten-free diets in patients with coeliac disease or dermatitis herpetiformis. However, in most of these instances disaccharidase deficiency occurs when the villus surface area is somewhat reduced, villi being shorter and altered in shape. We have now shown that there are several experimental situations and groups of patients in which discordance between crypt cell production rates and tissue disaccharidases is found. This militates against the hypothesis that enhanced

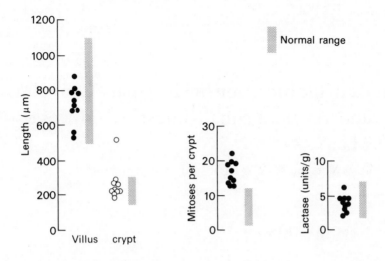

Figure 6.2.2 Tissue lactase activity and numbers of mitoses per crypt in a selected group of jejunal biopsies in which villi were of normal length. For clinical details see text

cell proliferation, due to immunological or other stimuli, results necessarily in the appearance of immature enterocytes on the surface of the villus and thereby produces a clinical state of enzyme deficiency with disaccharide intolerance. In animals with giardiasis, there appears to be a direct toxic effect of the parasites on the villus epithelial cells; perhaps of more interest is the fact that after recovery from rotavirus infection, a large and sustained increase in CCPR persists for more than a week after clinical and histological recovery. Though no enzyme deficiency was demonstrated in this post-infectious state, it remains to be shown whether this state of accelerated cell proliferation has any other adverse effects; if, for example, mucosal permeability to macromolecules is less efficient than normal, or whether the susceptibility to further infection is increased. Alternatively resistance to reinfection with the same or a different microorganism or parasite may even be increased.

ACKNOWLEDGEMENTS

This work has been supported by grants from the Medical Research Council and from the National Fund for Research into Crippling Diseases. I would like to thank my colleagues, particularly Dr D Snodgrass, for their cooperation.

6.3 Cell Proliferation in Normal, Convoluted and Avillous Small-intestinal Mucosae of Man

A J Watson, N A Wright and D R Appleton

6.3.1 INTRODUCTION

Coeliac disease is a condition in which susceptible individuals develop a malabsorption syndrome, with characteristic morphological and functional abnormalities of the small-intestinal mucosa, when their diet contains items based on the grain of wheat, rye, barley and probably oats (32). The starch fraction is entirely harmless and it is the protein fraction gluten which produces the deleterious effects. Of the two proteins which make up gluten, the alcohol-soluble gliadin (168) is the harmful agent and the property is still present in a water-soluble peptide fraction following peptic-tryptic digestion of wheat gliadin (238). However, precise definition of the responsible factor at molecular level has not as yet been achieved despite intensive efforts over a period of some two decades. The assumption that the small-intestinal mucosa in coeliac patients might lack an enzyme which would normally break down the harmful digestion product of gliadin was widely accepted at one time and cannot yet be entirely rejected on experimental evidence (310). An additional, or alternative, pathogenetic mechanism for the mucosal changes may be an abnormal immunological response involving an antigen-antibody reaction or a form of cell-mediated immune reaction (682).

There is good evidence that susceptibility to coeliac disease is genetically determined (444). Affected individuals are likely to be of northwestern-European, especially Irish, origin and there is a particularly high prevalence of the condition in the West of Ireland (492). Among first-degree relatives of patients coeliac disease is much more common than in the population at large and, even if asymptomatic, many relatives show coeliac-type mucosal abnormalities (588). There is a strong connection with the histocompatibility antigens HLA-B8 and HLA-DW3 which show linkage disequilibrium and may be linked to a separate coeliac-disease gene (682).

Other names used for coeliac disease include coeliac sprue, non-tropical sprue, idiopathic steatorrhoea and gluten-induced enteropathy. Like many other conditions defined initially in terms of signs and symptoms (syndromes) precise identification of coeliac disease as a specific nosological entity had to await discovery of the aetiological role of gluten. Towards the end of the Second World War the population of the Western Netherlands experienced a period of severe privation with shortages of foodstuffs including those based on wheat or rye. As adults grew lean, coeliac children thrived, and the incidence of the disease fell until conditions were restored to normal following the end of the war. The significance of these occurrences was elucidated by the Dutch paediatrician W K Dicke (167). With the subsequent introduction of the peroral biopsy technique (139, 232, 597, 644) the histopathology of the small-intestinal mucosa in untreated coeliac disease has been reported in great detail (1, 178, 600, 768), together with the sequence of changes by which normal morphology is restored during successful treatment, and the mode of reversion when treatment is discontinued (628). Valuable insights into the nature of the changes have also been provided by the use of additional techniques such as enzyme histochemistry (576), transmission electron microscopy (601, 645), and scanning electron microscopy (31, 454).

We can now define coeliac disease as a condition resulting from a probably permanent state of intolerance to dietary gluten associated with a flat avillous duodeno-jejunal mucosa on stereomicroscopy, usually with a mosaic pattern, and with characteristic histological changes, namely total villous atrophy, crypt hyperplasia, and a chronic inflammatory reaction. Strict adherence to a gluten-free diet leads to clinical and morphological improvement, but there is a liability to relapse following reintroduction of gluten.

The so-called animal models of coeliac disease are no more than morphological analogues of crypt-hyperplastic, villus-atrophic mucosae (271). Despite the limitations imposed by ethical and technical considerations there is no substitute for the direct study of the human disorder. Much can be learned about the proliferative status of normal and abnormal small-intestinal mucosae from the analysis of routine diagnostic biopsies, and the reasons for the increased numbers of mitotic cells in the crypts of coeliac mucosa can be investigated using stathmokinetic techniques in a small group of volunteers. We have already reported separately some of the results of these studies (768, 769, 814, 817, 820–823).

6.3.2 MATERIALS AND METHODS

6.3.2.1 BIOPSIES USED FOR DIAGNOSIS AND ANALYSIS OF MITOTIC INDICES

The biopsy specimens were obtained perorally from the vicinity of the duodeno-jejunal junction by means of a modified Crosby capsule; they were taken as near midday as possible to minimise the effect of circadian variation, retrieved without delay, and observed under the stereomicroscope at low magnification while being gently spread out for transfer, mucosal surface upwards, onto a small piece of glass. Primary fixation was in 10 percent neutral buffered formol-saline, and detailed inspection of the mucosal surface was best carried out after 24 h fixation when obscuring mucus and debris could safely be removed by gentle brushing. Post-fixation in a 5 percent solution of mercuric chloride in formol-saline was carried out to improve the quality of fixation and to give better nuclear staining, and the specimen was processed through to paraffin wax and embedded on edge. Some 200 serial sections 3 μm thick were cut, most of which were stained by Harris's haematoxylin and used for analysis of the crypts. For diagnostic assessment several sections were stained by haematoxylin and eosin and by the periodic-acid Schiff method after amylase digestion; flat coeliac mucosae were also routinely stained by the haematoxylin-van Gieson and by the picro-Mallory methods to detect collagen-isation of the lamina propria.

6.3.2.2 CLASSIFICATION OF BIOPSIES

The biopsy specimens studied were assigned to one of 3 main categories on the basis of their morphological appearances as seen on stereomicroscopic and histological examination. Although the value of stereomicroscopy has been disparaged (520, 599) both forms of examination are essential if errors are to be avoided. If stereomicroscopy has been neglected, the paraffin-embedded specimen can be processed back to 70 percent spirit without sustaining any harm.

Normal morphology. These specimens showed a normal villous appearance on stereomicroscopy and conformed to the conventional appearance of normality on histological examination. It is relatively unusual to find a specimen from the duodenojejunal region showing exclusively a population of tall finger-shaped villi, and narrow or broad leaf-shaped forms were accepted as normal; the presence of curved or angular leaves, of joined leaves, of straight ridges or sinuous ridges among the more regular leafy villi did not debar specimens from inclusion in this category. Specimens showing convolutions were invariably excluded.

Convoluted mucosae. The stereomicroscopic appearance of a small-intestinal biopsy is described as convoluted if individual villi have been wholly or largely replaced by a complex of intertwining tortuous ridge-like structures, so that there is a certain resemblance to the surface of the cerebral hemispheres (Figure 6.3.1). The height of the convolutions often appears comparable to that of normal villi, but frankly atrophic forms are sometimes encountered. The inexperienced observer may overlook isolated or scattered convolutions, but is

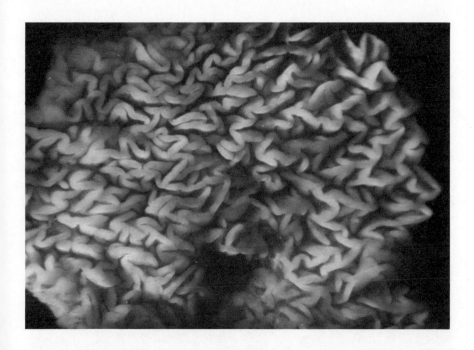

Figure 6.3.1 A peroral biopsy of proximal small-intestinal mucosa showing replacement of villi by so-called convolutions; this specimen would be assigned to group 3 (×16)

Table 6.3.1 Combinations of changes which characterise convoluted mucosae assigned to each of the three arbitrarily defined groups

Mucosal group	Stereomicroscopy	Histology
3	Surface completely or predominantly (over 70%) convoluted	Villi short and stubby; crypts obviously lengthened; surface epithelium abnormal; obvious increase in density of inflammatory cell infiltration
2	From 10 to 70% of surface occupied by convolutions	Some shortening of villi apparent on inspection; lengthening of crypts slight or inapparent; surface epithelium normal; density of inflammatory cell infiltration normal or just perceptibly increased
1	Not more than a few convolutions, distributed amongst leaves and ridges, and occupying less than 10% of surface	Normal or nearly so

more likely to misinterpret other angular, or sinuous formations as convolutions. The histological appearances of such specimens range from virtual normality to a state of severe villous atrophy with crypt hyperplasia and other changes approaching in severity those of untreated coeliac disease. For the purpose of analysis we have subdivided the convoluted mucosae into 3 groups on the basis of increasing severity of morphological abnormality according to the criteria set out in Table 6.3.1. In the event of a disparity between the severity of the stereomicroscopic and the histological changes, the more severe of the two assessments determined the group to which the specimen was assigned.

Flat avillous coeliac-type mucosae. The characteristic stereomicroscopic and histological appearances of the specimens assigned to this category are illustrated in Figures 6.3.2 and 6.3.3 and are so well established that further description is unnecessary.

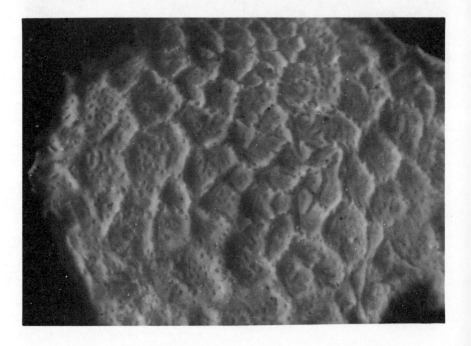

Figure 6.3.2 A peroral biopsy of proximal small-intestinal mucosa from a patient with untreated coeliac disease. This is a flat avillous mucosa showing the characteristic mosaic pattern. Some of the hyperplastic crypts open directly on to the surface, but it is more usual for several crypts to open into a short vestibular compartment just below the mucosal surface. The vestibular orifices are readily apparent on the surface of the mosaics (×16)

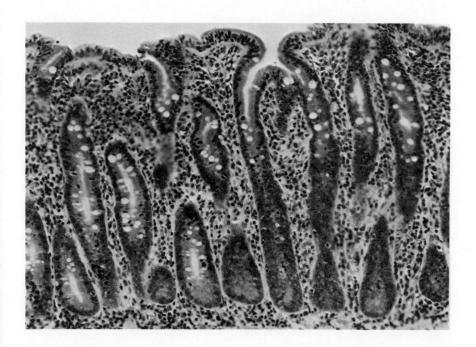

Figure 6.3.3 This shows the typical histological findings in the flat avillous mucosa from an untreated coeliac patient. There is total villous atrophy, but the crypts are hyperplastic and greatly elongated; dividing epithelial cells are plentiful and occur to a high level in the crypts; two crypts can be seen opening into a shared vestibule; the surface epithelium shows pseudostratification of nuclei and numerous intraepithelial lymphocytes; the lamina propria is heavily infiltrated by plasma cells, small and large mononuclear cells and eosinophils. (Haematoxylin and eosin ×150)

6.3.2.3 PATIENTS

The majority of patients had had a single biopsy sample of the proximal small-intestinal mucosa taken by the peroral route for diagnostic purposes. A large proportion of the samples were taken to exclude or confirm the diagnosis of coeliac disease. Many were taken from patients, with psoriasis or other dermatoses, who were possibly suffering from dermatogenic enteropathy (452, 650), and these investigations led to the discovery of the association between dermatitis herpetiformis (DH) and coeliac disease, the latter usually being subclinical (453, 651).

Our control patients, defined in terms of their having a morphologically normal biopsy, comprised 75 adults and 10 children less than 8 years old. There were 62 patients with flat coeliac-type mucosae; 13 adults and 29 children with untreated coeliac disease and 20 adults with DH. The 47 patients with convoluted mucosae constituted a heterogeneous group in terms of clinical diagnosis, though it is notable that there were 15 with DH and 2 more who were near relatives of DH patients. There were also 6 coeliac patients in various stages of remission or relapse, and 4 patients with giardiasis.

6.3.2.4 METHODS OF ANALYSIS

In all subjects the objective was to analyse 30 crypts, each of which had been axially sectioned so as to include the base, middle and mouth of the crypt in the plane of section. The 'left-hand' column of cells was enumerated from the bottom to the mouth of the crypt as seen in section. In villous mucosae this corresponds approximately to the junction of crypt and villus, whereas in avillous coeliac mucosae the mouth is represented by the apparent junction of the crypt with the surface epithelium; it is likely in some instances to include part of the crypt vestibule. The number of cells in this column will be referred to as the crypt length and provides a measure unaffected by tissue shrinkage resulting from fixation and processing. Within the crypt column the positions of all mitotic cells were recorded and the distribution of mitotic index (I_m) relative to a crypt of length equal to the mean of the appropriate group was determined by pooling data for all crypts examined in that group (82, 814).

We have explained elsewhere (28) how a useful description of the extent of proliferation up the crypt, the cut-off position (83, 84, 668), can be found from stathmokinetic experiments, provided an estimate of the cell cycle time is available. We are unable to apply this method to our human material because FLM studies cannot be undertaken, and instead have derived from the mitotic index distributions estimates of the cell position at which I_m falls to 50 percent of its maximum value (120); we term this the half-maximum position, HMP. If all cells below this position were proliferating with the same cell cycle time, the cut-off position would be half this distance from the bottom of the crypt.

6.3.2.5 STATHMOKINETIC STUDY

Five subjects took part in this study, having given their consent after being fully informed of the procedures involved. The cell birth rate (k_B) was measured by two stathmokinetic techniques, cells being arrested by rapid intravenous infusion of vincristine sulphate in a dosage of 0.045 mg per kg body weight.

In the first procedure a peroral biopsy of proximal small-intestinal mucosa was taken from the region of the duodeno-jejunal junction at 1330 h on day 1, using a modified Crosby capsule. On day 2 the capsule was passed to the same position under radiological monitoring and a further biopsy obtained at the same time as on the previous day, 2.5 h after the vincristine infusion. The birth rate for the crypt as a whole was estimated from the equation

$$k_B = \frac{I_m \text{ (day 2)} - I_m \text{ (day 1)}}{2.5}$$

and the crypt cell production rate (CCPR) by summing the birth rates at each cell position and multiplying by the column count.

In the second procedure the capsule of a Quinton multiple biopsy machine was passed to the same region as before; a biopsy was obtained, and after infusion of vincristine further biopsies were obtained at 15 minute intervals for about 2 h. The birth rate was estimated from the slope of a straight line fitted to the mitotic accumulation data, and the CCPR by considering once again the cumulative birth rates.

The handling, fixation, processing, and sectioning of the specimens was as in Section 6.3.2.1, and the method of counting as in Section 6.3.2.4, but with at least 3000 crypt-cell nuclei being counted for each biopsy specimen.

Three patients underwent the two-biopsy procedure:

AA, a male aged 61, suffered from rosacea and varicose ulcers of the legs. Both of his biopsy specimens were stereomicroscopically and histologically normal.

BB, a male aged 25, had a clinical diagnosis of DH but showed no clinical or biochemical evidence of malabsorption. Both of his biopsy specimens showed a completely convoluted mucosal surface on stereomicroscopy, while histological examination showed group-3-type changes.

CC, a male aged 37, had suffered from DH for over 10 years and had recently developed a megaloblastic anaemia due to folic acid deficiency; his skin condition was controlled by Dapsone and he was taking a normal diet. His mucosal biopsy specimens showed a flat avillous surface with a cobblestone appearance, and the histological changes were typical of untreated coeliac disease.

A further two patients were studied by the multiple biopsy procedure:

DD, a male aged 61, was being investigated to ascertain the cause of his chronic diarrhoea. Eleven biopsies, obtained over a period of 150 minutes, were considered to be morphologically normal.

EE, a female aged 55, had been diagnosed clinically as suffering from coeliac disease. Nine biopsies, obtained over 105 minutes, showed typical stereomicroscopic and histological appearances of untreated coeliac disease.

6.3.3 RESULTS

6.3.3.1 MORPHOMETRIC VARIABLES

The mean values for crypt length and column count in the 8 groups of patients studied are shown in Table 6.3.2 along with estimates of the total crypt-cell population obtained from the product of these two measurements. The most marked contrast in the values both for crypt length and column count is between the controls and the groups with flat mucosae; the crypt lengths in all 3 such groups are more than double control values and are very similar to one another. Crypts over 100 cells long were seen in all coeliac-type groups. The column count in the adult coeliac disease group, however, is greater than in the two similar groups. The estimates of total crypt cell population show a threefold increase or more compared with the controls.

All three groups with convoluted mucosae have increased mean crypt length; this is present even in group 1, but is most marked in group 3 as would be anticipated from the definition of the groups (Table 6.3.1). In group-3-convoluted the column count is also noticeably increased, leading to a doubling of total crypt cell population compared with controls.

Mitotic index distributions are shown in Figure 6.3.4; positions of the HMP are marked. From these have been calculated the total cells below and above the HMP; we shall call these the proliferation and maturation zones although we cannot be sure that all the cells in the proliferation zone are in fact in cycle. Their populations are given in Table 6.3.2. The proliferation zone increases in

Table 6.3.2 Morphometric data for crypts in different clinico-morphological groups. All figures are cells

Patient group	Crypt length	Column count	Total cells	Proliferation zone	Maturation zone
Adult controls	32	25	800	550	250
Childhood controls	34	25	850	600	250
Group 1 convoluted	37	26	950	750	200
Group 2 convoluted	39	27	1050	750	300
Group 3 convoluted	49	31	1500	1150	350
Adult coeliac disease	74	41	3050	1700	1350
Childhood coeliac disease	75	35	2650	1550	1100
Dermatitis herpetiformis	76	36	2700	1650	1050

size in absolute terms in the convoluted groups, and also appears to be slightly greater as a proportion of the total population. In the groups with flat mucosae it increases even more in terms of cell numbers, but it is the maturation zone which shows the greater increase, having some five times more cells than in controls.

The I_m data also enable the CCPRs to be estimated if certain assumptions are made. Table 6.3.3 shows the mean numbers of mitoses observed per crypt column; if the duration of mitosis is 1 h then these are also the numbers of cells produced by a column every hour, and multiplication by the column counts give the CCPRs. However, since mitoses migrate towards the lumen of the crypt, they are seen preferentially in longitudinal sections (702), and so we have

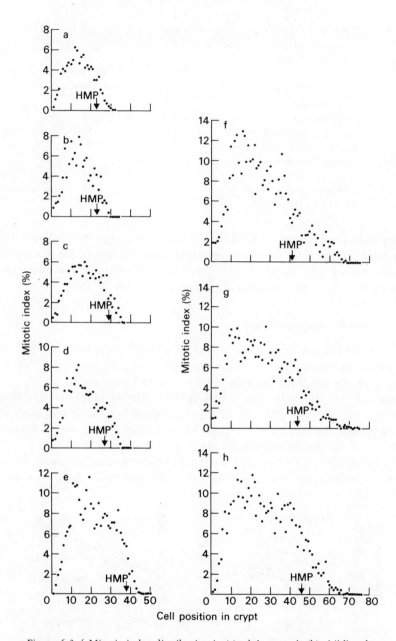

Figure 6.3.4 Mitotic index distribution in (a) adult controls (b) childhood controls (c) group 1 convoluted (d) group-2-convoluted (e) group-3-convoluted (f) adult coeliac disease (g) childhood coeliac disease and (h) dermatitis herpetiformis. Half-maximum positions are shown

Table 6.3.3 Observed number of mitoses per crypt column and estimated crypt cell production rate in different clinico-morphological groups

Patient group	Mitoses per column	CCPR (cells/crypt/h)
Adult controls	1.0	17
Childhood controls	1.2	21
Group 1 convoluted	1.3	23
Group 2 convoluted	1.5	28
Group 3 convoluted	2.7	59
Adult coeliac disease	3.9	110
Childhood coeliac disease	3.4	84
Dermatitis herpetiformis	4.1	105

multiplied the estimates of CCPR by 0.7 before entering them in Table 6.3.3. This value was obtained by examining crypt cross-sections in the samples from patients taking part in the stathmokinetic investigations; the effect of in-accuracy here or in the duration of mitosis can readily be seen.

6.3.3.2 STATHMOKINETIC STUDIES

The mitotic indices, corrected by multiplying by 0.7 as in Section 6.3.3.1, for the 3 patients subjected to the two biopsy procedure, are shown in Table 6.3.4 along with the cell birth rates and CCPRs derived from them.

Figure 6.3.5 illustrates the results of the multiple biopsy stathmokinetic technique on patients DD and EE, and Table 6.3.5 shows the birth rates calculated and the estimates of CCPR obtained from population sizes given in Table 6.3.2 for the appropriate groups.

The estimates of CCPR in all 5 stathmokinetic investigations show the same pattern between types of mucosa as do the estimates in Table 6.3.3 although

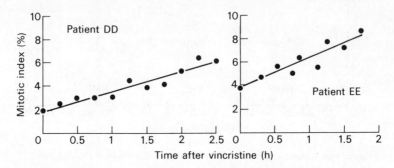

Figure 6.3.5 Stathmokinetic data from patients DD and EE

the stathmokinetic results are all slightly lower than would be expected from this table. A variety of reasons could account for this: failure of vincristine to arrest all cells in metaphase, degeneration of arrested metaphases, normal variability within or between individuals may all contribute to low values from stathmokinetic experiments. It is likely, however, that the values found by simple counting of mitoses are too high because the mitotic duration has been underestimated.

Table 6.3.4 Crypt size, mitotic index and cell production rate in 3 patients by a two-biopsy stathmokinetic technique

Patient	Patient group	Crypt cell population	Corrected $I_m(\%)$ Day 1	Day 2	k_B (cells/1000 cells/h)	CCPR (cells/crypt/h)
AA	Adult control	700	1.7	5.4	15	11
BB	Group 3 convoluted	1450	3.2	9.6	26	38
CC	Dermatitis herpetiformis	2050	3.6	10.4	27	55

Table 6.3.5 Birth rate in two patients by a multiple biopsy stathmokinetic technique. Crypt cell production rate is estimated from cell populations in Table 6.3.2

Patient	Patient group	k_B (cells/1000 cells/h)	CCPR (cells/crypt/h)
DD	Adult control	17	14
EE	Adult coeliac disease	25	76

6.3.4 DISCUSSION

6.3.4.1 MORPHOMETRIC PARAMETERS OF NORMAL VERSUS COELIAC CRYPTS

Simple inspection of well orientated histological sections suffices to show that coeliac crypts are longer than normal crypts, but it is less apparent that they are also increased in girth. If we compare the arithmetic means of the measurements for the two control groups and for the three coeliac groups respectively then we find that the mean crypt length is increased by a factor of 2.3 from 33 cells in the controls to 75 cells in the coeliacs. Similarly the mean column count is increased by a factor of 1.5 from 25 cells to 37 cells. The product of these two parameters gives a reliable estimate of the total crypt cell population (801) (Table 6.3.2), and if the mean values are compared we see that the total cell population of coeliac crypts is 3.4 times greater than in control crypts. The proliferation zone and the maturation zone both show an absolute increase in cell numbers, but the increase in size of the maturation zone is disproportionately greater than the increase in the size of the whole crypt.

6.3.4.2 PROLIFERATIVE PARAMETERS OF NORMAL VERSUS COELIAC CRYPTS

Despite the total atrophy and disappearance of villi from the proximal small-intestinal mucosa in untreated coeliac disease it is quite inappropriate to refer to the general state of the mucosa as one of atrophy; indeed the crypts are both hyperplastic and hyperproliferative. The assumption that this state constitutes a response to an abnormally high rate of cell loss, from the surface of the mucosa into the lumen of the bowel, was confirmed and quantified by Creamer and his colleagues (133, 526). They assessed the rate of cell loss by measuring the DNA content of the washings from perfused segments of small bowel and concluded that patients with untreated coeliac disease showed a sixfold increase over the normal rate of cell loss. Ordinarily the flat coeliac mucosa must achieve a new state of equilibrium to compensate for this change by a corresponding increase in the rate of cell production from the crypts. From the data in Table 6.3.3 it is evident that the CCPR from coeliac crypts is 5.2 times greater than from normal crypts. If the comparison is restricted to adult controls and adult coeliacs the increase in CCPR is 6.5 times, an estimate which matches closely the estimated increase in the rate of cell loss. These comparisons are valid only if we assume that there is no significant increase in the number of crypts per unit length of small bowel in coeliacs as compared with normals.

The increases in CCPR can be partly accounted for by the near trebling of cell number in the proliferation zone of the crypt, and for the rest by an approximately 50 percent reduction in cell cycle time, always assuming that t_m remains virtually constant. The results from the stathmokinetic studies are similar though lower (Tables 6.3.4 and 6.3.5) and possible explanations for this slight discrepancy have already been mentioned.

6.3.4.3 SIGNIFICANCE OF A CONVOLUTED MUCOSA

The duodeno-jejunal mucosa can assume a flat avillous appearance, with crypts opening directly or through shared vestibular chambers on to the surfaces of a mosaic of low plateaux, in conditions other than coeliac disease (358). Nevertheless, these changes are so characteristic as to be virtually diagnostic of untreated coeliac disease in appropriate clinical circumstances. On the other hand a convoluted appearance is often of unknown significance as an isolated finding even when all other aspects of the case have been taken into account (768, 817). In the context of coeliac disease a convoluted appearance represents an intermediate stage in the recovery or in the development of a flat mucosa. The distal limit of a flat coeliac mucosa may be separated from unaltered villous mucosa by an intermediate convoluted zone. Islands of convoluted mucosa may be found in an otherwise flat coeliac mucosa by multiple sampling. Convolutions may be a feature of various other disorders and the prevalence in apparently healthy subjects differs between population groups (33, 452, 817).

Our studies of the morphometric and proliferative parameters show that group-3-convoluted mucosae are in a hyperproliferative state intermediate between normal and flat mucosae; groups 1 and 2, on the other hand, differ little from normal controls. Our data are consistent with the hypothesis that group-3-convoluted mucosae represent a morphological adaptation to a moderately reduced population of villous enterocytes consequent upon increased cell loss and balanced by an appropriate increase in cell production. If the rate of cell loss increases further, the preservation of surface integrity entails loss of convolutions (so-called 'total villous atrophy') and further stepping-up of cell production perhaps to near maximum rates.

6.3.4.4 MECHANISMS FOR INCREASING CCPR IN RESPONSE TO INCREASED RATE OF LOSS OF MATURE ENTEROCYTES

In the light of present knowledge we can reasonably discard certain suggestions some of which are now of little more than historical interest. These include *mitotic arrest* as a cause of the increased mitotic index in coeliac crypts (598); though experimental models based on this concept show villous atrophy, there is also crypt atrophy (108). The concept of *enteroblastic hypoplasia* (131) is not in keeping with the usual finding of an increased mitotic index in flat coeliac mucosae; the patient shown by tritiated-thymidine (^{3}HTdR) studies to have a reduced output of cells from the crypts must be regarded as atypical (131). *Maturation arrest or delay* (131, 132) could in theory account for a reduction in CCPR even in the face of an increase in the rate of cell division within the proliferation zone. This would require loss or death of cells in the maturation zone and for this there is no morphological evidence (601). Furthermore, studies of coeliac mucosae maintained in organ culture have convincingly shown an increased labelling index when ^{3}HTdR was added to the culture medium, and an increase in the rate of migration from the crypts (724). In terms of Booth's analogy with the haemopoietic system (52, 53) our studies support the concept of *enteroblastic hyperplasia* comparable to erythroblastic hyperplasia in haemolytic anaemia. This reaction in the small-intestinal mucosa is mediated firstly by an increase in the size of the crypt with an absolute increase in the population of proliferating cells, and secondly by a reduction in T_c to about half its normal value. Whether these compensatory changes occur simultaneously or sequentially, and if the latter in what order, remains to be elucidated.

ACKNOWLEDGEMENT

The work reported in this paper was supported by a grant from the North of England Council of the Cancer Research Campaign. We are grateful to clinical colleagues, in particular to Dr. Janet Marks, for their collaboration.

6.4 Cell Differentiation in the Normal Colonic Mucosa and in Hyperplastic Polyps and Colonic Adenomas

G L Stoffels, A M Preumont and M de Reuck

6.4.1 INTRODUCTION

Controversy still exists concerning the relationships between colonic adenocarcinoma and the various sorts of polyps occurring in the colon. It is generally considered that the so-called hyperplastic polyps are not neoplastic in nature (307, 389), but that adenomatous and villous polyps represent true benign neoplasms (adenomas) (174, 311, 389). Some authors are of the opinion that while the majority of colonic carcinomas originate as such de novo, or as a result of malignant change in villous adenomas, such change does not occur to an appreciable extent in adenomatous polyps (90, 665). A further possibility is that malignant change may occur in hyperplastic polyps (137). The histopathological criteria which have been established for the diagnosis of neoplastic or hyperplastic polyps suggest that while both polypoid adenomas and villous polyps are composed of an immature-type epithelium, the epithelium of hyperplastic polyps shows features which suggest an overgrowth of mature or 'hypermature' cells.

Cell proliferation in various types of polyps has been investigated by a number of authors. In polypoid adenomas and villous polyps epithelial cells at the luminal surface have been shown to manifest tritiated thymidine (^{3}HTdR)-labelling activity (158, 423). In hyperplastic polyps on the other hand ^{3}HTdR-labelling is confined to the lower part of the crypt, as in the normal mucosa (307). We have used a technique involving ^{3}H-actinomycin (^{3}H-AM) to try to determine firstly what proportion of the different types of polyp show the abnormal surface-cell labelling pattern, and secondly, in those lesions which have abnormal surface cells what proportion of the surface cell population they represent.

Actinomycin in a cytotoxic drug binding specifically to DNA; when tritiated it is possible to detect its presence and quantify it in autoradiographic preparations of histological sections of tissues. It has been shown that the quantity of bound ^{3}H-AM is lower in non-cycling cells than in cycling cells (57). Actinomycin binding is a measure of the degree of complexing between DNA and chromosomal proteins (517, 518).

6.4.2 MATERIALS AND METHODS

The patients were prepared for colonoscopy and biopsy by a period of low-roughage diet and two soft enemas. Tissue samples were fixed in pure methanol for a 24 h period, then processed through to paraffin wax. Sections 3 μm thick were prepared and those used for routine histopathological diagnosis were stained with haematoxylin and erythrosin. Polyps of the colon and rectum were classified (303) as follows.

Hyperplastic polyps (synonyms: metaplastic polyps, focal polypoid hyperplasia) are composed of elongated, tortuous and often dilated crypts, with an uneven columnar epithelial lining often showing a serrated surface and retaining the basal localisation of its nuclei.

Polypoid adenomas (synonym; rubular adenomas) are benign tumours composed of branching glandular tubules often orientated perpendicularly to the muscularis mucosae and embedded in lamina propria.

Villous adenomas are sessile neoplasms consisting of epithelial fronds with scant supporting connective tissue.

Samples from nine of each of the above types of polyp were studied. Normal mucosal biopsies were provided for comparison from patients who had no evidence of colorectal disease either on radiological or on colonoscopic examination. Sections of normal mucosa were mounted on the same slides as the sections from the various types of polyp, to ensure that the treatment they were subjected to was precisely the same; sixteen slides were prepared for each case. The technique of actinomycin treatment has been described previously (675, 676); following this autoradiographs were prepared.

The grain count was measured in all cells where the nucleus was covered by one or more grains, since the presence of areas of cells completely unlabelled suggests an artefact. A minimum of 75 cells in each region was recorded, and counts were usually of 150 cells or more. The means and standard deviations were calculated for each count, and statistical differences between the means were calculated by Student's t-test.

6.4.3 RESULTS

In the normal colon practically all the cells in the lower two-thirds of the crypt were heavily labelled, the mean grain count being 27 grains per nucleus. In the

Table 6.4.1 Mean nuclear grain counts in different types of cells in various tissues, after labelling with tritiated actinomycin; 150 cells were counted except in two cases (†) where 75 were counted

| | Type of cell | | |
Tissue	Normal surface epithelium	Abnormal surface epithelium	Bottom of gland
Normal colon	3.8	—	27
Polypoid hyperplasia	2.2	—	29
Polypoid adenoma	3.5	20†	27
Villous adenoma	6.0†	34	36

upper third of the normal crypt there was an abrupt decrease in grain counts leading to a mean value of 3.8 in the most superficial cells (Table 6.4.1). Heavily labelled nuclei were very rarely seen in surface cells, there being only about two such nuclei per 150 cells counted.

In hyperplastic polyps, heavily labelled cells with a mean grain count of 29 again predominated in the middle and the lower parts of the crypt. Through the upper region of the crypt the grain count decreased progressively, and the mean value was 2.2 in superficial cells. As in the normal mucosa, heavily labelled nuclei were very infrequent at the surface.

In polypoid adenomas the cells in the lower three-quarters of the glands all showed heavy nuclear labelling with a mean grain count of 27. In the majority of glands there was a progressive decrease in grain count towards the surface, as had been observed in normal mucosa and in hyperplastic polyps. However in seven of the nine cases studied there were areas in which heavily labelled cells were present at the surface (Figure 6.4.1); in these 'abnormal' areas the mean grain count was 20. Abnormal areas of this sort accounted for only 10 percent of the surface region however.

In the villous adenomas, on the other hand, the mean grain count was similar in the surface region and in the deeper parts of the tumour (34 and 36 respectively), and glands showing the normal pattern of labelling were rare (Figure 6.4.2).

6.4.4 DISCUSSION

The binding of ^{3}H-AM depends on the degree of complexing between DNA and chromosomal proteins. In cycling cells binding is greatest during the S-phase (5 17). It is reduced when cells begin to differentiate and is very low in fully differentiated cells (57, 58).

The present results have shown that in the normal colon the distribution of ^{3}H-AM binding activity resembles closely the distribution of proliferating cells

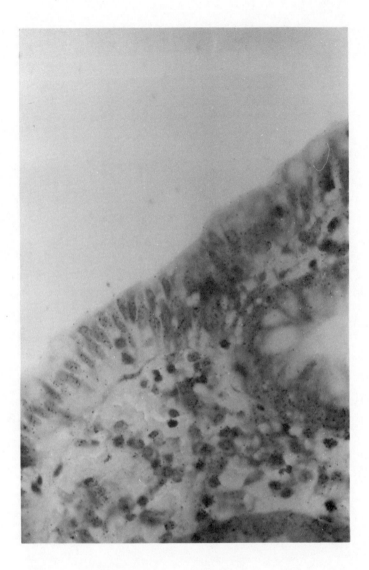

Figure 6.4.1 Polypoid adenoma showing surface epithelial cells with
increased ^{3}H-AM labelling ($\times 400$)

as revealed by conventional ^{3}HTdR labelling studies (423). In hyperplastic
polyps the pattern of ^{3}H-AM binding suggests that these lesions represent a
state of 'hypermaturation' of the epithelium, and this view is supported by
several studies using other techniques (307, 359, 389). Both in polypoid

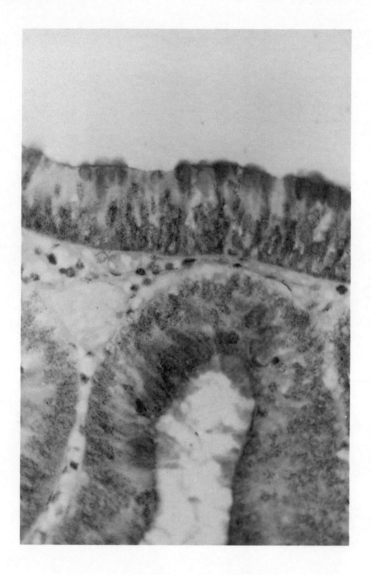

Figure 6.4.2 Villous adenoma showing as much ³H-AM labelling in surface
epithelial cells as in deeper cells (×400)

adenomas and in villous adenomas ^{3}HTdR incorporation has been observed in
the surface region (423) (see Section 6.5); our study has demonstrated that
heavy ^{3}H-AM binding too is seen at the surface of these lesions, demonstrating
the presence of poorly repressed cells. While this finding is not present in all

polypoid adenomas, and is of rather limited extent in those lesions which do show it, in the villous adenomas the presence of derepressed cells in the surface region is usual.

Therefore lesions which are relatively frequently complicated by carcinomatous transformation have derepressed cells in the surface epithelium; polypoid adenomas, less frequently complicated by carcinomatous transformation, show fewer derepressed surface cells; and hyperplastic polyps, which are not generally considered to be precarcinomatous, show none.

ACKNOWLEDGEMENTS

The authors are grateful to Prof J Brachet for his interest in this work. They wish to thank Prof Potvliege for his help throughout this study and Dr Salhadin and Dr Andre who made additional specimens available for study.

6.5 Aspects of Normal and Altered Epithelial Cell Proliferation in the Human Intestine

Eleanor E Deschner

6.5.1 INTRODUCTION

The range of disease states in the intestinal mucosa of man reflects the diversity of responses which can be elicited from the epithelial cell population, when normal genetic expression and homeostatic mechanisms are disturbed. When such conditions exist, knowledge concerning the activity of epithelial cells and clues about how to detect the presence of such disturbances before the full-blown disease manifests itself are goals much to be desired.

When gastrointestinal mucosa undergoing atrophy is examined, there is not only a reduction in the number of glands, but also a reduction in their size due to decreased numbers of component epithelial cells. What forces bring about this condition? How are growth restraints imposed? How are focal areas of stem cell destruction induced and these patchy alterations within the mucosa brought about?

The reverse obtains during the formation of hyperplastic foci and the development of neoplasms. Here an enlargement of the glands takes place and, at least in the latter instance, the number of glands is often greatly increased. Each of these pathological conditions represents a widely divergent response of the regulatory controls governing the epithelial cell population. Stages of altered regulation of cell proliferation have not only begun to be recognised, particularly in the large bowel, but they can be classified by their relative duration and their degree of neoplastic potential. They may even be considered as an index of the biological ageing phenomenon which is being expressed within the various portions of the digestive tract. Premature ageing or breakdown of tissues which secrete substances necessary for balanced function of the gastrointestinal mucosa may in fact contribute to the expression of altered cell behaviour and ultimately affect the induction time for disease more distally in the intestinal tract. Illustrations of a few of these concepts will be provided.

6.5.2 MUCOSAL ATROPHY

Mucosal atrophy of the small intestine occurs in a variety of conditions. The mucosa of patients with severe pernicious anaemia, for example, shows a shortening of villi, a decreased epithelial cell population and a decline in the number of mitoses (234). Patchy mucosal atrophy in biopsies of human ileum employed as a urinary conduit has also been reported (259).

Two patients with metastases from an epidermoid carcinoma of the bladder who had an ileal conduit constructed became available for cell proliferation studies after a period of 9 months in one case, and 19 months in the other (151, 152). These patients with limited life expectancy were injected with tritiated thymidine (^{3}HTdR) and multiple biopsies were collected over periods of 50 and 70 h respectively. One ileal mucosa appeared to have a normal histological appearance while the other was atrophic and superficially resembled large bowel mucosa.

The fraction of labelled mitoses (FLM) curves for both conduits are shown in Figure 6.5.1. In the normal-appearing conduit, few histological alterations

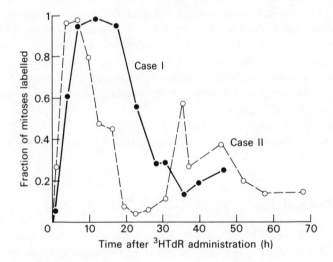

Figure 6.5.1 Fraction of labelled mitoses curves for 2 ileal conduits. Case 1 was of 9 months' duration and in an atrophic condition, and case 2 was of 19 months' duration and of normal histological appearance

were seen (152): the mean duration of G_2 was 2 h and of S-phase 11 h. A total cell cycle time (T_c) of 36 h was observed, so that the duration of G_1 was deduced as approximately 22 h. In the 9-month old conduit, in which the ileal mucosa appeared atrophic, the mean durations of both G_2 and S were almost twice as long: t_{G_2} was 4 h and t_s 20 h (151).

The average length of the crypt column in the normal-appearing mucosa was 38 cells, and at 1 h there were 2.4 labelled cells per crypt column (Table 6.5.1).

Table 6.5.1 Proliferative parameters in 2 human ileal conduits compared to those in normal ileum and colon (151, 152, 426, 428)

	Ileum	Colon	Ileal conduit A	Ileal conduit B
Cells/column	33	90	38	25
Labelled cells/column after 1 h	2.9	1.5	2.4	0.7
T_c(h)	>24	40	36	>47

In the atrophic mucosa, however, the number of labelled cells per column was 0.7, less than one third that seen in the histologically normal-appearing conduit, and the number of epithelial cells per crypt column was diminished to 25. The extended G_2, S and cell cycle durations in addition to the reduced numbers of DNA-synthesising cells of this atrophic mucosa, were closer to the values reported for normal large bowel (426) than normal ileum (428).

A number of possibilities have been suggested as causes of this atrophy. Chronic exposure to urine, which differs in composition and pH from the normal intestinal contents, and the different bacterial flora to which the mucosa is exposed, may account for some of the findings (2). Perhaps an equally important factor is that the mucosa is no longer in contact with the remaining portions of the gut where various gastrointestinal hormones or secretions may have a direct or modulating effect. Strong support for this latter possibility has emerged from several sources.

6.5.3 INTERNAL FACTORS AFFECTING THE MUCOSA

The influence of both bile and pancreatic secretions, as well as gastrointestinal hormones, has been the subject of much recent experimental and clinical investigation. Bile-acid feeding stimulates epithelial cell proliferation in the small intestine, accelerates migration up the villus, and reduces the cell cycle time (242). The influence of bile on the regulation of epithelial cell proliferation has been further elucidated by studies in which biliary flow was diverted away from the small and large bowel for two days (Table 6.5.2). Little effect on the labelling (I_s) or mitotic (I_m) indices was seen over 24 h in the jejunum, but in the colon there was a decrease in these indices, while in the ileum changes were of an intermediate degree (161).

Table 6.5.2 Labelling and mitotic indices in jejunal, ileal and colonic crypts, expressed as a percentage of values in sham-operated rats, of rats with a bile fistula 1 and 24 h after operation

Time after operation	Proliferative index (% of control)	Jejunum	Ileum	Colon
1 h	I_s	82	88	30
	I_m	87	98	46
24 h	I_s	87	75	55
	I_m	85	49	22

Investigations of the leading edge of labelled epithelial cells showed no measurable movement in the colon of bile-deprived rats, but migration was less affected as one proceeded proximally to the small bowel (Table 6.5.3). Grain

Table 6.5.3 Average position of the highest labelled cell in the jejunal, ileal, and colonic crypt columns of sham-operated and bile-fistula rats, 1 and 24 h after operation. All jejunal and ileal crypt columns were labelled; the percentage of unlabelled colonic crypt columns is shown

	Time after operation	Position of highest labelled cell			Unlabelled colonic crypt columns (%)
		Jejunum	Ileum	Colon	
Sham-operated	1 h	23	22	32	7
Bile-fistula		30	28	27	37
Sham-operated	24 h	55	44	32	26
Bile-fistula		45	39	27	56

density measurements remained relatively unchanged over 24 h in the colons of rats with a bile fistula, which suggests that a lengthening of the cell cycle time had occurred (161). An apparent loss of labelled epithelial cells took place in both sham-operated and bile-fistula rats. However, the phenomenon was of greater magnitude in the latter group, resulting in a shorter crypt column of 35.5 cells compared to 38.5 in sham-operated rats. There appear to be several mechanisms operating to regulate cell proliferation in this model, and the end point may very well be mucosal atrophy. The strong trophic effect of bile, not only on cell proliferation in the ileum, but more so on the colonic mucosa, has obvious significance in our understanding of the integrity of the digestive mucosa and its ultimate impact on colonic cancer.

In addition to the bile, secretions from the pancreas reaching the intestine through the duodenal papilla were found to influence the epithelial mucosa in general and the size of the villi in particular (17). A month after the duodenal papilla was transplanted to the ileum of the rat, villus size at this site had more than doubled. Diversion of bile into the ileum also induced villus enlargement, but this was moderate by comparison with the effect created by the pancreatic secretions. Enhanced mitotic activity in the crypts and reduced exfoliation at the villus tips were offered as provisional explanations for the observed effect.

It appears reasonable to state that the integrity of the normal mucosa is dependent on the controlled discharge and flow of bile, pancreatic secretions and gastrointestinal hormones, with each of them and their constituents appearing in balanced proportions. The consequences of interruption in or alterations to concentration or composition of these secretions may thus be important in such widely disparate conditions as mucosal atrophy and neoplastic growth.

6.5.4 EXTERNAL FACTORS AFFECTING THE MUCOSA

That proper nutrition is responsible for general good health and a balanced internal environment for cells and tissues has always been widely accepted. But only recently has the nature of the profound effects of diet been demonstrated; for example, diet can influence the colonic concentration of sterols, bile acids, and their bacterial metabolites (266, 564, 569, 646). The effect of these substances on cell proliferation has just begun to be appreciated. When compared with a control population, patients with colonic cancer as well as those with adenomatous polyps have a higher faecal concentration of the secondary bile acids, lithocholic and deoxycholic acids. Similarly, patients at high risk of developing colonic cancer, such as those with ulcerative colitis and familial polyposis, excrete increased amounts of cholesterol or its metabolites (559).

There are marked differences between these high risk groups and strict vegetarians, in whom there is a low incidence of large bowel cancer. Plant sterols comprise a substantial portion of vegetarian diets, the most common components being β-sitosterol, campesterol, and stigmasterol. Volunteers fed 5 to 10 g per day β-sitosterol for 2 weeks demonstrated a 20 to 40 percent decrease in plasma cholesterol concentrations (529), whereas hypercholesterolaemic subjects fed 9 g per day for 2 to 3 months revealed only a 10 to 25 percent decrease in serum cholesterol (646).

Rats given 4 intrarectal instillations of 2 mg of the carcinogen N-methyl-N-nitrosourea (MNU), while fed a diet supplemented with β-sitosterol at a dose of 0.2 percent, showed a decrease from 49 to 33 percent in the number of animals with a colorectal tumour (124). Preliminary evidence suggests a reduction in I_s in the colons of rats fed the plant sterol; this would presumably reduce the opportunity for expression of malignant transformation.

In contrast, intrarectal administration of secondary bile acids, ie, lithocholic acid and taurodeoxycholate, significantly increased the incidence of colonic cancer induced by N-methyl-N'-nitro-N-nitrosoguanidine in rats (494). Moreover, a dietary ingestion of cholic acid at a dose level of 0.2 percent enhanced MNU-induced tumour formation from 49 to 69 percent (125). Cholic-acid feeding also increased the faecal concentration of bile acids between two- and three-fold, which is similar to the difference between human populations with a high incidence of colorectal cancer and populations with a low incidence of the disease. Although the concentration of individual bile acids was increased, only the deoxycholic acid constituent was increased significantly (125). Deoxycholic acid may be acting as a tumour promotor or co-carcinogen. On a cellular level, the effect of cholic acid on colonic cell proliferation was noticeable after as short a time as 5 weeks' treatment (Figure 6.5.2).

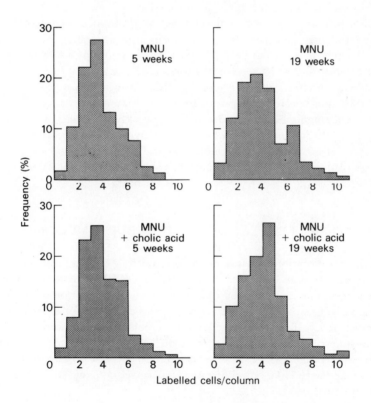

Figure 6.5.2 The number of labelled epithelial cells in crypt columns in the distal colonic mucosa of rats 5 and 19 weeks after the first of 4 intrarectal instillations of 2 mg of MNU. The animals were given 0.2% cholic acid in their diet concurrently starting with the first instillation

Examination of the distribution of labelled cells in groups given MNU alone or MNU plus cholic acid indicated a shift toward higher labelling indices in the rodents fed the bile acid. Nineteen weeks after the beginning of the experiment, differences between the groups were further intensified (125). The mechanisms by which this occurred are believed to involve either a shortening of the generation time, as has been suggested (460), or an increase in the rate of cell proliferation (125), or a combination of both (125). These alterations in cell proliferation are believed to allow for expression of MNU-induced malignancy earlier and with greater frequency in the cholic-acid treated rats.

Removal of the gallbladder, the normal storage site of bile, causes a more continuous flow of the secretion into the duodenum and changes the composition of faecal bile acids. Recent evidence has indicated that the secondary bile acid, deoxycholic acid, the same faecal constituent presumed to be the tumour promotor primarily responsible for elevated MNU-induced neoplasia in cholic-acid-fed rodents, becomes the predominant bile acid after cholecystectomy (530). Furthermore, it has been observed that in a group of 638 patients with recent colonic cancer, 10 percent had had a cholecystectomy in the previous 10 years (781). In contrast, absence of a gallbladder was observed in only 5 to 6 percent of non-selected autopsies (267). Experimentally, a four-fold higher incidence of colonic tumours induced by 10 weekly injections of 15 mg per kg 1,2-dimethylhydrazine was found in mice following cholecystectomy (70 versus 16 percent at 20 weeks). Epidemiological analyses of larger populations are in progress to determine the significance of this observation.

6.5.5 ALTERED REGULATION IN COLORECTAL MUCOSA

An early manifestation of loss of regulatory control over cell proliferation in the large bowel of man has been recognised since 1963. Different groups of investigators, one applying the technique of in-vivo injection of ^{3}HTdR to a familial polyposis patient with limited life expectancy (126) and the other using an in-vitro labelling procedure (153) reported the presence of DNA-synthesising cells at the surface of colorectal crypts. This observation was confirmed by others (49, 459) and was found to occur at high frequency among many groups with large bowel disease (163) as well as a few with no detectable gastrointestinal disease (155).

More recently, an additional fact has been brought to light in a study conducted in Louvain and New York (459). Thirty biopsies of histologically normal colorectal mucosa from 26 patients were used for ^{3}HTdR-incorporation studies. Thirteen patients were being treated for large bowel cancer and 13 were controls. The mean labelling indices were 7.9 $\pm$ 0.9 for control patients and

9.8 ± 1.2 for the cancer patients; because of wide variability these values are not significantly different.

Among the control population the constant proliferative pattern observed was of labelling predominantly in the lower third of the crypts. However, six of 17 specimens from cancer patients demonstrated labelling principally in the middle or middle and upper third. A comparison of the labelling distribution and the relative position of labelled cells in colonic crypts of cancer and control patients from New York is presented in Figure 6.5.3. In 3 of the 6 cancer patients an upward shift of the major zone of DNA synthesis toward the surface was seen.

Labelling in the upper third of the crypt and along the surface was more frequent in the cancer group than in the control population (Table 6.5.4), significantly so in the New York series.

When the overall labelling distributions of cancer and control patients were compared, a difference was also found (Table 6.5.4), which was doubtless

Table 6.5.4 Labelling index and site of predominant labelling in the crypts of normal-appearing colorectal mucosa in 13 control subjects and 13 patients with colorectal tumours in New York and Louvain

	Labelling index (%)			
	Lower crypt	Mid crypt	Upper crypt	Total
Controls	15.1	7.9	0.8	7.9
Cancer patients	15.2	12.7	1.6	9.8
	Predominant labelling (% of total)			
	Lower crypt	Mid crypt	Upper crypt	
Controls	64	33	3	
Cancer patients	52	43	5	

related to the increased I_s in the middle and upper crypt present in some of the cancer patients. The I_s for each third of the crypt was not significantly different between groups since only 6 out of 17 specimens exhibited this abnormal labelling pattern (459).

This shift in the major zone of cell renewal can be thought of as a more severe defect in regulatory control and a stage which still precedes the development of a visible colonic lesion.

6.5.6 HIGH RISK GROUPS

Asymptomatic (control) patients over the age of 45 had biopsy material labelled

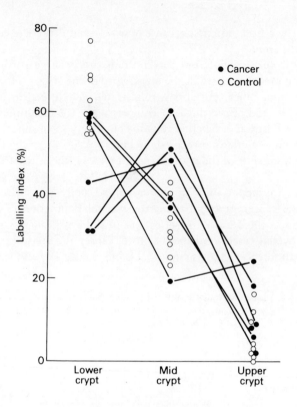

Figure 6.5.3 The percentage of labelled cells distributed in the 3 regions of colonic crypts for 8 controls and 6 cancer patients. Three cancer patients exhibited an upward shift of the major proliferation compartment

Table 6.5.5 Numbers and percentages of subjects with abnormal patterns of cell proliferation in normal-appearing colorectal mucosa for different disease groups

Disease group	Number of patients	Upper labelling number (percentage)	Zone shift number (percentage)
Control	8	6 (75)	0 (0)
Familial polyposis	15	10 (67)	6 (40)
Non-symptomatic relatives of familial polyposis patients	12	11 (92)	5 (42)
Isolated polyps	18	15 (83)	12 (67)
Colonic cancer	15	11 (73)	5 (33)
Total high risk	60	47 (78)	28 (47)

with [3]HTdR and evaluated for disturbed cell proliferation (Table 6.5.5). Data from such patients as well as those distributed among several groups at high risk for colonic cancer are presented. These groups include familial polyposis patients, non-symptomatic relatives of patients with familial polyposis, patients with a previous history of colonic cancer, and patients with a previous history of isolated adenomatous polyps.

In each series only a relatively small percentage of patients had biopsy specimens characterised by what we would regard as totally normal [3]HTdR incorporation. Instead, a large percentage showed DNA-synthesising cells in the upper third of colorectal crypts, indicating expansion of the proliferation compartment with loss of regulatory controls which normally suppress DNA synthesis in this region. This was seen in approximately 80 percent of high risk patients. A notably smaller percentage in each of the groups expressed the second abnormality, a shift in the major zone of cell renewal away from the lower crypt; this smaller frequency is thought to provide support for the concept that the displacement of the major zone of cell proliferation is a later stage in the evolution of the mucosa toward the neoplastic state.

Additional support for this statement can be obtained by an examination of two diverse sets of data. One relates to the DMH model in mice and the other to the labelling distribution within adenomatous polyps.

Mice injected weekly with DMH at a dose of 20 mg per kg body weight form microadenomas or areas of focial atypism as early as 22 days after the initiation of carcinogen treatment (149). This coincides with the time when DNA-synthesising cells and mitoses are recognised in the upper regions of crypts. The distribution of labelled epithelial cells was examined in a small group of CF-1 mice studied for the acute effect of the carcinogen. The two mice killed after five DMH injections both showed an abnormal distribution of labelled cells, with the major zone of proliferation shifted to the middle and upper third of the crypts (150). The incidence of focal atypias was increased in frequency and was followed within a further 10 weeks by the macroscopic appearance of adenomas. Only later did colonic carcinomas arise (160). Thus, the finding of the predominant middle and upper crypt labelling in DMH-treated colonic mucosa prior to the appearance of polyps and cancer would suggest that it is an important preneoplastic event.

Additional supportive evidence that this observation bears on the development of colonic neoplasia can be derived from labelled cell distribution studies of adenomatous polyps (156). When longitudinal sections of adenomas removed from a patient with a variant of familial polyposis (Gardner's syndrome) were examined, cell renewal was found principally along the upper surface, although it also occurred along the entire length of the crypt column. A similar pattern has been confirmed by other investigators (389, 458). This would suggest that cells capable of DNA synthesis move up the crypt wall, continue to adhere to the basement membrane, and collect at the mucosal surface where new cells and new glands are formed.

Normally new crypts are formed at the base of existing glands; this is the method whereby colonic crypts develop during postnatal growth (457), and involves bifurcation or fission of the preexisting gland. Whenever crypts atrophy because of stem-cell degeneration, whether induced by a single injection of DMH (150) or by neutron irradiation (85), the mechanism for repopulation of crypts involves bifurcation at the base of glands.

However, repeated treatment with DMH induces not only this normal type

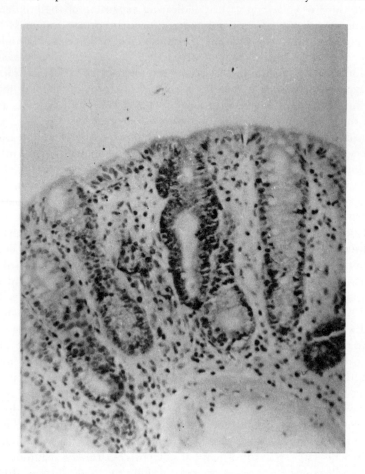

Figure 6.5.4 Mucosa of distal colon of mouse after 38 days of DMH treatment showing bud or pocket arising from the upper region of one crypt (×225)

of gland development, but a second type which occurs closer to the surface. Budding or branching arises from the middle or upper regions of the crypt, the zones where the abnormally distributed DNA-synthesising cells accumulate. This unusual gland development is a further event in the sequence leading to the formation of an adenomatous polyp. Mid and upper crypt bulging and branching has been recognised after as few as three weekly injections of DMH (Figure 6.5.4) (149), and, together with the mode of cell proliferation described in adenomatous polyps, provides strong support for the importance of recognising the altered distribution of DNA-synthesising cells and the concomitant shift of the major zone of cell renewal in colonic crypts.

6.5.7 SUMMARY

We believe that a number of observations have been made which provide greater understanding of the finely balanced regulatory mechanisms which guide and maintain the gastrointestinal mucosa. Alteration in the mucosal environment through diet, loss of contact with normal secretions, or changes in their critical concentrations, may induce no immediate obvious changes in the histological appearance or proliferative behaviour of epithelial cells. However, chronic disturbances over a period of 10 to 20 years may ultimately induce expression of a recognisable disease state. One such manifestation of diseased mucosa, namely the formation of adenomatous polyps has, perhaps more clearly than other syndromes, allowed the sequence of steps and the degrees of diminished control to be best described. Regulation of certain disease states in such a way as to reduce the risk of cancer is a distinct possibility now that the effect of diet and its impact on the physiological environment of intestinal epithelial cells is better appreciated.

References

1. Abrams G D. Microbial effects on mucosal structure and function. *Am J Clin Nutr* 1977; 30: 1880–1886   2.7

2. Abrams G D, Bauer H, Sprinz H. Influence of the normal flora on mucosal morphology and cellular renewal in the ileum. A comparison of germ-free and conventional mice. *Lab Invest* 1963; 12: 355–364   5.5, 6.5

3. Abt A B, Carter S L. Goblet cell carcinoid of the appendix. An ultrastructural and histochemical study. *Arch Pathol Lab Med* 1976; 100: 301–306   3.2

4. Ader R. Early experiences accelerate maturation of the 24-hour adrenocortical rhythm. *Science* 1969; 163: 1225–1226   2.6

5. Al-Dewachi H S, Appleton D R, Watson A J, Wright N A. Variation in the cell cycle time in the crypts of Lieberkühn of the mouse. *Virchows Archiv (Cell Pathol)* 1979; 31: 37–44   1.1

6. Al-Dewachi H S, Wright N A, Appleton D R, Watson A J. The cell cycle time in the rat jejunal mucosa. *Cell Tissue Kinet* 1974; 7: 587–594   1.1, 1.3, 1.4, 2.1, 3.1, 3.2, 4.2, 5.1, 5.5

7. Al-Dewachi H S, Wright N A, Appleton D R, Watson A J. Cell population kinetics in the mouse jejunal crypt. *Virchows Archiv (Cell Pathol)* 1975; 18: 225–242   2.3, 3.1, 3.2

8. Al-Dewachi H S, Wright N A, Appleton D R, Watson A J. The effect of starvation and refeeding on cell population kinetics in the rat small bowel mucosa. *J Anat* 1975; 119: 105–121   1.1, 2.2

9. Al-Dewachi H S, Wright N A, Appleton D R, Watson A J. Studies on the mechanism of diurnal variation of proliferative indices in the small bowel mucosa of the rat. *Cell Tissue Kinet* 1976; 9: 459–467   1.1, 2.2, 3.2

10. Al-Dewachi H S, Wright N A, Appleton D R, Watson A J. The effects of a single injection of hydroxyurea on cell population kinetics in the small bowel mucosa of the rat. *Cell Tissue Kinet* 1977; 10: 203–213   1.1, 4.2

11. Al-Dewachi H S, Wright N A, Appleton D R, Watson A J. The effects of a single injection of cytosine arabinoside on cell population kinetics in the mouse small intestine. *Virchows Archiv (Cell Pathol)* (In Press)   2.5, 4.3

12. Allen C, Kendall J W. Maturation of the circadian rhythm of plasma corticosterone in the rat. *Endocrinology* 1967; 80: 926–930   2.6

13. Allen E. The estrus cycle in the mouse. *Am J Anat* 1922; 30: 297–371   4.5

14. Alm, T, Licznerski G. The intestinal polyposes. *Clin Gastroenterol* 1973; 2: 577–602   6.1

15. Alper T, Hornsey S, Pike M C, Smith P. In: *Effects of Radiation on Cellular Proliferation and Differentiation*, IAEA, Vienna 1968; 515   4.3

16. Al-Thamery D M, Ferguson A. The effects of giardia infection on small   6.2
    intestinal disaccharidases in mice. Acta Paediat Belg 1979; 32: 152
17. Altmann G G. Influence of bile and pancreatic secretions on the size of   2.1, 2.2, 4.4,
    the intestinal villi in the rat. Am J Anat 1971; 132: 167–178   5.5, 6.5
18. Altmann G G. Influence of starvation and refeeding on mucosal size and   4.4, 5.5
    epithelial renewal in the rat small intestine. Am J Anat 1972; 133:
    391–400
19. Altmann G G. Factors involved in the differentiation of the epithelial   2.2
    cells in the rat small intestine. In: Cairnie A B, Lala P K, Osmond D G.
    eds. Stem Cells of Renewing Cell Populations. New York: Academic Press
    1976; 51–65
20. Altmann G G, Enesco M. Cell number as a measure of distribution and   2.1, 2.6
    renewal of epithelial cells in the small intestine of growing and adult
    rats. Am J Anat 1967; 121: 319–336
21. Altmann G G, Leblond C P. Factors influencing villus size in the small   2.2, 4.4
    intestine of adult rats as revealed by transposition of intestinal segments.
    Am J Anat 1970; 127: 15–36
22. Amacher D E, Alarif A, Epstein S S. The effects of ingested chrysotile on   5.5
    DNA synthesis in the gastrointestinal tract, liver and pancreas of the rat.
    Environ Health Perspect 1974; 9: 319–324
23. Amacher D E, Alarif A, Epstein S S. The dose-dependant effects of   5.5
    ingested chrysotile on DNA synthesis in the gastrointestinal tract, liver
    and pancreas of the rat. Environ Res 1975; 10: 208–216
24. Anderson C M. Histological changes in the duodenal mucosa in coeliac   6.3
    disease. Reversibility during treatment with a wheat gluten free diet.
    Arch Dis Child 1960; 35: 419–427
25. Annison E F. In: Dougherty R W. ed. Physiology of Digestion in the   2.7
    Ruminant. Washington DC: Butterworth 1965; 185–197
26. Annison E F, Armstrong D G. Volatile fatty acid metabolism and energy   2.7
    supply. In: Phillipson A T. ed. Physiology of Digestion and Metabolism in
    the Ruminant. Newcastle upon Tyne: Oriel Press 1970: 422–437
27. Appleton D R, Sunter J P. Estimating the proportion of proliferating   1.4
    cells in a population. Virchows Archiv (Cell Pathol) 1979; 32: 69–73
28. Appleton D R, Sunter J P, Watson A J. The cut-off position in the   1.4, 5.5, 6.3
    intestinal crypt. Cell Tissue Kinet (In Press)
29. Appleton D R, Wright N A, Dyson P. The age distribution of cells in   1.4
    stratified squamous epithelium. J Theor Biol 1977; 65: 769–779
30. Asano T, Pollard M, Madsen D C. Effects of cholestyramine on   5.4
    1,2-dimethylhydrazine-induced enteric carcinoma in germfree rats
    (39124). Proc Soc Exp Biol Med 1975; 150: 780–785
31. Asquith P, Johnson A G, Cooke W T. Scanning electron microscopy of   6.3
    normal and coeliac jejunal mucosa. Am J Dig Dis 1970; 15: 511–521
32. Baker P G, Read A E. Oats and barley toxicity in coeliac disease. Postgrad   6.3
    Med J 1976; 52: 264–268
33. Baker S J. Geographical variations in the morphology of the small   6.3
    intestinal mucosa in apparently healthy individuals. Pathol Microbiol
    (Basel) 1973; 39: 222–237
34. Barros D'Sa A A B, Buchanan K D. Role of gastrointestinal hormones in   2.2
    the response to massive resection of the small bowel. Gut 1977; 18:
    877–881

35. Barthold S W. Autoradiographic cytokinetics of colonic hyperplasia in mice. *Cancer Res* 1979; **39**: 24–29   2.1

36. Barthold S W, Jonas A M. Morphogenesis of early 1,2-dimethylhydrazine induced lesions and latent period reduction of colon carcinogenesis in mice by a variant of *Citrobacter freundii*. *Cancer Res* 1977; **37**: 4352–4360   5.1, 5.4

37. Bassett J M. Diurnal patterns of plasma insulin, growth hormone, corticosteroid and metabolite concentrations in fed and fasted sheep. *Aust J Biol Sci* 1974; **27**: 167–181   2.7

38. Baundry M, Martres M P, Swartz J C. H_1 and H_2-receptors in the histamine induced accumulation of cyclic AMP in guinea pig brain slices. *Nature* 1975; **253**: 362–363   5.3

39. Behnke O, Moe H. An electron microscopic study of mature and differentiating Paneth cells in the rat especially of their endoplasmic reticulum and lysosomes. *J Cell Biol* 1964; **22**: 633–652   3.2

40. Bellinger L L, Williams F E, Bernardis L L. Effects of hypophysectomy, thyroidectomy, castration and adrenalectomy on diurnal food and water intake in rats. *Proc Soc Exp Biol Med* 1979; **161**: 162–166   2.2

41. Beremblum I, Haran N, Rosin A. The carcinogenic action in the mouse of 20-methylcholanthrene by rectal administration. *Am J Pathol* 1956; **32**: 579–589   5.1

42. Berlinger N T, Lopez C, Vogel J, Lipkin M, Good R A. Defective recognitive immunity in family aggregates of colon carcinoma. *J Clin Invest* 1977; **59**: 761–769   6.1

43. Bertalanffy F D. Mitotic rates and renewal times of the digestive tract epithelia in the rat. *Acta Anat (Basel)* 1960; **40**: 130–148   2.1

44. Bielschowsky F. Distant tumours produced by 2 amino and 2 acetyl-amino-fluorene. *Br J Exp Pathol* 1944; **25**: 1–4   5.1

45. Bielschowsky F. Comparison of the tumours produced by 2 acetylamino-fluorene in piebald and Wistar rats. *Br J Exp Pathol* 1946; **27**: 135–139   5.1

46. Birkett D P. Epidemiology of cancer of the colon and rectum. *Cancer* 1971; **28**: 3–13   6.1

47. Bizzozero G. Über die Regeneration der Elemente der schlauchförmigen Drüsen und des Epithels des Magendarmkanals. *Anat Anz* 1888; **3**: 781–784   2.1

48. Blackwell J N, Barneston R St C, Gilmour H M, Ferguson A, Heading R C. What is the role of gluten in dermatitis herpetiformis? *Scott Med J* 1979; **24**: 326   6.2

49. Bleiberg H, Mainguet P, Galand P. Cell renewal in familial polyposis. Comparison between polyps and adjacent healthy mucosa. *Gastroenterology* 1972; **63**: 240–245   6.1, 6.5

50. Boarder T A, Blackett N M. The poliferative status of intestinal epithelial clonogenic cells: sensitivity to S phase specific cytotoxic agents. *Cell Tissue Kinet* 1976; **9**: 589–596   3.1, 4.2, 4.3

51. Bolton R E, Davis J M G. The short term effects of chronic asbestos ingestion in rats. *Ann Occup Hyg* 1976; **19**: 121–128   5.5

52. Booth C C. Enteropoiesis: structural and functional relationships of the enterocyte. *Postgrad Med J* 1968; **44**: 12–16   6.3

53. Booth C C. Enterocytes in coeliac disease. *Br Med J* 1970; **3**: 725–31; **4**: 14–17   6.3

54. Both N J de, Dongen J M van, Hofwegen B van, Keulemans J, Visser W   2.1, 3.2
    J, Galjaard H. The influence of various cell kinetic conditions on
    functional differentiation in the small intestine of the rat. A study of
    enzymes bound to subcellular organelles. *Dev Biol* 1974; **38**: 119–137

55. Both N J de, Kamp A W M van der, Dongen J M van. The influence of   3.2
    changing crypt cell kinetics on functional differentiation in the small
    intestine of the rat. Nucleotide and protein synthesis. *Differentiation*
    1975; **4**: 175–182

56. Both N J de, Plaisier H M. The influence of changing cell kinetics on   2.1, 3.2, 6.2
    functional differentiation in the small intestine of the rat. A study of
    enzymes involved in carbohydrate metabolism. *J Histochem Cytochem*
    1974; **22**: 352–360

57. Brachet J, Hulin N. Binding of tritiated actinomycin and cell differenti-   6.4
    ation. *Nature* 1969; **222**: 481–482

58. Brachet J, Hulin N. Actinomycin binding in differentiating and   6.4
    dividing cells. *Exp Cell Res* 1970; **59**: 486–488

59. Brandt J, Cooper J W, Osborne J W. Migration rates of duodenal and   2.2
    colonic epithelial cells after X-irradiation of exteriorized jejunum and
    ileum. *Radiat Res* 1972; **51**: 440

60. Brimblecombe R W, Owen D A A, Parsons M E. The cardiovascular   5.3
    effects of histamine in laboratory animals. *Agents Actions* 1974; **4**:
    191–192

61. Bruce W R, Meeker, B E. Comparison of the sensitivity of normal   4.2
    hematopoietic and transplanted lymphoma colony-forming cells to
    tritiated thymidine. *J Natl Cancer Inst* 1965; **34**: 849–856

62. Brugal G. Presence of intestinal chalones. In: Cairnie A B, Lala P K,   2.2, 3.2
    Osmond D G eds. *Stem Cells of Renewing Populations*. New York:
    Academic Press 1976; 41–50

63. Brugal G, Garbay C, Giroud F, Adelh D. A double scanning micro-   2.3
    photometer for image analysis: hardware, software and biomedical
    applications. *J Histochem Cytochem* 1979; **27**: 144–152

64. Brugal G, Pelmont J. Existence of two chalone-like substances in   2.3
    intestinal extract from the adult newt inhibiting embryonic intestinal
    cell proliferation. *Cell Tissue Kinet* 1975; **8**: 171–188

65. Buchanan K D (Ed) *Gastrointestinal hormones. Clinics in Endocrinology and*   2.2
    Metabolism. London: Saunders 1979

66. Buchholtz T W, Malamud D, Ross J S, Malt R A. Onset of cell   4.4
    proliferation in the shortened gut: growth after subtotal colectomy.
    Surgery 1976; **80**: 601–607

67. Bullock F D, Rohdenburg G L. Spontaneous tumours of the rat. *J Cancer*   5.1
    Res 1917; **2**: 39–60

68. Bullough H F. Cyclical Changes in the skin of the mouse during the   4.5
    oestrous cycle. *J Endocrinol* 1943; **3**: 380–387

69. Bullough W S. Mitotic activity in the adult female mouse, *Mus*   4.5
    musculus L. A study of its relation to the oestrous cycle in normal and
    abnormal conditions. *Philos Trans R Soc Lond (Biol)* 1946; **231**: 453–516

70. Bullough W S. The control of epidermal thickness. *Br J Dermatol* 1972;   2.3
    87: 187–199

71. Bullough W S. Chalone control mechanisms. *Life Sci* 1975; **16**: 323–330   2.3

72. Burek J D. *Pathology of Aging Rats. A morphological and experimental study*   5.5

of the age-associated lesions in aging BN/Bi, WAG/Wij and (WAG x BN)F₁
rats. West Palm Beach, Fla; CRC Press Inc 1978

73. Burgess D R. Morphogenesis of intestinal villi. II. Mechanisms of   1.2
    formation of previllous ridges. *J Embryol Exp Morphol* 1975; 34: 723–740

74. Burholt D R, Schultze B, Baurer W. Mode of growth of the jejunal crypt   1.1, 3.2
    cells of the rat: an autoradiographic study using double labelling with
    ^{3}H- and ^{14}C-thymidine in lower and upper parts of the crypts. *Cell Tissue
    Kinet* 1976; 9: 107–117

75. Burns F J, Tannock I F. On the existence of a G_0 phase in the cell cycle. *Cell*   1.3
    Tissue Kinet 1970; 3: 321–334

76. Burton K. A study of the conditions and mechanisms of the   5.5
    diphenylamine reaction for the colorometric estimation of DNA. *Biochem
    J* 1956; 62: 315–322

77. Bussey H J R. *Familial polyposis coli*. Baltimore: The Johns Hopkins   6.1
    University Press 1975

78. Cairnie A B. Cell proliferation studies in the intestinal epithelium of the   1.1, 2.1, 3.2
    rat: response to continuous irradiation. *Radiat Res* 1967; 32: 240–264

79. Cairnie A B. Further studies on the response of the small intestine to   3.2
    continuous irradiation. *Radiat Res* 1969; 38: 82–94

80. Cairnie A B. Renewal of goblet and Paneth cells in the small intestine.   3.1, 3.2
    Cell Tissue Kinet 1970; 3: 35–45

81. Cairnie A B. Homeostasis in the small intestine. In: Cairnie A B, Lala P   1.1, 2.2
    K, Osmond D G. eds. *Stem Cells of Renewing Cell Populations*. New York
    and London, Academic Press 1976; 67–77

82. Cairnie A B, Bentley J. Cell proliferation studies in the intestinal   1.1, 1.3, 1.4,
    epithelium of the rat. Hyperplasia during lactation. *Exp Cell Res* 1967;   3.3, 5.1, 5.5,
    46: 428–440   6.3

83. Cairnie A B, Lamerton L F, Steel G G. Cell proliferation studies in the   1.1, 1.3, 2.1,
    intestinal epithelium of the rat. I Determination of the kinetic paramet-   2.3, 3.2, 4.2,
    ers. *Exp Cell Res* 1965; 39: 528–538   6.3

84. Cairnie A B, Lamerton L F, Steel G G. Cell proliferation studies in the   1.1, 1.4, 3.2,
    intestinal epithelium of the rat. II Theoretical aspects. *Exp Cell Res* 1965;   5.2, 5.5, 6.3
    39: 539–553

85. Cairnie A B, Millen B H. Fission of crypts in the small intestine of the   2.1, 2.2, 2.5,
    irradiated mouse. *Cell Tissue Kinet* 1975; 8: 189–196   3.1, 6.5

86. Cairns J. Mutation, selection and the natural history of cancer. *Nature*   3.1
    1975; 225: 197–200

87. Campbell R L, Singh D V, Nigro N D. Importance of the fecal stream on   5.4
    the induction of colon tumors by azoxymethane in rats. *Cancer Res* 1975;
    35: 1369–1371

88. Carrière R M. The influence of thyroid and testicular hormones on   2.2
    epithelium of crypts of Lieberkühn in the rat's intestine. *Anat Rec* 1966;
    156: 423–432

89. Castleden W M, Shilkin K B. Diet, liver function and dimethylhyd-   5.1
    razine induced gastrointestinal tumours in male Wistar rats. *Br J Cancer*
    1979; 39: 731–739

90. Castleman B, Krickstein H I. Do adenomatous polyps of the colon   5.2, 6.4
    become malignant? *New Engl J Med* 1962; 267: 469–475

91. Chan L, O'Malley B W. Mechanism of action of the sex steroid hor-   4.5
    mones. *N Engl J Med* 1976; 294: 1322–1328, 1372–1381, 1430–1437

92. Chan P C, Cohen L A, Narisawa T, Weisburger J H. Early effects of a single intrarectal dose of 1,2-dimethylhydrazine in mice. *Cancer Res* 1976; 36: 13–17   5.1, 5.2

93. Chang W W L. Renewal of the epithelium in the descending colon of the mouse. III Diurnal variation in the proliferative activity of epithelial cells. *Am J Anat* 1971; 131: 111–119   1.4, 2.2, 3.3, 4.5

94. Chang W W L. Histogenesis of symmetrical 1,2-dimethylhydrazine induced neoplasms of the colon in the mouse. *J Natl Cancer Inst* 1978; 60: 1405–1418   5.1, 5.2, 6.1

95. Chang W W L, Leblond C P. Renewal of the epithelium in the descending colon of the mouse. I Presence of three cell populations: vacuolated-columnar, mucous and argentaffin. *Am J Anat* 1971; 131: 73–100   1.4, 4.5, 5.2

96. Chang W W L, Leblond C P. A unitarian theory of the origin of the three populations of epithelial cells in the mouse large intestine. *Anat Rec* 1971; 169: 293   5.2

97. Chang W W L, Mak K M, MacDonald P D M. Cell population kinetics of 1,2 dimethylhydrazine induced colonic neoplasms and their adjacent colonic mucosa in the mouse. *Virchows Archiv (Cell Pathol)* 1979; 30: 149–361   5.1, 5.2

98. Chang W W L, Nadler N J. Renewal of the epithelium in the descending colon of the mouse. IV Cell population kinetics of vacuolated-columnar and mucous cells. *Am J Anat* 1975; 144: 39–56   1.3, 1.4, 3.3, 4.5, 5.2

99. Cheng H. Origin, differentiation and renewal of the four main epithelial cell types in the mouse small intestine. II Mucous cells. *Am J Anat* 1974; 141: 481–502   3.1, 3.2

100. Cheng H. Origin, differentiation and renewal of the four main epithelial cell types in the mouse small intestine. IV Paneth cells. *Am J Anat* 1974; 141: 521–536   3.1, 3.2

101. Cheng H, Leblond C P. Origin, differentiation and renewal of the four main epithelial cell types in the mouse small intestine. I Columnar cells. *Am J Anat* 1974; 141: 461–480   3.2, 4.2

102. Cheng H, Leblond C P. Origin, differentiation and renewal of the four main epithelial cell types in the mouse small intestine. III Entero-endocrine cells. *Am J Anat* 1974; 141: 503–520   3.2

103. Cheng H, Leblond C P. Origin, Differentiation and renewal of the four main epithelial cell types in the mouse small intestine. V Unitarian theory of the origin of the four epithelial cell types. *Am J Anat* 1974; 141: 537–562   3.1, 3.2, 4.2, 4.3, 5.2

104. Cheng H, Merzel J, Leblond C P. Renewal of Paneth cells in the small intestine of the mouse. *Am J Anat* 1969; 126: 507–526   3.1, 3.2

105. Christophers E. Eine neue Methode zur Darstellung des Stratum Corneum. *Arch Klin Exp Derm* 1970; 237: 7171–722   4.2

106. Chomchai C, Bhadrachari N, Nigro N D. The effect of bile on the induction of experimental intestinal tumors in rats. *Dis Colon Rectum* 1974; 17: 310–312   5.4

107. Clapperton J L, Czerkawski J W. Metabolism of propane-1:2-diol infused into the rumen of the sheep. *Br J Nutr* 1972; 27: 348–356   2.7

108. Clark P A, Harland W A. Experimental malabsorption with jejunal atrophy induced by colchicine. *Br J Exp Pathol* 1963; 44: 520–523   6.3

109. Clarke R M. Mucosal architecture and epithelial cell production rate in   1.1, 2.5, 6.2
     the small intestine of the albino rat. *J Anat* 1970; **107**: 519–529

110. Clarke R M. The effect of growth and of fasting on the number of villi   1.1, 2.1, 2.2,
     and crypts in the small intestine of the albino rat. *J Anat* 1972; **112**:   5.5
     27–33

111. Clarke R M. Progress in measuring epithelial turnover in the villus of the   1.1
     small intestine. *Digestion* 1973; **8**: 161–175

112. Clarke R M. Control of intestinal epithelial replacement: lack of evidence   2.1, 2.2
     for a tissue-specific blood-borne factor. *Cell Tissue Kinet* 1974; **7**:
     241–250

113. Clarke R M. Morphological description of intestinal adaptation: meas-   2.1
     urements and their meaning. In: Dowling R H, Riecken E O eds.
     Intestinal Adaptation. New York: Schattauer Verlag 1974; 11–17

114. Clarke R M. Diet, mucosal architecture and epithelial cell production in   2.1, 2.2
     the small intestine of specified-pathogen-free and conventional rats. *Lab*
     Anim 1975; **9**: 201–209

115. Clarke R M. Evidence for both luminal and systemic factors in the   4.4
     control of rat intestinal epithelial replacement. *Clin Sci Mol Med* 1976;
     50: 139–144

116. Clarke R M. The effects of age on mucosal morphology and epithelial cell   2.1, 5.5
     production in rat small intestine. *J Anat* 1977; **123**: 805–811

117. Clarke R M. 'Luminal nutrition' versus 'functional work-load' as   2.2
     controllers of mucosal morphology and epithelial replacement in the rat
     small intestine. *Digestion* 1977; **15**: 411–424

118. Clarke R M, Hardy R N. The use of (^{125}I) polyvinyl pyrrolidone K.60 in   2.6
     the quantitative assessment of the uptake of macromolecular substances
     by the intestine of the young rat. *J Physiol (Lond)* 1969; **204**: 113–125

119. Clarke R M, Hardy R N. An analysis of the mechanism of cessation of   2.6
     uptake of macromolecular substances by the intestine of the young rat
     ('closure'). *J Physiol (Lond)* 1969; **204**: 127–134

120. Cleaver J E. *Thymidine Metabolism and Cell Kinetics*. Amsterdam: North   1.1, 1.4, 2.6,
     Holland Publishing Company, 1967   6.3

121. Cleveland J C, Cole J W. Relationship of experimentally induced   5.1
     intestinal tumours to laxative ingestion. *Cancer* 1969; **23**: 1200–1203

122. Coffey R G, Middleton E. In: Haddem J W, Coffey R C, Spreadfico F   5.3
     eds. *Immunopharmacology*. New York: Plenum Medical Book Company
     1977; 203–225

123. Coggle J E, Gordon M Y. Quantitative measurements on the haemopoei-   4.2
     tic systems of three strains of mice. *Hematol* 1975; **3**: 181–186

124. Cohen B I, Raicht R F, Deschner E E, Fazzini E, Takahashi M, Sarwel A   6.5
     N. Effect of β-sitosterol on MNU induced colon cancer in rats.
     Submitted for publication 1979

125. Cohen B I, Raicht R F, Deschner E E, Takahashi M, Sarwal A N, Fazzini   6.5
     E. Biochemical and cell kinetic alterations following cholic acid feeding on
     MNU induced colon tumours in rats. *J Natl Cancer Inst* 1979 (In Press)

126. Cole J W, McKalen A. Studies on the morphogenesis of adenomatous   6.1, 6.5
     polyps in the human colon. *Cancer* 1963; **16**: 998–1002

127. Comline R S, Silver I A, Steven D H. In: Code C F, ed. *Handbook of*   2.7
     Physiology. Section 6: *Alimentary Canal*. Vol. V. Washington D.C.:
     American Physiological Society 1968: 2647–2671

128. Coulombre A J, Coulombre J L. Intestinal development. I Mor-   1.2
     phogenesis of the villi and musculature. *J Embryol Exp Morphol* 1958; 6:
     403–411

129. Cox A J, Wilson R H, De Eds F. The carcinogenic activity of 2   5.1
     acetaminofluorene. Characteristics of the lesions in albino rats. *Cancer Res*
     1947; 7: 647–657

130. Crafts R C. The effect of endocrines on the formed elements of the blood.   4.5
     II. The effect of estrogens in the dog and monkey. *Endocrinology* 1941;
     29: 606–618

131. Creamer B. Dynamics of the mucosa of the small intestine in idiopathic   6.3
     steatorrhoea. *Gut* 1962; 3: 295–300

132. Creamer B. The turnover of the epithelium of the small intestine. *Br Med*   6.3
     Bull 1967; 23: 226–230

133. Creamer B, Croft D N. Losses from the gut in the coeliac syndrome. In: 6.3
     Booth C C, Dowling R H, eds. *Coeliac disease*. London and Edinburgh:
     Churchill Livingstone 1970

134. Creamer B, Shorter R G, Bamforth J. The turnover and shedding of   1.1
     epithelial cells. II. The shedding in the small intestine. *Gut* 1961; 2:
     117–118

135. Crean G P. A comparison between the effects of hypophysectomy and   2.2
     adrenalectomy on the gastric mucosa of the rat. *Gut* 1968; 9: 343–347

136. Crean G P, Rumsey R D E, Wheeler S M. Further observations   2.2
     concerning the effects of hypophysectomy on the gastric mucosa of the
     rat. *Gut* 1971; 12: 721–726

137. Crocker D W, Veith F W. Focal primary mucosal hyperplasia of the   6.4
     colon: the case for its importance in the pathogenesis of cancer. *Ann Surg*
     1964; 160: 215–225

138. Cronkite E O, Bond V P, Fleidner T M, Rubini J R. The use of tritiated   4.2
     thymidine in the study of DNA synthesis and cell turnover in hemopoie-
     tic tissues. *Lab Invest* 1959; 8: 263–277

139. Crosby W H, Kugler H W. Intraluminal biopsy of the small intestine: 6.3
     the intestinal biopsy capsule. *Am J Dig Dis* 1957; 2: 236–241

140. Cruse J P, Lewin M R, Ferulano G P, Clark C G. Co-carcinogenic effects   5.1
     of dietary cholesterol in experimental colon cancer. *Nature* 1978; 276:
     822–825

141. Cunningham H M, Pontefract R D. Asbestos fibres in beverages and   5.5
     drinking water. *Nature* 1971; 232: 332–333

142. Cunningham H M, Pontefract R D. Asbestos fibres in beverages,   5.5
     drinking water and tissue, their passage through the intestinal wall and
     movement through the body. *J Assoc Off Anal Chem* 1973; 56: 976–981

143. Dahlqvist A. Method for assay of intestinal disaccharidases. *Anal Biochem*   6.2
     1964; 7: 18–25

144. Danes B S, Krush A J. Brief communication: the Gardner syndrome: a   6.1
     family study in cell culture. *J Natl Cancer Inst* 1977; 58: 771–775

145. Davies M G, Marks R, Nuki G. Dermatitis herpetiformis—a skin   6.3
     manifestation of a generalised disturbance in immunity. *Q J Med* 1978; 47
     (186): 221–248

146. DeCosse J J, Condon R E, Adams M B. Surgical and medical measures in   6.1
     prevention of large bowel cancer. *Cancer* 1977; 40: 2549–2552

147. Della Porta G. Induction of intestinal mammary and ovarian tumours in   5.1

hamsters with oral administration of 20-methylcholanthrene. *Cancer Res* 1961; 21: 575–579

148. DeRubertis F R, Craven P A. Activation of the guanylate cyclase-guanosine 3′5′-monophosphate system of rat colonic mucosa by N-methyl-N′-nitro-N-nitrosoguanidine. *Cancer* 1977; 40: 2600–2608   5.3

149. Deschner E E. Experimentally induced cancer of the colon. *Cancer* 1974; 34 (suppl): 824–828   5.1, 5.2, 6.5

150. Deschner E E. Early proliferative defects induced by six weekly injections of 1,2 dimethylhydrazine in epithelial cells of mouse distal colon. *Z Krebsforsch* 1978; 91: 205–216   5.2, 6.5

151. Deschner E E, Goldstein M J, Melamed M R, Sherlock P. A histological and kinetic study of an ileal conduit. *Gastroenterology* 1973; 64: 920–925   6.5

152. Deschner E E, Goldstein M J, Melamed M R, Sherlock P. Radioautographic observation of a 19-month-old ileal conduit. *Gastroenterology* 1976; 71: 832–834   6.5

153. Deschner E E, Lewis C M, Lipkin M. In-vitro study of human rectal epithelial cells. I. Atypical zone of H^3-thymidine incorporation in mucosa of multiple polyposis. *J Clin Invest* 1963; 42: 1922–1928   6.1, 6.5

154. Deschner E E, Lipkin M. Study of human rectal epithelial cells in vitro. III. RNA, protein, and DNA synthesis in polyps and adjacent mucosa. *J Natl Cancer Inst* 1970; 44: 175–185   6.1

155. Deschner E E, Lipkin M. Proliferative patterns in colonic mucosa in familial polyposis. *Cancer* 1975; 35: 413–418   2.1, 6.4, 6.5

156. Deschner E E, Lipkin M. Proliferation and differentiation of gastrointestinal cells in health and disease. In: Lipkin M, Good R A, eds. *Gastrointestinal Tract Cancer*. New York: Plenum Medical Book Company 1978: 3–27   6.1, 6.5

157. Deschner E E, Lipkin M, Peterson A, Cooper M. Cell proliferation kinetics in DMH induced neoplasms of mouse. *Proc Amer Assn for Cancer Res* 1975; 16: 139   6.1

158. Deschner E E, Lipkin M, Solomon C. Study of human rectal epithelial cells in vitro. II. H^3-thymidine incorporation into polyps and adjacent mucosa. *J Natl Cancer Inst* 1966; 36: 849–857   6.4

159. Deschner E E, Long F C. Colonic neoplasms in mice produced with six injections of 1,2-dimethylhydrazine. *Oncology* 1977; 34: 255–257   6.1

160. Deschner E E, Long F C, Maskens A P. Relationship between dose, time and tumour yield in mouse dimethylhydrazine-induced colon tumorigenesis. *Cancer Lett* 1979; 8: 23–28   6.5

161. Deschner E E, Raicht R F. Influence of bile on kinetic behaviour of colonic epithelial cells of the rat. *Digestion* 1979; 19: 322–327   6.5

162. Deschner E E, Winawer S, Lipkin M. Patterns of nucleic acid and protein synthesis in normal human gastric mucosa and atrophic gastritis. *J Natl Cancer Inst* 1972; 48: 1567–1574   6.1

163. Deschner E E, Winawer S J, Long F C, Boyle C C. Early detection of colonic neoplasia in patients at high risk. *Cancer* 1977; 40: 2625–2631   6.5

164. Deschodt-Lanckman M, Robberecht P, Camus J, Baya C, Christophe J. Hormonal and dietary adaptation of rat pancreatic hydrolases before and after weaning. *Am J Physiol* 1974; 226: 39–44   2.6

165. Desjeux J F, Sassier P, Tichet J, Sarrut S, Lestradet H. Sugar absorption by flat jejunal mucosa. *Acta Paediatr Scand* 1973; 62: 531–537   2.3

166. Dethlefsen L A, Ohlsen J D, Roti Roti J L. Cell synchronization in-vivo: 4.2
fact of fancy? In: *Growth Kinetics and Biochemical Regulation of Normal and
Malignant cells*. Baltimore: Williams and Wilkins Co 1977: 481–488

167. Dicke W K, Coeliakie, een onderzoek naar de nadelige invloed van   6.3
sommige graansorten op de lijder aan coeliakie. MD Thesis, University
of Utrecht. Cited in 'Coeliac disease and wheat', *Lancet* 1952; 1:
857–858 (leading article)

168. Dicke W K, Weijers H A, Kamer J H van de. Coeliac disease; presence   6.3
in wheat of a factor having deleterious effect in cases of coeliac disease.
Acta Paediatr 1953; 42: 34–42

169. Dicker S E. Inhibition of compensatory renal growth by substances from   2.3
the kidney in rats. *J Physiol (Lond)* 1971; 218: 62–63

170. Diwan B A, Meier H, Blackman K E. Genetic differences in the   5.1
induction of colorectal tumours by 1,2 dimethylhydrazine in inbred
mice. *J Natl Cancer Inst* 1977; 59: 455–458

171. Dobson A. Active transport through the epithelium of the reticulo-   2.7
rumen sac of sheep. *J Physiol (Lond)* 1959; 146: 235–251

172. Dobson A, Phillipson A T. The influence of the contents of the rumen   2.7
and of adrenalin upon its blood supply. *J Physiol (Lond)* 1956; 133:
76–77

173. Dobson A, Phillipson A T. Absorption from the ruminant forestomach.   2.7
In: Code C F, ed. *Handbook of Physiology, Section 6: Alimentary Canal, Vol.
V*. Washington D.C. American Physiological Society 1968; 2761–2774

174. Docherty M. Pathologic aspects in control of spread of colonic car-   6.4
cinoma. *Proc Staff Meet Mayo Clin* 1958; 33: 157–163

175. Dockray G J. Molecular evolution of gut hormones: application of   2.2
comparative studies on the regulation of digestion. *Gastroenterology* 1977;
72: 344–358

176. Dongen J M van, Kooyman J, Visser W J, Holt S J, Galjaard H. The   2.1
effect of increased crypt cell proliferation on the activity and subcellular
localisation of esterases and alkaline phosphatase in the rat small
intestine. *Histochem J* 1977; 9: 61–75

177. Dongen J M van, Visser W J, Daems W Th, Galjaard H. The relation   3.2
between cell proliferation, differentiation and ultrastructural development in rat intestinal epithelium. *Cell Tissue Kinet* 1976; 174: 183–199.

178. Doniach I, Shiner M. Duodenal and jejunal biopsies. II. Histology.   6.3
Gastroenterology 1957; 33: 71–86

179. Dowling R H. The influences of luminal nutrition on intestinal   4.4
adaptation after small bowel resection and bypass. In: Dowling R H,
Riecken E O, eds. *Intestinal Adaptation*. Stuttgart: Schattauer Verlag
1975: 35–46

180. Dowling R H, Booth C C. Functional compensation following small   2.3
intestinal resection in the rat. *Clin Sci* 1966; 32: 139–149

181. Dowling R H, Gleeson M H. Cell turnover following small bowel   2.1
resection and by-pass. *Digestion* 1973; 8: 176–190

182. Draser B S, Bone E S, Hill M F, Marks C G. Colon cancer and bacterial   6.1
metabolism in familial polyposis. *Gut* 1975; 16: 824–825

183. Dresden M H, Heilman S A, Schmidt J D. Collagenolytic enzymes in   5.2
human neoplasms. *Cancer Res* 1972; 32: 993–996

184. Druckrey H. Production of colonic carcinomas by 1,2 dialkylhydrazines   5.1, 5.4

and azoxyalkanes. In: Burdette J W, ed. *Carcinoma of the Colon and Antecedent Epithelium*. Springfield, Illinois: Charles C Thomas 1970: 367–279

185. Druckrey H, Preussman R, Matzkies F, Ivankovic S. Selektive Erzeugung von Darmkrebs bei Ratten durch 1,2 Dimethylhydrazin. *Naturwissenschaften* 1967; 54: 285–286   5.1, 5.2, 5.3

186. Druckrey H, Steinhoff D, Preussman R, Ivankovic S. Erzeugung von Krebs durch eine einmalige Dosis von Methylnitroso-Harnstoff und verschiedenen Dialkylnitrosaminen an Ratten. *Z Krebsforsch* 1964; 66: 1–10   5.1

187. Duffill M, Appleton D R, Dyson P, Shuster S, Wright N A. The measurement of the cell cycle time in squamous epithelium using the metaphase arrest technique with vincristine. *Br J Dermatol* 1977; 96: 493–502   1.1

188. Dukes P P, Goldwasser E. Inhibition of erythopoiesis by estrogen. *Endocrinology* 1961; 69: 21–29   4.5

189. Dunham E W, Haddox M K, Goldberg N D. Alteration of vein cyclic $3':5'$ nucleotide concentration during changes in contractility. *Proc Natl Acad Sci USA* 1974; 71: 815–819   5.3

190. Dupont J R, Biggers D C, Sprinz H. Intestinal renewal and immunosympathectomy. *Arch Path* 1965; 80: 357–362   2.6

191. Durrant G J, Ganellin C R, Owen D A A, Parsons M E. S-{3-(N,N-dimethylamino)propyl} isothiourea (dimaprit) a highly specific histamine H_2-receptor agonist. *Proc European Branch of the Histamine Club* 1976: 31–32   5.3

192. Dworkin L D, Levine G M, Garber N J, Spector M H. Small intestinal mass of the rat is partially determined by indirect effects of intraluminal nutrition. *Gastroenterology* 1976; 71: 626–630   2.2, 4.4

193. Eastwood G L. Small bowel morphology and epithelial proliferation in intravenously alimented rabbits. *Gastroenterology* 1976; 70: A24/882   2.2, 2.7

194. Eastwood G L. Gastrointestinal epithelial renewal. *Gastroenterology* 1977; 72: 962–975   2.1, 2.2, 2.7

195. Eastwood G L, Trier J S. Epithelial cell renewal in cultured rectal biopsies in ulcerative colitis. *Gastroenterology* 1973; 64: 383–390   5.4, 6.1

196. Eastwood G L, Trier J S. Epithelial cell proliferation during organogenesis of rat colon. *Anat Rec* 1974; 179: 303–310   1.2

197. Ecknauer R, Clarke R M, Meyer H. Acute distal intestinal obstruction in gnotobiotic rats: intestinal morphology and cell renewal. *Virchows Archiv (Cell Pathol)* 1977; 25: 151–160   2.1

198. Elgjo K. Reversible inhibition of epidermal G_1 cells by repeated injections of aqueous skin extracts (chalone). *Virchows Archiv (Cell Pathol)* 1974; 15: 157–163   2.3

199. Elgjo K, Loerum O D, Edgehill W. Growth regulation in mouse epidermis. I. G_2 inhibitor present in the basal layer. *Virchows Archiv (Cell Pathol)* 1971; 8: 277–283   2.3

200. Elias E, Dowling R H. The mechanism for small-bowel adaptation in lactating rats. *Clin Sci Mol Med* 1977; 51: 427–433   2.2

201. Elkind M M. Sublethal x-ray damage and its repair in mammalian cells. I. In: Silini G, ed. *Proceedings of the Third International Congress of Radiation Research, Cortina, 1966*. Amsterdam: North Holland Publishing Co. 1967: 558–586   4.3

202. Elmes P C, Simpson M J C. Insulation workers in Belfast. 3. Mortality   5.5
     1940–1966. *Br. J Ind Med* 1971; 28: 226–236
203. Elson C O, Reilly R W, Rosenberg I H. Small intestinal injury in the   6.2
     graft-versus-host reaction: an innocent bystander phenomenon. *Gastro-*
     enterology 1977; 72: 886–889
204. Emery R S, Brown R E, Black A L. Metabolism of D1-1,2-   2.7
     propanediol-2-^{14}C in a lactating cow. *J Nutr* 1967; 92: 348–356
205. Enoch M R, Johnson L R. Effect of hypophysectomy and growth   2.2
     hormone on serum and antral gastrin levels in the rat. *Gastroenterology*
     1976; 70: 727–732
206. Enterline H T, Evans G W, Mercado-Lugo R, Miller L, Fitts W Y.   5.2
     Malignant potential of adenomas of colon and rectum. *JAMA* 1962; 179:
     322–330
207. Epifanova O I. Mitotic cycles in estrogen-treated mice: a radioauto-   4.5
     graphic study. *Exp Cell Res* 1966; 42, 562–577
208. Epifanova O I. Effects of hormones on the cell cycle. In: Baserga R, ed.   4.5
     The Cell Cycle and Cancer. New York: Marcel Dekker Inc. 1971: 145–190
209. Epifanova O I, Tchoumak M G. The action of adrenalin upon the mitotic   5.3
     cycle of the intestinal epithelium in mice. *Tsitologiia* 1963; 5: 455–458
210. Evans J T, Hauschka T S, Mittelman A. Differential susceptibility of   5.1
     four mouse strains to induction of multiple large bowel neoplasms by
     1,2-dimethylhydrazine. *J Natl Cancer Inst* 1974; 52: 999–1000
211. Evans J T, Lutman G, Mittelman A. The induction of multiple large   5.2
     bowel neoplasms in mice. *J Med (Basel)* 1972; 3: 212–215
212. Evans J T, Shaws T B, Sproul E E, Prolini N S, Mittelman A, Hauschka   6.1
     T. Genetics of colon carcinogenesis in mice treated with 1,2-
     dimethylhydrazine. *Cancer Res* 1977; 37: 134–136
213. Eyre P and Chand N. Preliminary evidence for two sub-classes of   5.3
     histamine H$_2$-receptors. *Agents Actions* 1979; 9: 1–3
214. Farmer R G, Hawk W A, Turnbull R B Jr. Carcinoma associated with   5.4
     mucosal ulcerative colitis and with transmural colitis and enteritis
     (Crohn's disease). *Cancer* 1971; 28: 289–292
215. Feldman E J, Dowling R H, McNaughton J, Peters T J. Effect of oral   4.4
     versus intravenous nutrition on intestinal adaptation after small bowel
     resection in the dog. *Gastroenterology* 1976; 70: 712–719
216. Fell B F, Campbell R M, Mackie W S, Weekes T E C. Changes   2.7
     associated with pregnancy and lactation in some extra-reproductive
     organs of the ewe. *J Agric Sci Camb* 1972; 79: 397–407
217. Fell B F, Kay M, Whitelaw F G, Boyne R. Observations on the   2.7
     development of ruminal lesions in calves fed on barley. *Res Vet Sci* 1968;
     9: 458–466
218. Fell B F, Weekes T E C. In: McDonald I W, Warner A C I, eds.
     Digestion and Metabolism in the Ruminant. Armidale: The University of
     New England Publishing Unit 1975; 101–118
219. Fenoglio C M, Kaye G I, Lane N. Distribution of human colonic   5.2
     lymphatics in normal, hyperplastic and adenomatous tissue. Its relation-
     ship to metastasis from small carcinomas in pedunculated adenomas,
     with two case reports. *Gastroenterology* 1973; 64: 51–66
220. Fenyö G. Morphological changes of the adapting small intestine under   2.1
     various conditions. *Acta Chir Scand suppl* 1976; 469: 1–31

221. Fenyö G, Hallberg D, Soda M, Roos K A. Morphological changes in the 4.4
small intestine following jejuno-ileal shunt in parenterally fed rats. *Scand J Gastroenterol* 1976; 11: 635–640

222. Ferguson A. Lymphocytes and cell-mediated immunity in the small 6.2
intestine. In: Weatherall D, ed. *Advanced Medicine 14*, Tunbridge Wells;
Pitman Medical Publishing Co Ltd. 1978; 278–293

223. Ferguson A, Carr K E, MacDonald T T, Watt C. Hypersensitivity 6.2
reactions in the small intestine. 4. Influence of allograft rejection on
small intestinal mucosal architecture: a scanning and transmission
electron microscope study. *Digestion* 1978; 18: 56–63

224. Ferguson A, Jarrett E E E. Hypersensitivity reactions in the small 6.2
intestine. 1. Thymus dependence of experimental 'partial villous atrophy'. *Gut* 1975; 16: 114–117

225. Ferguson A, MacDonald T T. Effects of local delayed hypersensitivity on 6.2
the small intestine. *Ciba Found Symp* 1977; 46: 305–327

226. Ferguson A, Parrott D M V. Histopathology and time course of rejection 6.2
of allografts of mouse small intestine. *Transplantation* 1973; 15: 546–554

227. Ferguson A, Paul F, Snodgrass D M. Lactose tolerance in lamb rotavirus 6.2
infection. *Gut* (Submitted for publication)

228. Ferguson A, Sutherland A, MacDonald T T, Allan F. Technique for 6.2
microdissection and measurement in biopsies of human small intestine. *J Clin Pathol* 1977; 30: 1068–1073

229. Fiala E S. Investigations into the metabolism and mode of action of the 5.1
colon carcinogen 1:2 dimethylhydrazine. *Cancer* 1975; 36: 2407–2412

230. Fiala E S, Kulakis C, Bobotas G, Weisburger J H. Detection and 5.1
estimation of azomethane in expired air of 1,2 dimethylhydrazine treated
rats. *J Natl Cancer Inst* 1976; 56: 1271–1273

231. Fishman P H, Brady R O, Henneberry R C, Freese E. Alterations of 2.7
surface glyconjugates and cell morphology induced by butyric acid. In:
Cell Surface Carbohydrate Chemistry. New York: Academic Press 1978:
153–180

232. Flick A L, Quinton W E, Rubin C E. Hydraulic biopsy tube for external 6.3
delivery of multiple biopsies from any level of the gastrointestinal tract.
Gastroenterology 1960; 38: 964

233. Folkman J. Tumor angiogenesis factor. *Cancer Res* 1974; 34: 2109– 5.2
2113

234. Foroozan P, Trier J S. Mucosa of the small intestine in pernicious 6.5
anaemia. *N Engl J Med* 1967; 277: 553–559

235. Forrester J M. The number of villi in rat's jejunum and ileum: effect of 2.1
normal growth, partial enterectomy and tube feeding. *J Anat* 1972; 111:
283–291

236. Foulds L. The induction of tumours in mice of the R_3 strain by 2 5.1
acetylaminofluorene. *Br J Cancer* 1947; 1: 172–176

237. Frankfurt O S. Effect of hydrocortisone, adrenalin and actinomycin D on 4.5
transition of cells to the DNA synthesis phase. *Exp Cell Res* 1968; 52:
220–232

238. Frazer A C, Fletcher R F, Shaw B, Ross C A C, Sammons H G, 6.3
Schneider R. Gluten-induced enteropathy. The effect of partially
digested gluten. *Lancet* 1959; ii: 252–255

239. Frindel E, Croizat H, Vassort F. Stimulating factors liberated by treated 4.2

bone marrow: in-vitro effect on CFU kinetics. *Exp Hematol* 1976; 4: 56–61

240. Frindel E, Guigon M, Dumenil D, Fache M P. Stimulating factors and   4.2
cell recruitment in murine bone marrow stem cells and EMT6 tumours.
Cell Tissue Kinet 1978; 11: 393–403

241. Fry R J M, Lesher S, Kohn H. Age effect on cell transit time in mouse   5.5
jejunal epithelium. *Am J Physiol* 1961; 201: 213–216

242. Fry R J M, Staffeldt E. Effect of a diet containing sodium deoxycholate   6.5
on the intestinal mucosa of the mouse. *Nature* 1964; 203: 1396–1398

243. Fuji R. Quantitation of the number of villi and crypts in the intestine of   2.1
rodent animals. *Experientia* 1972; 28: 1209–1210

244. Galand P, Rodesch F, Leroy F, Chrétien J. Altered duration of DNA   1.4, 4.5
synthesis and cell cycle in non-target tissues of mice treated with
oestrogen. *Nature* 1967; 216: 1211–1212

245. Galjaard H, Bootsma D. The regulation of cell proliferation and   2.3
differentiation in intestinal epithelium. II. A quantitative histochemical
and autoradiographic study after low doses of X-irradiation. *Exp Cell Res*
1969; 58: 79–92

246. Galjaard H, Buys J, Duuren M van, Giesen J. A quantitative histochemical study of intestinal mucosa after X-irradiation. *J Histochem Cytochem*
1970; 18: 291–301

247. Galjaard H, Meer-Fieggen W van der, Giesen J. Feedback control by   1.3, 2.1
functional villus cells on cell proliferation and maturation in intestinal
epithelium. *Exp Cell Res* 1972; 73: 197–207

248. Gardner E J. A genetic and clinical study of intestinal polyposis, a   6.1
predisposing factor for carcinoma of the colon and rectum. *Am J Hum
Genet* 1951; 3: 167–176

249. Gelfant S. A new concept of tissue and tumour cell proliferation. *Cancer*   1.1
Res 1977; 37: 2845–2862

250. Gennaro A R, Villaneuva R, Sukonthaman Y, Vathanophas V,   5.1, 5.4
Rosemond G P. Chemical carcinogenesis in transposed intestinal segments. *Cancer Res* 1973; 33: 536–541

251. Gilbert C W. The labelled mitoses curve and the estimation of the   1.4, 5.1
parameters of the cell cycle. *Cell Tissue Kinet* 1972; 5: 53–63

252. Gillette E L, Withers H R, Tannock I. The age sensitivity of epithelial   4.2, 4.3
cells of mouse small intestine. *Radiology* 1970; 96: 639–643

253. Ginsburg F, Salomon D, Sreevalsan T, Freese E. Growth inhibition and   2.7
morphological changes caused by lipophilic acids in mammalian cells.
Proc Natl Acad Sci USA 1973; 70: 2457–2461

254. Gleeson M H, Dowling R H, Peters T J. Biochemical changes in   2.1
intestinal mucosa after experimental small bowel by-pass in the rat. *Clin
Sci* 1972; 43: 743–757

255. Goedbloed J F. The embryonic and postnatal growth of rat and mouse. I.   1.2
The embryonic and early postnatal growth of the whole embryo. A model
with exponential growth and sudden changes in growth rate. *Acta Anat*
1972; 82: 305–336

256. Goldberg N D, Haddox M K, Hartle D K, Hadden J W. The biological   5.3
role of cyclic 3'.5'-guanosine monophosphate. *Proc 5th Internat Congr
Pharmacol* Basel, Karger 1973; vol 5. 146–169

257. Goldberg N D, Haddox M K, Nicol S E et al. Biological regulation   5.3

through opposing influences of cyclic GMP and cyclic AMP: the Yin-Yang hypothesis. *Adv Cyclic Nucleotide Res* 1975; 5: 307–330

258. Goldberg N D, O'Dea R E, Haddox M K. Cyclic GMP. *Adv Cyclic Nucleotide Res* 1973; 3: 155–223   5.3

259. Goldstein M J, Melamed M R, Grabstald H, Sherlock P. Progressive villous atrophy of the ileum used as a urinary conduit. *Gastroenterology* 1967; 52: 859–864   6.5

260. Goodrum P J, Sowell J G, Cardoso S S. Characterisation of the circadian rhythm of mitosis in the corneal epithelium of the immature rat. In: Scheving L E, Halberg F, Pauly J E, eds. *Chronobiology*. Tokyo: Igahu Shoin Ltd. 1974; 29–32   2.6

261. Gordon H A, Pesti L. The gnotobiotic animal as a tool in the study of host microbial relationships. *Bacteriol Rev* 1971; 35: 390–429   2.7

262. Gorski J, Noteboom W D, Nicolette J A. Estrogen control of the synthesis of RNA and protein in the uterus. *J Cell Comp Physiol* 1965; 66: 91–109   4.5

263. Gospodarowicz D, Mescher A L, Birdwell C R. Control of cellular proliferation by the fibroblast and epidermal growth factors. *Natl Cancer Inst Monogr* 1978; 48: 109–130   2.2

264. Grahn D, Ainsworth E J, Williamson F S, Fry R J M. A program to study fission neutron-induced chronic injury in cells, tissues and animal populations utilizing the Janus reactor of the Argonne National Laboratory. In: *Radiobiological Applications of Neutron Irradiation*, IAEA, Vienna 1972; 211–228   4.2

265. Greenstein A J, Sachar D, Pucillo A et al. Cancer in Crohn's disease after diversionary surgery. A report of seven carcinomas occurring in excluded bowel. *Am J Surg* 1978; 135: 86–90   5.4

266. Grega O, Taman R, Prusora F. Gastrointestinal cancer and nutrition. *Gut* 1969; 10: 1031–1034   6.5

267. Gronemeyer R, Bässler R. Pathologic der Gallenowegserkrankungen. *Klinikarzt* 1975; 4: 361–368   6.5

268. Gushchin V A. Branching of the G_1-phase in the mitotic cycle of guinea pig colon crypt cells (in Russian). *Tsitologiia* 1976; 18: 1455–1463   1.3

269. Haase P, Cowen D M, Knowles J C, Cooper E H. Evaluation of dimethylhydrazine induced tumours in mice as a model system for colorectal cancer. *Br J Cancer* 1973; 28: 530–543   5.1, 5.2

270. Haeger K, Jacobson D, Kahlson G. Atrophy of the gastrointestinal mucosa following hypophysectomy or adrenalectomy. *Acta Physiol Scand* 1953; 111: 161–169   2.2

271. Haeney M R, Ferguson R, Asquith P. Animal models for coeliac disease and inflammatory bowel disease. In: Asquith P, ed. *Immunology of the Gastrointestinal Tract*. London and Edinburgh: Churchill Livingstone 1979: 129–151   6.3

272. Hagemann R F. Intestinal cell proliferation during fractionated abdominal irradiation. *Br J Radiol* 1976; 49: 56–61   4.1

273. Hagemann R F. Compensatory proliferative response of the colonic epithelium to multifraction irradiation. *Int J Radiat Oncol Biol Phys* 1979; 5: 69–71   4.1

274. Hagemann R F, Concannon J P. Mechanism of intestinal radiosensitization by actinomycin D. *Br J Radiol* 1973; 46: 302–308   4.1

275. Hagemann R F, Concannon J P. Time/dose relationships in abdominal   4.1
      irradiation: a definition of principles and experimental evaluation. *Br J
      Radiol* 1975; 48: 545–555

276. Hagemann R F, Lesher S. Intestinal crypt survival and total and per   3.3, 4.2
      crypt levels of proliferative cellularity following irradiation: age response
      and animal lethality. *Radiat Res* 1971; 47: 159–167

277. Hagemann R F, Lesher S. Irradiation of the GI tract: compensatory   4.1
      response of stomach, jejunum and colon. *Br J Radiol* 1971; 44: 599–602

278. Hagemann R F, Lesher S. Intestinal cytodynamics: adductions from drug   4.2
      and radiation studies. In: Zimmerman A M, Padilla G M, Cameron I L,
      eds. *Drugs and the Cell Cycle*. New York: Academic Press 1973: 195–217

279. Hagemann R F, Sigdestad C P, Lesher S. A method for quantitation of   2.2
      proliferative intestinal mucosal cells on a weight basis. Some values for
      C57B1/6. *Cell Tissue Kinet* 1970; 3: 21–26

280. Hagemann R F, Sigdestad C P, Lesher S. Intestinal crypt survival and   4.1
      total and per crypt levels of proliferative cellularity following irradiation:
      single X-ray exposures. *Radiat Res* 1971; 46: 533–546

281. Hagemann R F, Stragand J J. Fasting and refeeding: cell kinetic response   1.1, 1.4, 2.1,
      of jejunum, ileum and colon. *Cell Tissue Kinet* 1977; 10: 3–14   2.2, 4.4, 5.4

282. Halliday R. The absorption of antibodies from immune sera by the gut of   2.6
      the young rat. *J Endocrinol* 1955; 18: 56–66

283. Haltmeyer G C, Deneberg V H, Thatcher J, Zarrow M X. Response of   2.6
      the adrenal cortex of the neonatal rat after subjection to stress. *Nature*
      1966; 212: 1371–1373

284. Hamada T. Effect of 1,2-propanediol on the rumen mucosal growth of   2.7
      kids. *J Dairy Sci* 1975; 58: 1352–1359

285. Hamada T. Stimulatory effects of 1,2-propanediol on relative growth of   2.7
      liver and rumen mucosa of kids. *Bull Natl Inst Anim Indust Japan* 1978;
      34: 19–27

286. Hamilton A I, Blackwood H J J. Insulin deficiency and cell proliferation   2.7
      in oral mucosal epithelium of the rat. *J Anat* 1977; 124: 757–763

287. Hamilton E. Diurnal variation in proliferative compartments and their   1.4, 3.3
      relation to cryptogenic cells in the mouse colon. *Cell Tissue Kinet* 1979;
      12: 91–100

288. Hamilton E. Induction of radioresistance in mouse colon crypts by   3.3
      X-rays. *Int J Radiat Biol* 1979; 36: 537–545

289. Hamilton J R, Gall D G, Butler D G, Middleton P J. Viral   6.2
      gastroenteritis: recent progress, remaining problems. *Ciba Found Symp*
      1976; 42: 209–219

290. Hamilton T H. Control by estrogen of genetic transcription and   4.5
      translation. *Science* 1968; 161: 649–661

291. Hampton J C Further evidence for the presence of a Paneth cell   3.2
      progenitor in mouse intestine. *Cell Tissue Kinet* 1968; 1: 309–317

292. Hansen O H, Pederson T, Larsen J K, Rehfeld J F. Effect of gastrin on   2.2
      gastric mucosal cell proliferation in man. *Gut* 1976; 17: 536–541

293. Hanson W R, Fry R J M. The effect of hydroxyurea or high specific   4.2
      activity tritiated thymidine in combination with colcemid on intestinal
      cell survival in B6CF$_1$/Anl mice. *Radiat Res* 1978; 74: 525

294. Hanson W R, Fry R J M, Sallese A R. The effect of ^{3}H-thymidine and   4.2
      colcemid suicide on clonogenic cell survival in the intestinal mucosa of

B6CF$_1$ mice. *Radiat Res* 1976; 67: 602–603

295. Hanson W R, Henninger D L, Fry R J M. Time dependence of intestinal proliferative cell risk versus stem cell risk to radiation or colcemid cytotoxicity following hydroxyurea. *Int J Radiat Oncol Biol Phys* 1979; 5: 1685–1690 — 4.2

296. Hanson W R, Osborne J W. Epithelial cell kinetics in the small intestine of the rat 60 days after resection of 70 percent of the ileum and jejunum. *Gastroenterology* 1971; 60: 1087–1097 — 1.3, 2.1, 2.2, 2.3

297. Hanson W R, Osborne J W, Sharp J G. Compensation by the residual intestine after intestinal resection in the rat. I. Influence of amount of tissue removed. *Gastroenterology* 1977; 72: 692–700 — 2.1, 2.2, 4.4

298. Hanson W R, Osborne J W, Sharp J G. Compensation by the residual intestine after intestinal resection in the rat. II. Influence of postoperative time interval. *Gastroenterology* 1977; 72: 701–705 — 2.1, 2.2, 4.4

299. Hanson W R, Rijke R P C, Plaisier H M, Ewijk W van, Osborne J W. The effect of intestinal resection on Thiry-Vella fistulae of jejunal and ileal origin: evidence for a systemic control mechanism of cell renewal. *Cell Tissue Kinet* 1977; 10: 543–555 — 2.1, 2.2, 4.4

300. Harding J D, Cairnie A B. Changes in intestinal cell kinetics in the small intestine of lactating mice. *Cell Tissue Kinet* 1975; 8: 135–144 — 1.1, 2.1, 2.2

301. Hartmann N R, Gilbert C W, Jansson B, MacDonald P D M, Steel G G, Valleron A-J. A comparison of computer methods for the analysis of fraction labelled mitoses curves. *Cell Tissue Kinet* 1975; 8: 119–124 — 1.4

302. Hasegawa I L, Matsumira Y, Tojo S. Cellular kinetics and histological changes in experimental cancer of the uterine cervix. *Cancer Res* 1976; 36: 359–364 — 6.1

303. Haubrich W S, Berk J E. In: Bockus H L, ed. *Gastroenterology*. Philadelphia: Saunders 1976 Chap 86; 1058 — 6.4

304. Hawks A, Hicks R M, Holsman J W, Magee P N. Morphological and biochemical effects of 1,2 dimethylhydrazine and 1 methylhydrazine in rats and mice. *Br J Cancer* 1974; 30: 429–439 — 5.1

305. Hawks A, Magee P N. The alkylation of nucleic acids of rat and mouse in vivo by the carcinogen 1,2 dimethylhydrazine. *Br J Cancer* 1974; 30: 440–446 — 5.1

306. Hayashi I, Sato G H. Saibo-baiyo-eki ni okeru kessei no yakuwari. *Kaguku* 1978; 48: 33–41 — 2.7

307. Hayashi T, Yatani R, Apostol J, Stemmermann G N. Pathogenesis of hyperplastic polyps of the colon: A hypothesis based on ultrastructure and in-vitro cell kinetics. *Gastroenterology* 1974; 66: 347–356 — 6.4

308. Heaton K W. Cancer of the large bowel: dietary factors. In: Truelove S C, Lee E, eds. *Topics in Gastroenterology* 5. Oxford: Blackwell 1977: 29–44 — 5.4

309. Heird W C, Tsang H L, MacMillan R, Kaplan R, Rosenweig N S. Comparative effects of total parenteral nutrition, oral feeding and starvation on rat small intestine. *Gastroenterology* 1974; 66: A55/709 — 2.7

310. Hekkens W Th J M. The toxicity of gliadin, a review. In: McNicholl B, McCarthy C F, Fottrell P F, eds. *Perspectives in coeliac disease*. Lancaster: MTP Press Ltd 1978: 3–14 — 6.3

311. Helwig E. The evaluation of adenomas of the large intestine and their relation to carcinoma. *Surg Gynecol Obstet* 1947; 87: 36–49 — 6.4

312. Hendry J H. Diurnal variations in radiosensitivity of mouse intestine. *Br*   3.3, 4.2
J Radiol 1975; 48: 312–314

313. Hendry J H. Regeneration of stem-cells in intestinal epithelium after   3.1
irradiation. In: Okada F, et al, eds. *Proc VI Int Congress Radiat Res Tokyo*
1979; 664–669

314. Hendry J H, Potten C S. Cryptogenic cells and proliferative cells in   3.1, 3.3, 4.2
intestinal epithelium. *Int J Radiat Biol* 1974; 25: 583–588

315. Henning S J, Sims J M. Delineation of the glucocorticoid-sensitive   2.2
period of intestinal development in the rat. *Endocrinology* 1979; 104:
1158–1163

316. Herbst J J, Sunshine P. Postnatal development of the small intestine of   2.6
the rat. Changes in mucosal morphology at weaning. *Pediatr Res* 1969; 3:
27–33

317. Hernandez F J, Reid J D. Mixed carcinoid and mucus-secreting   3.2
intestinal tumours. *Arch Path* 1969; 88: 489–496

318. Heslop B. Cystic adenocarcinoma of the ascending colon in rats occurring   5.1
as a self limiting outbreak. *Lab Anim* 1969; 3: 185–195

319. Hietanen E, Hänninen O. Effect of chyme on mucosal enzyme levels in   2.1
small intestine of the rat. *Metabolism* 1972; 21: 991–1000

320. Hill M J. The effect of some factors on the faecal concentration of acid   6.1
steroids, neutral steroids and urobilins. *J Pathol* 1971; 104: 239–245

321. Hill M J. The role of colon anaerobes in the metabolism of bile acids and   5.4
steroids and its relation to colon cancer. *Cancer* 1975; 36: 2387–2400

322. Hill M J, Aries V C. Faecal steroid composition and its relationship to   5.1
cancer of the large bowel. *J Pathol* 1971; 104: 129–139

323. Hill M J, Crowther J S, Drasar B S, Hawksworth G, Aries V, Williams   5.1
R E O. Bacteria and aetiology of cancer of large bowel. *Lancet* 1971; i:
95–100

324. Hill M J, Drasar B S, Williams R E O et al. Faecal bile-acids and   5.4
clostridia in patients with cancer of the large bowel. *Lancet* 1975; i:
535–539

325. Hillarp N. The construction and functional organisation of the auton-   2.6
omic innervation apparatus. *Acta Physiol Scand* 1959; 46 (Suppl 157);
1–38

326. Hinni J B, Watterson R L. Modified development of the duodenum of   1.2
chick embryos hypophysectomised by partial decapitation. *J Morphol*
1963; 113; 381–426

327. Hinrichs H R, Peterson R O, Baserga R. Incorporation of thymidine   4.4
into DNA of mouse organs. *Arch Path* 1964; 78: 245–253

328. Hoff M B. *The effect of estrogen on cell proliferation and differentiation in*   4.5
colonic epithelium of the mouse, Mus musculus L. Ph D Thesis, The City
University of New York, New York 1978

329. Hoff M B, Chang W W L. The effect of estrogen on epithelial cell   4.4.5
proliferation and differentiation in the crypt of the descending colon of
the mouse. A radioautographic study. *Am J Anat* 1979; 155: 507–516

330. Hofmann R R. *The Ruminant Stomach*. Nairobi: East African Literature   2.7
Bureau 1973

331. Homburger F, Hsueh S S, Kerr C S, Russfield A B. Inherited   5.1
susceptibility of inbred strains of Syrian hamsters to induction of
subcutaneous sarcomas and mammary and gastrointestinal carcinomas by

subcutaneous and gastric administration of polynuclear hydrocarbons. *Cancer Res* 1972; 32: 360–366

332. Hooper C E S. Use of colchicine for the measurement of mitotic rate in the intestinal epithelium. *Am J Anat* 1961; 108: 231–244   5.2

333. Hopper A F, Rose P M, Wannamacher R W. Cell population changes in the intestinal mucosa of protein depleted or starved rats. II. Changes in cellular migration. *J Cell Biol* 1972; 53: 225–230   1.1

334. Hopper A F, Wannamacher R W, McGovern P A. Cell population changes in the intestinal epithelium of the rat following starvation and protein depletion. *Proc Soc Exp Biol Med* 1968; 128: 695–698   1.1

335. Horava A, Haam E von. Experimental cancer of the colon. *Cancer Res* 1958; 18: 764–767   5.1

336. Horikoshi H, Suzuki Y. On circulating sex steroids during the estrous cycle and the early pseudopregnancy in the rat with special reference to its luteal action. *Endocrinol Jpn* 1974; 21: 69–79   4.5

337. Hornsey S. The effectiveness of fast neutrons compared with low LET radiation on cell survival measures in the mouse jejunum. *Radiat Res* 1973; 55: 58–68   3.1, 4.3

338. Houck J C. *Chalones*. Amsterdam, Oxford: North Holland Publishing Company; New York: American Elsevier Publishing Co Inc. 1976   2.5

339. Houck J C, Hennings H. Chalones. Specific endogenous mitotic inhibitors. *FEBS Lett* 1973; 32: 1–6   2.3

340. Houpt T R. Transfer of urea and ammonia to the rumen. In: Phillipson A T, ed. *Physiology of Digestion and Metabolism in the Ruminant*. Newcastle upon Tyne: Oriel Press 1970; 119–131   2.7

341. Hughes C A, Bates T, Dowling R H. Cholecystokinin and secretin prevent the intestinal mucosal hypoplasia of total parenteral nutrition in the dog. *Gastroenterology* 1978; 75: 34–41   4.4

342. Hume I D, Warner A C I. Evolution of microbial digestion in mammals. In: *Proceedings of 5th International Symposium of Ruminant Physiology*, Clermont-Ferrand, September 1979.   2.7

343. Hungate R. E. The *Rumen and its Microbes*. London: Academic Press 1966   2.7

344. Imondi A R, Balis M E, Lipkin M E. Nucleic acid metabolism in the gastrointestinal tract of the mouse during fasting and restraint stress. *Exp Mol Pathol* 1968; 9: 339–348   2.2

345. Iwana T, Utsunomiya J, Sasaki J. Epithelial cell kinetics in the crypts of familial polyposis of the colon. *Jpn J Surg* 1977; 7: 230–234   6.1

346. Jacobs M M. Inhibitory effects of selenium on dimethylhydrazine and methylazoxymethanol colon carcinogenesis. *Cancer* 1977; 40: 2557–2564   6.1

347. Jacobs R, Dodgson K S, Richards R J. A preliminary study of biochemical changes in rat small intestine following long term ingestion of chrysotile asbestos. *Br J Exp Path* 1977; 58: 541–548   5.5

348. Jacobs R, Weinzweig M, Dodgson K S, Richards R J. Nucleic acid metabolism in the rat following short-term and prolonged ingestion of chrysotile asbestos or cigarette smoke condensate. *Br J Exp Path* 1978; 59: 594–600   5.5

349. Jensen E V, DeSombre E R. Estrogen-receptor interaction. *Science* 1973; 182: 126–134   4.5

350. Jensen R, Connell W E, Deem A W. Parakeratosis of the rumen of lambs fattened on pelleted feed. *Am J Vet Res* 1958; 19: 277–282   2.7

351. Johnson E M, Cantor E, Douglas J R. Biochemical and functional   2.6
      evaluation of the sympathectomy produced by administration of
      guanethidine to newborn rats. *J Pharmacol Exp Ther* 1975; 193: 503–512
352. Johnson L R. The trophic action of gastrointestinal hormones. *Gastroen-*   2.2, 4.4
      terology 1976; 70: 278–288
353. Johnson L R. New aspects of the trophic action of gastrointestinal   2.2
      hormones. *Gastroenterology* 1977; 72: 788–792
354. Johnson L R, Guthrie P D. Secretin inhibition of gastrin stimulated   2.3
      deoxyribonucleic acid synthesis. *Gastroenterology* 1974; 67: 601–606
355. Johnson L R, Guthrie P D. Effect of cholecystokinin and 16-16   2.3
      dimethylprostaglandin E_2 on RNA and DNA of gastric and duodenal
      mucosa. *Gastroenterology* 1976; 70: 59–65
356. Jordan H N, Phillips R W. Effects of fatty acids on isolated ovine   2.7
      pancreatic islets. *Am J Physiol* 1978; 234: E162–E167
357. Jung-Testas I, Bayard F, Baulien E E. Two sex steroid receptors in mouse
      fibroblasts in culture. *Nature* 1976; 259: 136–138
358. Katz A J, Grand R J. All that flattens is not 'sprue.' *Gastroenterology*   6.3
      1979; 76: 375–377
359. Kaye G I, Fenoglio C M, Pascal R R, Lane N. Comparative electron   5.2, 6.4
      microscopic features of normal, hyperplastic and adenomatous human
      colonic epithelium. *Gastroenterology* 1973; 64: 926–945
360. Keating R J, Tcholakian R K. In vivo patterns of circulating steroids in   2.2
      adult male rats. I. Variations of testosterone during 24- and 48-hour
      standard and reverse light/dark cycles. *Endocrinology* 1979; 104: 184–188
361. Keynes R D, Harrison F A. Transport of inorganic ions across the rumen   2.7
      epithelium. In: Phillipson A T, ed. *Physiology of Digestion and Metabolism*
      in the Ruminant. Newcastle upon Tyne: Oriel Press 1970; 113–118
362. Kikkawa N. Experimental studies of polypogenesis of the large intestine.   6.1
      Med J Osaka Univ 1974; 24: 293–314
363. Kimura H, Murad F. Two forms of guanylate cyclase in mammalian   5.3
      tissues and possible mechanisms of their regulation. *Metabolism* 1975; 24:
      439–445
364. King E S J, Varasdi G. Experimentally induced tumours of the intestine.   5.1
      Aust NZ J Surg 1959; 29: 38–53
365. Kirchner F R, Osborne J W. Failure to find a humoral factor which   2.1, 2.2, 4.4
      influences the compensatory response after resection of the rat small
      bowel. *Cell Tissue Kinet* 1978; 11: 227–234
266. Klein H Z. Mucinous carcinoid tumour of the vermiform appendix.   3.2
      Cancer 1974; 33: 770–777
367. Klein R M. Alteration of cellular proliferation in the ileal epithelium of   2.2, 2.6, 5.3
      suckling and weaned rats: the effects of isoproterenol. *Cell Tissue Kinet*
      1977; 10: 353–364
368. Klein R M. Alteration of neonatal rat parotid gland acinar cell
      proliferation by guanethidine-induced sympathectomy. *Cell Tissue Kinet*
      1979; 12: 411–426
369. Klein R M. Analysis of intestinal cell proliferation after guanethidine-   2.6
      induced sympathectomy. II. Percent labelled mitoses studies. *Cell Tissue*
      Kinet 1979; 12: 649–658
370. Klein R M. Analysis of intestinal cell proliferation after guanethidine-   2.6
      induced sympathectomy. III. Effects of chemical sympathectomy on

circadian variation in mitotic activity. *Cell Tissue Kinet* 1980; 13: 153–162

371. Klein R M, Harrington D B, Piliero S J. Isoproterenol-induced changes   2.6
in cell cycle kinetics of parotid gland acinar cells in 8-day old rats. *J Dent Res* 1976; 55: 611–616

372. Klein R M, Torres J. Analysis of intestinal cell proliferation after   2.2
guanethidine-induced sympathectomy. *Cell Tissue Res* 1978; 195: 239–250

373. Klein R M, Torres J. Analysis of intestinal cell proliferation after   2.6
guanethidine-induced sympathectomy. I. Stathmokinetic, labelling index, mitotic index, and cellular migration studies. *Cell Tissue Res* 1978; 195: 239–250

374. Knudston K P, Priest R E, Jacklin A J, Jesseph J E. Effects of partial   2.3
resection on mammalian small intestine. I. Initial radioautographic studies in the dog. *Lab Invest* 1962; 11: 433–439

375. Kobayashi A, Matsumoto H. Studies on methylazoxymethanol the   5.1
aglycone of cycasin: isolation, biological and chemical properties. *Arch Biochem* 1965; 110: 373–380

376. Koldovsky O, Sunshine P, Kretchmer M. Cellular migration of intesti-   2.6
nal epithelia in suckling and weaned rats. *Nature* 1966; 212: 1389–1390

377. Kopelovich L, Conlon S, Pollack R. Defective organisation of actin in   6.1
cultured skin fibroblasts from patients with inherited adenocarcinoma. *Proc Natl Acad Sci USA* 1977; 74: 3019–3022

378. Kovacs L, Potten C S. An estimation of proliferative population size in   1.4
stomach, jejunum and colon of DBA-2 mice. *Cell Tissue Kinet* 1973; 6: 125–134

379. Kuehl F A. Prostaglandins, cyclic nucleotides and cell function. *Prostag-   5.3
landins* 1974; 5: 325–340

380. Kunos G. Thyroid hormone-dependent interconversion of myocardial   2.2
and adrenoreceptors in the rat. *Br J Pharmacol* 1977; 59: 177–189

381. Kuo J F, Kuo W N. Regulation by β-adrenergic receptor and muscarinic   5.3
cholinergic receptor activation of intracellular cyclic AMP and cyclic GMP levels in rat lung slices. *Biochem Biophys Res Comnun* 1973; 55: 660–665

382. Lachat J-J, Goncalves R P. Influence of autonomic denervation upon the   2.6
kinetics of the ileal epithelium of the rat. *Cell Tissue Kes* 1978; 192: 285–297

383. Lahiri S K, Putten L M van. Location of the G_o-phase in the cell cycle of   4.2
the mouse haemopoietic spleen colony forming cells. *Cell Tissue Kinet* 1972; 5: 365–369

384. Lamerton L F. Cell proliferation under continuous irradiation. *Radiat Res*   3.2
1966; 27: 119–138

385. Lamerton L F. Cell proliferation and the differential response of normal   1.1
and malignant tissues. *Br J Radiol* 1972; 45: 161–175

386. LaMont J T, O'Gorman T A. Experimental colon cancer. *Gastroenterology*   5.1
1978; 75: 1157–1169

387. Lanciault G, Johnson E D. The gastrointestinal circulation. *Gastroenterol-   2.2
ogy* 1976; 71: 851–873

388. Land P C, Bruce W R. Fecal mutagens: a possible relationship with   6.1
colorectal cancer. *Proc Amer Assn for Cancer Res* 1978; 19: 167

389. Lane N, Kaplan H, Pascal R R. Minute adenomatous and hyperplastic   5.2, 6.4, 6.5
      polyps of the colon: divergent patterns of epithelial growth with specific
      associated mesenchymal changes. *Gastroenterology* 1971; 60: 537–551
390. Lane N, Lev R. Observations on the origin of adenomatous epithelium of   5.2, 6.1
      the colon: serial section studies of minute polyps in familial polyposis.
      Cancer 1963; 16: 751–764
391. Laplace J-P. Sur l'existence éventuelle d'un facteur circulant, intervenant   4.4
      dans le déterminisme de l'augmentation pondérale du tissu intestinal
      restant après une resection limitée d'intestin grêle. Étude chez le
      porcelete par circulation sanguine croisée. *Rec Méd Vét* 1972; 147:
      931–947
392. Laqueur G L. Carcinogenic effects of cycad meal and cycasin methylazoxy-   5.1
      methanol glycoside in rats, and effects of cycasin in germ free rats. *Fed
      Proc* 1964; 23: 1386–1388
393. Laqueur G L. The induction of intestinal neoplasms in rats with the   5.1, 5.2
      glycoside cycasin and its aglycone. *Virchows Archiv (Pathol Anat)* 1965;
      340: 151–163
394. Laqueur G L, Matsumoto H. Neoplasms in female Fischer rats following   5.1
      intraperitoneal injection of methylazoxymethanol. *J Natl Cancer Inst*
      1966; 37: 217–232
395. Laqueur G L, McDaniel E G, Matsumoto H. Tumor induction in   5.1
      germfree rats with methylazoxymethanol (MAM) and synthetic MAM
      acetate. *J Natl Cancer Inst* 1967; 39: 355–371
396. Laqueur G L, Mickelsen O, Whiting M G, Kurland L T. Carcinogenic   5.1
      properties of nuts from *Cycas circinalis* indigenous to Guam. *J Natl Cancer
      Inst* 1963; 31: 919–951
397. Laqueur G L, Spatz M. Toxicology of cycasin. *Cancer Res* 1968; 28:   5.1
      2262–2267
398. Lauwers H. *Morfologische bijdrage tot de kennis van het resorberend vermogen*   2.7
      van rundervoormagen. PhD Dissertation. Rijksuniversiteit: Ghent 1973
399. Leaver D D, Swann P F, Magee P N. Induction of tumours in the rat by a   5.1
      single oral dose of N-nitrosomethylurea. *Br J Cancer* 1969; 23: 177–187
400. Leblond C P. In: Price D, ed. *Conference on dynamics of proliferating tissues*.   4.4
      Chicago: University of Chicago Press 1958
401. Leblond C P. In: Strohlman F, ed. *The Kinetics of Cellular Proliferation*.   1.3
      New York and London: Grune and Stratton 1959; 31–47
402. Leblond C P, Carriere R M. Effect of growth hormone and thyroxine on   2.2
      mitotic rate of intestinal mucosa of rat. *Endocrinology* 1955; 56: 261–266
403. Leblond C P, Cheng H. Identification of stem cells in the small intestine   1.1, 1.3, 2.1,
      of the mouse. In: Cairnie A B, Lala P K, Osmond D G, eds. *Stem Cells of*   3.2
      Renewing Populations. New York: Academic Press 1976; 7–31
404. Leblond C P, Clermont Y, Nadler N J. The pattern of stem cell renewal   3.2
      in three epithelia (esophagus, intestine and testis). In: *Proceedings of the
      Canadian Cancer Research Conference*. Oxford: Pergamon Press 1967; 7:
      3–30
405. Leblond C P, Messier B. Renewal of chief cells and goblet cells in the   3.2
      small intestine as shown by radioautograph after injection of ^{3}H-
      thymidine into mice. *Anat Rec* 1958; 132: 247–259
406. Leblond C P, Stevens C E. The constant renewal of the intestinal   2.1, 2.3, 2.6,
      epithelium in the albino rat. *Anat Rec* 1948; 100: 357–377   3.2

407. Leblond C P, Walker B E. Renewal of cell populations. *Physiol Rev* 1956;   2.1
36: 257–276

408. Lee A E, Rogers L A. Cell division in the mouse vagina during   4.5
continuous oestrogen stimulation. *J Endocrinol* 1972; 54: 357–358

409. Lehnert S. Changes in growth kinetics of jejunal epithelium in mice   5.5
maintained on an elemental diet. *Cell Tissue Kinet* 1979; 12: 239–248

410. Lenaz L, Sternberg S S, Philips F S. Cytotoxic effects of 1-β-D-   4.3
arabinofuranosylcytosine and 1-β-D-arabinofuranosyl-5-fluorocytosine
in proliferating tissues in mice. *Cancer Res* 1969; 29: 1790–1798

411. Lesher J, Lesher S. Effect of single-dose partial-body X-irradiation on cell   2.1
proliferation in the mouse small intestinal epithelium. *Radiat Res* 1974;
57: 148–157

412. Lesher S. Compensatory reactions in intestinal crypt cells after 300   3.2
roentgens of cobalt-60 gamma irradiation. *Radiat Res* 1967; 32:
510–519

413. Lesher S, Bauman J. Cell kinetic studies of the intestinal epithelium;   1.1
maintenance of the intestinal epithelium in normal and irradiated
animals. In: *Human Tumor Cell Kinetics*. Washington D.C.: National
Cancer Institute Monograph. 30. 1969: 185–198

414. Lesher S, Fry R J M, Kohn H. Age and generation time of the mouse   5.5
duodenal epithelial cells. *Exp Cell Res* 1961; 24: 334–343

415. Lesher S, Lamerton L F, Sacher G A, Fry R J M, Steel G G, Roylance P   2.1, 2.3
J. Effect of continuous gamma irradiation on the generation cycle of the
duodenal crypt cells of the mouse and rat. *Radiat Res* 1966; 29: 57–70

416. Lesher S, Walburg H E, Sacher G A. Generation cycle in the duodenal   2.3
crypt cells of germ free and conventional mice. *Nature* 1964; 202:
884–886

417. Levin R J. The effects of hormones on the absorption, metabolic and   2.2
digestive functions of the small intestine. *J Endocrinol* 1969; 45:
315–348

418. Levine G M, Deren J J, Steiger E, Zinno R. Role of oral intake in   2.7
maintenance of gut mass and disaccharide activity. *Gastroenterology* 1974;
67: 975–982

419. Levine G M, Deren J J, Yezdimir E. Small-bowel resection: oral intake is   4.4
the stimulus for hyperplasia. *Dig Dis* 1976; 21: 542–546

420. Lightdale C, Lipkin M. Cell division and tumor growth. In: Becker F   6.1
F, ed. *Cancer vol 3*. New York: Plenum Publishing Co 1977: 201–215

421. Lindström C G, Rosengren J E, Ekberg O. Experimental colonic   5.1
tumours in the rat. III. Induction time, distribution and appearance of
induced tumours. *Acta Radiol Diag* 1978; 19: 799–816

422. Lipkin M. Proliferation and differentiation of gastrointestinal cells.   2.1
Physiol Rev 1973; 53: 891–915

423. Lipkin M. Phase 1 and phase 2 proliferative lesions of colonic epithelial   2.1, 5.4, 6.1,
cells in premalignant diseases leading to colonic cancer. *Cancer* 1974; 34:   6.4
878–888

424. Lipkin M. Growth kinetics of normal and premalignant gastrointestinal   6.1
epithelium. In: *Growth Kinetics and Biochemical Regulation of Normal and
Malignant Cells*. Baltimore: Williams and Wilkins 1977: 562–589

425. Lipkin M. Susceptibility of human population groups to colon cancer. *Adv*   6.1
Cancer Res 1978; 27: 281–304

426. Lipkin M, Bell B. Cell Proliferation. In: Code C F, ed. *Handbook of*   6.1, 6.5
      Physiology. Section 6: Alimentary Canal Vol V Washington D.C. American
      Physiological Society 1967; 2861–2879

427. Lipkin M, Quastler H. Cell population kinetics in the colon of the mouse. *J*   1.3, 1.4
      Clin Invest 1962; 4: 141–146

428. Lipkin M, Sherlock P, Bell B. Cell proliferation kinetics in the   6.5
      gastrointestinal tract of man. *Gastroenterology* 1963; 45: 721–729

429. Lipkin M, Sherlock P, DeCosse J. *Current Problems on Cancer* (In   6.1
      Press)

430. Lipscomb H L, Gardner P J, Sharp J G. The effect of neonatal thymectomy   2.2
      on the induction of autoimmune orchitis in rats. *J Reprod Immunol* 1979;
      1: 209–218

431. Loehry C A, Croft D N, Singh A K, Creamer B. Cell turnover in the small   5.5
      intestinal mucosa. *Gut* 1969; 10: 13–18

432. Loehry C A, Grace R. The dynamic structure of a flat small intestinal mucosa   5.1
      studied in the explanted rat jejunum. *Gut* 1974; 15: 289–293

433. Löhrs U, Wiebecke B, Eder M. Morphologische und Autoradiog-   5.2
      raphische Untersuchung der Darmschleimhautveränderungen nach ein-
      maliger injektion von 1,2-Dimethylhydrazin. *Z Ges Exp Med* 1969; 151:
      297–307

434. Loran M R, Carbone J V. The humoral effect of intestinal resection on   4.4
      cellular proliferation and maturation in parabiotic rats. In: Sullivan M R,
      ed. *Gastrointestinal Radiation Injury.* Amsterdam: Excerpta Medica 1968:
      127–139

435. Loran M R, Crocker T T. Population dynamics of intestinal epithelia in the   2.3, 2.6, 4.4
      rat 2 months after partial resection of the ileum. *J Cell Biol* 1963; 19:
      285–291

436. Loran M R, Crocker T T, Carbone J V. The humoral effect of intestinal   2.3
      resection on cellular proliferation and maturation in parabiotic rats. *Fed Proc*
      1964; 23: 407

437. Lorenz E, Stewart H L. Tumors of the alimentary tract induced in mice by   5.1
      feeding olive oil emulsions containing carcinogenic hydrocarbons. *J Natl*
      Cancer Inst 1947; 7: 227–238

438. Lowenfels A B. Why are small-bowel tumours so rare? *Lancet* 1973;   5.4
      i: 24–26

439. MacDonald P D M. Statistical inference from the fraction labelled mitoses   5.2
      curve. *Biometrika* 1970; 57: 489–503

440. MacDonald P D M. Stochastic models for cell proliferation. In: Driessche   5.2
      P van den, ed. *Mathematical Problems in Biology.* New York, Springer-
      Verlag 1974: 155–163

441. MacDonald T T, Ferguson A. Hypersensitivity reactions in the small   6.2
      intestine. 2. Effects of allograft rejection on mucosal architecture and
      lymphoid cell infiltrate. *Gut* 1976; 17: 81–91

442. MacDonald T T, Ferguson A. Hypersensitivity reactions in the small   6.2
      intestine. 3. The effects of allograft rejection and of graft-versus-host
      disease on epithelial cell kinetics. *Cell Tissue Kinet* 1977; 10: 301–312

443. MacDonald T T, Ferguson A. Small intestinal epithelial cell kinetics and   6.2
      protozoal infection in mice. *Gastroenterology* 1978; 74: 496–500

444. MacDonald W C, Dobbins W O, Rubin C E. Studies of the familial   6.3
      nature of celiac sprue using biopsy of the small intestine. *N Engl J Med*
      1964; 272: 448–456

445. Macher B A, Lockey M, Fung Y K, Seeley C C. Studies on the 2.7
mechanisms of butyrate-induced morphological changes in KB cells. *Exp Cell Res* 1978; 117: 95–102

446. MacKenzie I C. Ordered structure of the stratum corneum of mammalian 4.2
skin. *Nature* 1969; 222: 881–882

447. Mak K M, Chang W W L. Pentgastrin stimulates epithelial cell 2.2
proliferation in duodenal abd colonic crypts in fasted rats. *Gastroenterology* 1976; 71: 1117–1120

448. Mancuso T F, El Attar A A. Carcinogenic risk and duration of 5.5
employment among asbestos workers. In Holstein and Anspach, eds.
International Konferenz über die Biologische Wirkungen des Asbestos. Dresden
1973: 161–166

449. Mandel M, Ichinotsubo D, Mower H. Nitroso group exchange as a way 6.1
of activation of nitrosamines by bacteria. *Nature* 1977; 267: 248–249

450. Manns J G, Boda J M. Insulin release by acetate, propionate butyrate 2.7
and glucose in lambs and adult sheep. *Am J Physiol* 1967; 212: 747–755

451. Manns J G, Boda J M, Willes R F. Probable role of propionate and 2.7
butyrate in control of insulin secretion in sheep. *Am J Physiol* 1967; 212:
756–764

452. Marks J M, Shuster S. Small-intestinal mucosal abnormalities in various 6.3
skin diseases—fact or fancy? *Gut* 1970; 11: 281–291

453. Marks J, Shuster S, Watson A J. Small-bowel changes in dermatitis 6.3
herpetiformis. *Lancet* 1966; ii: 1280–1282

454. Marsh M N, Brown A C, Swift J A. The surface ultrastructure of the 6.3
small intestinal mucosa of normal control human subjects and of patients
with untreated and treated coeliac disease using the scanning electron
microscope. In: Booth C C, Dowling R H, eds. *Coeliac Disease*:
Edinburgh and London, Churchill Livingstone 1970: 26–44

455. Martin M S, Martin F, Michiels R et al. An experimental model for 5.1, 5.2
cancer of the colon and rectum. *Digestion* 1973; 8: 22–34

456. Maskens A P. Histogenesis and growth pattern of 1,2 dimethylhydrazine 2.1, 5.1, 5.2,
induced rat colon adenocarcinoma. *Cancer Res* 1976; 36: 1585–1592 6.1

457. Maskens A P. Histogenesis of colon glands during postnatal growth. 6.5
Acta Anat 1978; 100: 17–26

458. Maskens A P. Histogenesis of adenomatous polyps in the human large 6.5
intestine. *Gastroenterology* 1979; 77: 1245–1251

459. Maskens A P, Deschner E E. Tritiated thymidine incorporation into 6.5
epithelial cells of normal-appearing colorectal mucosa of cancer patients.
J Natl Cancer Inst 1977; 58: 1221–1224

460. Mastromarino A J, Wilson R. Increased intestinal turnover and radiosen- 6.5
sitivity to supralethal whole-body irradiation resulting from cholic
acid-induced alterations of the intestinal microecology of germfree CFW
mice. *Radiat Res* 1976; 66: 393–400

461. Masuda K, Withers H R, Mason K A, Chen K Y. Single dose-response 3.1, 4.2
curves of murine gastrointestinal crypt stem cells. *Radiat Res* 1977; 69:
65–75

462. Mathan M, Moxey P C, Trier J S. Morphogenesis of fetal rat duodenal 1.2
villi. *Am J Anat* 1976; 146: 73–92

463. Matsubara N, Mori H, Hirono I. Effect of colostomy on intestinal 5.1
carcinogenesis by methylazoxymethanol acetate in rats. *J Natl Cancer Inst*
1978; 61: 1161–1164

464. Matsumoto H, Higa H H. Studies on methylazoxymethanol the   5.1
     aglycone of cycasin: methylation of nucleic acids in vitro. *Biochem J* 1966;
     98: 20c–22c

465. McCoy G W. A preliminary report of tumours found in wild rats. *J Med*   5.1
     Res 1909; 21: 285–296

466. McDermott F T, Roundnew B. Ileal crypt cell population kinetics after   2.1
     40 percent small bowel resection. *Gastroenterology* 1976; 70: 707–711

467. McDonald G S A, Hourihane D O'B. Mucinous carcinoid tumour of the   3.2
     appendix containing Paneth cells. *Ir J Med Sci* 1977; 146: 386

468. McEwen B S. Interactions between hormones and nerve tissue. *Sci Am*   4.5
     1976; 235 (1): 45–58

469. McGilliard A D, Jacobson N L, Sutton J D. In: Dougherty R W, ed.   2.7
     Physiology of Digestion in the Ruminant. Washington D.C. Butterworth
     1965; 39–50

470. Menge H, Gräfe M, Lorenz-Meyer H, Riecken E O. The influence of   2.1
     food intake on the development of structural and functional adaptation
     following ileal resection in the rat. *Gut* 1975; 16: 468–472

471. Merzel J. Some histophysical aspects of Paneth cells of mice as shown by   3.2
     histochemical and radioautographic studies. *Acta Anat* 1967; 66:
     603–630

472. Messier B, Leblond C P. Cell proliferation and migration as revealed by   1.4
     autoradiography after injection of thymidine H^3 into male rats and mice.
     Am J Anat 1960; 106: 247–265

473. Miller L J, Gorman C A, Go V L W. Gut-thyroid interrelationships.   2.2
     Gastroenterology 1978; 75: 901–911

474. Miwa M, Takenaka S, Ito K et al. Spontaneous colon tumors in rats. *J*   5.1
     Natl Cancer Inst 1976; 56: 615–621

475. Miyake I. Interrelationship between the release of pituitary luteinizing   4.5
     hormone and the secretions of ovarian estrogen and progestin during
     estrus cycle in the rat. In: Itoh S, ed. *Integrative Mechanisms of Neuroendoc-*
     rine Systems. Sapporo: Hokkaido University of Medicine 1968; 139–149

476. Moe H. A quantitative study of the occurrence of goblet cells in the small   1.3
     intestine of the cat. *Ann NY Acad Sci* 1963; 106: 518–544

477. Moir R J. Ruminant digestion and evolution. In: Code C F, ed.   2.7
     Handbook of Physiology. Section 6: Alimentary Canal Vol V. Washington
     D.C. American Physiological Society 1968: 2673–2694

478. Møller U, Larsen J K, Faber M. The influence of injected tritiated   3.3
     thymidine on the mitotic circadian rhythm in the epithelium of the
     hamster cheek pouch. *Cell Tissue Kinet* 1974; 7: 231–239

479. Moog F. The functional differentiation of the small intestine. III. The   2.6
     influence of the pituitary-adrenal system on the differentiation of
     phosphatase in the duodenum of the suckling mouse. *J Exp Zool* 1953;
     124: 329–346

480. Moog F, Yeh K-Y. Pinocytosis persists in the ileum of hypophysecto-   2.6
     mised rats unless closure is induced by thyroxine or cortisone. *Dev Biol*
     1979; 69: 159–169

481. Moolten F L, Bucher N L R. Regeneration of rat liver: transfer of   4.4
     humoral agent by cross-circulation. *Science* 1967; 158: 272–274

482. Moon K H, Bunge R G. Silastic testosterone capsules. I. Observations in   2.2
     the castrated male rat. *Invest Urol* 1968; 6: 329–333

483. Moore J V. Ablation of murine jejunal crypts by alkylating agents. *Br J Cancer* 1979; 39: 175–181   3.1

484. Mori Y, Akedo H, Tanigawa Y, Okada M. Effect of sodium butyrate on granulopoiesis of mastocytoma cells. *Exp Cell Res* 1979; 118: 15–22   2.7

485. Morin C L, Ling V. Effect of pentagastrin on the rat small intestine after resection. *Gastroenterology* 1978; 75: 224–229   2.2, 4.4

486. Morson B C. Some peculiarities in the histology of intestinal polyps. *Dis Colon Rectum* 1962; 5: 337–344   5.2

487. Morson B C. The pathogenesis of colorectal cancer. In: *Major Problems in Pathology (10)*. London Toronto Philadelphia: Saunders 1978   5.1

488. Morson B C, Bussey H J R. Predisposing causes of intestinal cancer. *Curr Probl Surg* 1970; 7: 1–50   5.2, 6.1

489. Musso F, Lachat J-J, Cruz A R, Goncalves R P. Effect of denervation on the mitotic index of the intestinal epithelium of the rat. *Cell Tissue Kinet* 1975; 163: 395–402   2.6

490. Muto T, Bussey H J R, Morson B C. The evolution of cancer of the colon and rectum. *Cancer* 1975; 36: 2251–2270   5.2

491. Mutt V, Joupes J E. Hormonal peptides of the upper intestine. *Biochem J* 1971; 125: 57–58   2.2

492. Mylotte M, Egan-Mitchell B, McCarthy C F, McNicholl B. Incidence of coeliac disease in the West of Ireland. *Br Med J* 1973; 1: 703–705   6.3

493. Nagasawa F T, Shirota F N. Decomposition of methylazoxymethanol, the aglycone of cycasin in D_2O. *Nature* 1972; 236: 234–235   5.1

494. Narisawa T, Magadia N E, Weisburger J H, Wynder E L. Promoting effect of bile acids on colon carcinogenesis after intrarectal instillation of N-methyl-N'-nitro-N-nitrosoguanidine in rats. *J Natl Cancer Inst* 1974; 53: 1093–1097   5.4, 6.5

495. Navarrette A, Spjut H J. Effect of colostomy on experimentally induced neoplasms of the colon in the rat. *Cancer* 1967; 20: 1466–1472   5.1

496. Necas E, Neuwirt J. Proliferation rate of haemopoietic stem cells after damage by several cytostatic agents. *Cell Tissue Kinet* 1976; 9: 479–487   4.2

497. Necas E, Neuwirt J. Control of haemopoietic stem cell proliferation by cells in DNA synthesis. *Br J Haematol* 1976; 33: 395–400   4.2

498. Negro-Vilar A, Saad W A, McCann S M. Evidence for the role of prolactin in prostate and seminal vesicle growth in immature male rats. *Endocrinology* 1977; 100: 729–737   2.2

499. Nomura K, Schlake W, Grundmann E. New aspects of intestinal carcinogenesis by 1,2 dimethylhydrazine dihydrochloride (DMH) and the influence of antilymphocytic globulin (ALG) on its progress. *Z Krebsforsch* 1978; 92: 17–33   5.1

500. Nordstrom C, Dahlqvist A. Quantitative distribution of some enzymes along the villi and crypts of human small intestine. *Scand J Gastroenterol* 1973; 8: 407–416   6.2

501. Nundy S, Malamud D, Obertop H, Sczerban J, Malt R A. Onset of cell proliferation in the shortened gut: colonic hyperplasia after ileal resection. *Gastroenterology* 1977; 72: 263–266   2.2, 4.4, 5.4

502. Obertop H, Nundy S, Malamud D, Malt R A. Onset of cell proliferation in the shortened gut: rapid hyperplasia after jejunal resection. *Gastroenterology* 1977; 72: 267–270   4.4

503.   O'Connor T M. Cell dynamics in the intestine of the mouse from late   1.2, 2.6
       fetal life to maturity. *Am J Anat* 1966; 118: 525–536
504.   O'Farrell M K, Clingan D, Rudland P S, Asua L J de. Stimulation of the   2.7
       initiation of DNA synthesis and cell division in several cultured mouse
       cell types. *Exp Cell Res* 1979; 118: 311–321
505.   Office of Population Censuses and Surveys: *1977 Mortality Statistics*   5.1
       HMSO 1978
506.   Ong S H, Whitley T H, Stowe N W, Steiner A L. Immunohistochemi-   5.3
       cal localisation of 3'.5' cyclic AMP and 3'.5' cyclic GMP in rat liver,
       intestine and testis. *Proc Natl Acad Sci USA* 1975; 72: 2022–2026
507.   Ørskov E R. The effect of processing on digestion and utilization of   2.7
       cereals by ruminants. *Proc Nutr Soc* 1976; 35: 245–252
508.   Osborne J W, Kirchner F R, Sharp J G. Preliminary evidence against a   2.2
       circulating humoral factor having control of the compensatory response
       observed following X-irradiation or resection of the rat small bowel.
       Radiat Res 1977; 70: 641–642
509.   Osborne J W, Nicholson D P, Prasad K N. Induction of intestinal   5.4
       carcinoma in the rat by X-irradiation of the small intestine. *Radiat Res*
       1963; 18: 76–85
510.   Oscarson J E A, Veen H F, Ross J S, Malt R A. Ileal resection potentiates   5.4
       1,2 dimethylhydrazine-induced colonic carcinogenesis. *Ann Surg* 1979;
       189: 503–508
511.   Oscarson J E A, Veen H F, Williamson R C N, Ross J S, Malt R A.   2.2, 4.4
       Compensatory postresectional hyperplasia and starvation atrophy in small
       bowel: dissociation from endogenous gastrin levels. *Gastroenterology*
       1977; 72: 890–895
512.   Padykula H A. Recent functional interpretations of intestinal morphol-   1.3
       ogy. *Fed Proc* 1962; 21: 873–879
513.   Paesi F J A, De Gough S E. Growth inhibition by oestrogen in   4.5
       hypophysectomised immature rats. *Acta Physiol Pharmacol Neerl* 1954; 3:
       227–231
514.   Pansu D, Berard A, Dechelette M A, Lambert R. Influence of secretin   2.2
       and pentagastrin on the circadian rhythm of cell proliferation in the
       intestinal mucosa in rats. *Digestion* 1974; 11: 266–274
515.   Pearse A G E. Peptides in brain and intestine. *Nature* 1976; 262:   2.2
       92–94
516.   Pearse A G E, Polak J L, Bloom S R. The new gut hormones: cellular   2.2
       sources, physiology, pathology and clinical aspects. *Gastroenterology*
       1977; 72: 746–761
517.   Pederson T. Chromatin structure and the cell cycle. *Proc Natl Acad Sci*   6.4
       USA 1972; 69: 2224–2228
518.   Pederson T, Robbins E. Chromatin structure and the cell division cycle.   6.4
       Actinomycin binding in synchronised Hela cells. *J Cell Biol* 1972; 55:
       322–327
519.   Pegg A E, Hawks A. Increased transfer nucleic acid methylase activity in
       tumors induced in the mouse colon by the administration of 1,2   5.1
       dimethylhydrazine. *Biochem J* 1971; 122: 121–123
520.   Perera D R, Weinstein W M, Rubin C. Small intestinal biopsy. *Hum*   6.3
       Pathol 1975; 6: 157–217
521.   Perry P M. Intestinal absorption following small bowel resection. *Ann R*   5.4

Coll Surg Engl 1976; 57: 139–147

522. Pfeffer L, Lipkin M, Stutman O, Kopelovich L. Growth abnormalities in   6.1
     cultured human skin fibroblasts. *J Cell Physiol* 1976; 89: 29–37

523. Phelps T A, Blackett N M. Protection of intestinal damage by   4.3
     pretreatment with cytosine arabinoside (Ara-C). In: Conference on
     Combined Modalites: Chemotherapy/Radiotherapy. *Int J Radiat Onc Biol
     Phys* 1978.

524. Phillips T L, Wharam M D, Margolis L W. Modification of radiation   4.2
     injury to normal tissues by chemotherapeutic agents. *Cancer* 1975; 35:
     1678–1684

525. Pietras R J, Szego C M. Specific binding sites for estrogen on the outer   4.5
     surface of isolated endometrial cells. *Nature* 1977; 265: 69–72

526. Pink I J, Croft D N, Creamer B. Cell loss from small intestinal mucosa: a   6.3
     morphological study. *Gut* 1970; 11: 217–222

527. Pishva B, Mann M, Djahanguiri B, Abtahi F S. Decreased mitotic   2.2
     activity in the stomach, duodenum and colon of rats treated with high
     doses of histamine. *Pharmacology* 1975; 13: 1–4

528. Poleski M H, Blattner W A, Chait M et al. CEA in colonic lavage of   6.1
     individuals at high risk of large bowel cancer. *Gastroenterology* 1978; 74:
     1140

529. Pollak D J. Reduction of blood cholesterol in man. *Circulation* 1953; 7:   6.5
     702–706

530. Pomare E W, Heaton K W. The effect of cholecystectomy on bile salt   6.5
     metabolism. *Gut* 1973; 14: 753–762

531. Post J, Wilson R, Sklarew R J, Pachter B, Hoffman J. Replication of   2.6
     spleen lymphocytes and ileal crypt cells in conventional and germ-free
     young rats. *Proc Soc Exp Biol Med* 1972; 140: 553–555

532. Potten C S. Further observations on the late labelling associated with   3.1
     stimulus-responsive cells in skin. *Cell Tissue Kinet* 1973; 6: 553–566

533. Potten C S. The epidermal proliferative unit: the possible role of the   4.2
     central basal cell. *Cell Tissue Kinet* 1974; 7: 77–88

534. Potten C S. Small intestinal crypt stem cells. In: Cairnie A B, Lala P K,   1.1, 2.1, 3.2
     Osmond D G, eds. *Stem Cells of Renewing Cell Populations*. New York:
     Academic Press, 1976: 79–84

535. Potten C S. Extreme sensitivity of some intestinal crypt cells to X and γ 3.1
     irradiation. *Nature* 1977; 269: 518–521

536. Potten C S. Epithelial proliferative subpopulations. In: Lord B I, Potten   3.2
     C S, Cole R J, eds. *Stem Cells and Tissue Homeostasis*. Cambridge:
     Cambridge University Press, 1978: 335–358

537. Potten C S, Shlemon E, Al-Barwari S E, Hume W J, Searle J. Circadian   2.2, 3.1, 3.3
     rhythms of presumptive stem cells in three different epithelia of the
     mouse. *Cell Tissue Kinet* 1977; 10: 557–568

538. Potten C S, Al-Barwari S E, Searle J. Differential radiation response   3.1, 3.2
     amongst proliferating epithelial cells. *Cell Tissue Kinet* 1978; 11:
     149–160

539. Potten C S, Allen T D. Ultrastructure of cell loss in intestinal mucosa. *J*   1.1
     Ultrastruct Res 1977; 60: 272–277

540. Potten C S, Hendry J H. Differential regeneration of intestinal prolifera-   3.1, 3.2, 4.2
     tive cells and cryptogenic cells after irradiation. *Int J Radiat Biol* 1975;
     27: 413–424

541. Potten C S, Hume W J, Reid P, Cairns J. The segregation of DNA in epithelial stem cells. *Cell* 1978; 15: 899–906   3.1

542. Potten C S, Kovacs L, Hamilton E. Continuous labelling studies on mouse skin and intestine. *Cell Tissue Kinet* 1974; 7: 271–283   1.4, 3.1, 4.2

543. Potten C S, Schofield R, Lajtha L G. A comparison of cell replacement in bone marrow, testes and three regions of surface epithelium. *Biochim Biophys Acta* 1979; 560: 281–299   3.1

544. Pouillart P, Hoang Thi Hoang T. Putting mouse cells into cycle (CFUs) by diverse agents: radiations, cytostatics, androgens and BCG. *Exp Haematol* 1973; 1: 263–271   4.2

545. Poulakos L, Osborne J W. The kinetics of cellular recovery in locally X-irradiated rat ileum. *Radiat Res* 1973; 53: 402–413   2.2

546. Pound A W, McGuire L J. Repeated partial hepatectomy as a promoting stimulus for carcinogenic response of liver to nitrosamines in rats. *Br J Cancer* 1978; 37: 586–594   5.4

547. Pozharrisski K M. Tumours of the intestines. In: *Pathology of Tumours in Laboratory Animals*. Vol. 1. *Tumours of the Rat. Part 1.* International Agency for Research on Cancer, Lyon 1973: 119–140   5.1

548. Pozharisski K M. The significance of nonspecific injury for colon carcinogenesis in rats. *Cancer Res* 1975; 35: 3824–3830   5.4

549. Pozharisski K M. Morphology and morphogenesis of experimental epithelial tumors of the intestine. *J Natl Cancer Inst* 1975; 54: 1115–1135   5.1, 5.2

550. Pozharisski K M, Kapustin Y M, Likhachev A J. The mechanisms of carcinogenic action of 1,2-dimethylhydrazine (SDMH) in rats. *Int J Cancer* 1975; 15: 673–683   5.1

551. Pozharisski K M, Klimashevski V F. Comparative morphological and histoautoradiographic study of multiple experimental intestinal tumours. *Exp Pathol (Jena)* 1974; 9: 88–98   5.1, 5.2

552. Pozharissky K M, Klimashevsky V F, Gushchin V A. Peculiarity of the kinetics of the enterocyte population in various segments of the alimentary tract as a factor determining the tumor development (In Russian). *Dokl Akad Nauk USSR* 1975; 220: 216–219   1.3

553. Pozharissky K M, Klimashevsky V F, Gushchin V A. The comparative analysis of cell population of enterocytes in different parts of the small and large intestine in rats. I. Parameters of the mitotic cycle and heterogeneity of the proliferating enterocyte population. (In Russian). *Tsitologiia* 1977; 19: 303–317   1.3

554. Prasad K N, Sakamoto A. Effect of sodium butyrate in combination with prostaglandin E and inhibitors of cyclic nucleotide phosphodiesterase on human amelanotic melanoma cells in culture. *Experientia* 1978; 34: 1575–1576   2.7

555. Quastler H. The nature of intestinal radiation death. *Radiat Res* 1956; 4: 303–320   3.2

556. Quastler H, Bensted, J P M, Lamerton L F, Simpson S M. Adaptation to continuous irradiation: observations on the rat intestine. *Br J Radiol* 1959; 32: 501–512   3.2

557. Quastler H, Sherman F G. Cell population kinetics in intestinal epithelium of the mouse. *Exp Cell Res* 1959; 17: 420–438   1.3, 2.3, 2.6, 3.2, 4.5, 5.2, 5.3

558. Redhun L I. Cyclic nucleotides, calcium and cell division. *Int Rev Cytol* 5.3
1977; 9: 1–54

559. Reddy B S, Martin C W, Wynder E L. Fecal bile acids and cholesterol 6.5
metabolites of patients with ulcerative colitis, a high risk group for
development of colon cancer. *Cancer Res* 1977; 37: 1697–1701

560. Reddy B S, Mastromarino A, Gustafson C, Lipkin M, Wynder, E L. 6.1
Fecal bile acids and neutral sterols in patients with familial polyposis.
Cancer 1976; 38: 1694–1698

561. Reddy B S, Narisawa T, Weisburger J H. Effect of a diet with high 5.1
levels of protein and fat on colon carcinogenesis in F344 rats treated with
1,2 dimethylhydrazine. *J Natl Cancer Inst* 1976; 57: 567–569

562. Reddy B S, Weisburger J H, Narisawa T, Wynder E L. Colon 5.1
carcinogenesis in germ-free rats with 1,2 dimethylhydrazine and
N-methyl-N'-nitro-N-nitrosoguanidine. *Cancer Res* 1974; 34:
2368–2372

563. Reddy B S, Weisburger J H, Wynder E L. Effects of dietary fat level and 5.4
dimethylhydrazine on fecal acid and neutral sterol excretion and colon
carcinogenesis in rats. *J Natl Cancer Inst* 1974; 52: 507–511

564. Reddy B S, Weisburger J H, Wynder E L. Effects of high risk and low 6.1, 6.5
risk diets for colon carcinogenesis on fecal microflora and steroids in man.
J Nutr 1975; 105: 878–884

565. Reddy B S, Wynder E L. Large bowel Carcinogenesis: fecal constituents 5.1, 6.1
of populations with diverse incidence rates of colon cancer. *J Natl Cancer
Inst* 1973; 50: 1437–1442

566. Reddy B S, Wynder E L. Large bowel carcinogenesis: fecal constituents 5.4
bile acids and neutral sterols in colon cancer patients and patients with
adenomatous polyps. *Cancer* 1977; 39: 2533–2539

567. Redman R S, Sreebny L M. Changes in patterns of feeding activity, 2.6
parotid secretory enzymes and plasma corticosterone in developing rats. *J
Nutr* 1976; 106: 1295–1306

568. Redman R S, Sweney L R. Changes in diet and patterns of feeding 2.6
activity of developing rats. *J Nutr* 1976; 106: 615–626

569. Reid J T. The future role of ruminants in animal production. Phillipson 2.7
A T, ed. *Physiology of Digestion and Metabolism in the Ruminant*. Newcastle
upon Tyne: Oriel Press, 1970: 1–22

570. Reid R L. Studies on the carbohydrate metabolism of sheep. I. The range 2.7
of blood sugar values under several conditions. *Aust J Agr Res* 1950; 1:
182–199.

571. Reiskin A B, Mendelsohn M L. A comparison of the cell cycle in induced 5.2
carcinomas and their normal counterpart. *Cancer Res* 1964; 24:
1131–1136

572. Rendall R E G. The data sheets on the chemical and physical properties 5.5
of the UICC standard reference samples. In: Shapiro H A, ed.
Pneumoconiosis Proc Intl Conf Johannesburg, 1969. Capetown, Oxford
University Press 1970: 23–27

573. Rey J, Schmitz J, Rey F, Jos J. Cellular differentiation and enzymatic 6.2
defects. *Lancet* 1971; ii: 218

574. Richards T C. Early changes in the dynamics of crypt cell populations in 1.3, 1.4, 5.1
mouse colon following administration of 1,2 dimethylhydrazine. *Cancer
Res* 1977; 37: 1680–1685

575. Riches A G, Cork M J, Thomas D B. Humoral factors controlling the   2.2
growth fraction of hematopoietic stem cells. *J Anat* 1979; 129: 873

576. Riecken E O. Histochemistry of the small intestine in various malabsorp-   6.3
tion states. In: Card W I, Creamer B, eds. *Modern Trends in Gastroenterology—4*. London: Butterworth 1970: 20–41

577. Riecken E O, Menge H. Nutritive effects of food constituents on the   2.1
structure and function of the intestine. *Acta Hepatogastroenterol* 1977; 24:
389–399

578. Rijke R P C. *Control Mechanisms of Cell Proliferation in Intestinal*   2.1
Epithelium. Thesis, Erasmus University, Rotterdam 1977

579. Rijke R P C, Dongen J M van. Control mechanisms of crypt cell   1.1, 2.1
production in the small intestinal epithelium. *Acta Histochem (Jena)* 1980
Suppl; 21: 81–99

580. Rijke R P C, Gart R. Epithelial cell kinetics in the descending colon of   2.1
the rat. I. The effect of ischaemia-induced epithelial cell loss. *Virchows
Archiv (Cell Pathol)* 1979; 31: 15–22

581. Rijke R P C, Gart R, Langendoen N J. Epithelial cell kinetics in the   2.1
descending colon of the rat. II. The effect of experimental bypass.
Virchows Archiv (Cell Pathol) 1979; 31: 23–30

582. Rijke R P C, Hanson W R, Plaisier H M. The effect of transposition to   2.1, 4.4
jejunum on epithelial cell kinetics in an ileal segment. *Cell Tissue Kinet*
1977; 10: 399–406

583. Rijke R P C, Hanson W R, Plaisier H M, Osborne J W. The effect of   1.1, 2.1, 3.2
ischemic villus cell damage on crypt cell proliferation in the small
intestine: evidence for a feedback control mechanism. *Gastroenterology*
1976; 71: 786–792

584. Rijke R P C, Meer-Fieggen W van der, Galjaard H. Effect of villus   2.1
length on cell proliferation and migration in small intestinal epithelium.
Cell Tissue Kinet 1974; 7: 577–586

585. Rijke R P C, Plaisier H, Hoogeveen A T, Lamerton L F, Galjaard H.   1.1, 2.1, 3.2
The effect of continuous irradiation on cell proliferation and maturation
in small intestinal epithelium. *Cell Tissue Kinet* 1975; 8: 441–453

586. Rijke R P C, Plaisier H M, Ruiter H de, Galjaard H. The influence of   2.1, 2.2
experimental bypass on cellular kinetics and maturation of small
intestinal epithelium in the rat. *Gastroenterology* 1977; 72: 896–901

587. Rijke R P C, Plaisier H M, Langendoen N J. Epithelial cell kinetics in   2.1
the descending colon of the rat. *Virchows Archiv (Cell Pathol)* 1979; 30:
85–94

588. Robinson D C, Watson A J, Wyatt E H, Marks J M, Roberts D F.   6.3
Incidence of small-intestinal mucosal abnormalities and of clinical coeliac
disease in the relatives of children with coeliac disease. *Gut* 1971; 12:
789–793

589. Rodriguez M S B de, Sunter J P, Watson A J, Wright N A, Appleton D   1.4
R. Cell population kinetics in the mucosal crypts of the descending colon
of the mouse. *Virchows Archiv (Cell Pathol)* 1979; 29: 351–361

590. Rogers K J, Pegg A E. Formation of O^6 methylguanine by alkylation of   5.1
rat liver, colon and kidney DNA following administration of 1,2
dimethylhydrazine. *Cancer Res* 1977; 37: 4082–4087

591. Rosenberg I L. The aetiology of colonic suture line recurrence. *Ann R*   5.4
Coll Surg Engl 1979; 61: 251–257

592. Roti Roti J L, Dethlefsen L A. Matrix simulation of duodenal crypt cell   4.2
kinetics. I. The steady state. *Cell Tissue Kinet* 1975; 8: 321–333

593. Rowinski J, Nowak M, Sawicki W. Proliferation kinetics in epithelium   1.3
of guinea pig. III. Distribution of blood capillaries along the crypt. *Cell
Tissue Kinet* 1972; 5: 237–243

594. Rowinski J, Sawicki W. Proliferation kinetics in epithelium of guinea-   1.3
pig colon. V. The question of a diurnal rhythm of mitoses. *Bull Acad Pol
Sci* 1972; 20: 443–446

595. Rowinski J, Sawicki W. Relationship between the cell cycle and cell   1.3
localisation in crypts of the guinea pig ascending colon. *Am J Anat* 1972;
135: 537–538

596. Rowlatt U M. Neoplasms of the alimentary canal of rats and mice. In: 5.1
Cotchin C, Roe F J C, eds. *Pathology of Laboratory Rats and Mice*.
Oxford: Blackwell Scientific Publications 1967: 57–84

597. Royer M, Croxatto O, Biempica L, Balcazar Morrison A J. Biopsie   6.3
duodenal por aspiracion bajo control radioscopico. *Prensa Med Argen*
1955; 42: 2515–2519

598. Rubin C E, Brandborg L L, Phelps P C, Taylor H C Jr. Studies of celiac   6.3
disease. I. The apparent identical and specific nature of the duodenal and
proximal jejunal lesion in celiac disease and idiopathic steatorrhea.
Gastroenterology 1960; 38: 28–49

599. Rubin C E, Eidelman S, Weinstein W M. Sprue 'by any other name'.   6.3
Gastroenterology 1970; 58: 409–413

600. Rubin W. Celiac disease. *Am J Clin Nutr* 1971; 24: 91–111   6.3

601. Rubin W, Ross L L, Sleisenger M H, Weser E. An electron microscopic   6.3
study of adult celiac disease. *Lab Invest* 1966; 15: 1720–1747

602. Rundell J O, Lecce J G. Independence of intestinal epithelial cell   2.6
turnover from cessation of absorption of macromolecules (closure) in the
neonatal mouse, rabbit, hamster and guinea pig. *Biol Neonate* 1972; 20:
51–57

603. Rutter W J, Pictet R L, Morris W. Toward molecular mechanism of   1.3
developmental processes. *Ann Rev Biochem* 1973; 42: 601–646

604. Saetren H. A principle of autoregulation of growth. *Exp Cell Res* 1956;   2.3
11: 229–232

605. Sakata T, Hikosaka K, Shiomura Y, Tamate H K. Stimulatory effect   2.7
of insulin on ruminal epithelial cell mitosis in adult sheep. *Br J Nutr*
(Submitted for publication)

606. Sakata T, Tamate H. Effect of the intermittent feeding on the mitotic   2.7
index and the ultrastructure of basal cells of the ruminal epithelium in
the sheep. *Tohoku J Agr Res* 1974; 25: 156–163

607. Sakata T, Tamate H. Light and electron microscopic observations of the   2.7
forestomach mucosa in the golden hamster. *Tohoku J Agr Res* 1976; 27:
26–39

608. Sakata T, Tamate, H. Presence of circadian rhythm in the mitotic index   2.7
of the ruminal epithelium in sheep. *Res Vet Sci* 1978; 24: 1–3

609. Sakata T, Tamate H. Rumen epithelial cell proliferation accelerated by   2.7
rapid increase in intraruminal butyrate. *J Dairy Sci* 1978; 61:
1109–1113

610. Sakata T, Tamate H. Influence of butyrate on microscopic structure of   2.7
ruminal mucosa in adult sheep. *Jap J Zootech Sci* 1978; 49: 687–696

611. Sakata T, Tamate H. Rumen epithelium cell proliferation accelerated by   2.7
      propionate and acetate. *J Dairy Sci* 1979; 62: 49–52

612. Sakata T, Tamate H. Postnatal development of the forestomach and its   2.7
      epithelium in the golden hamster. *Jap J Zootech Sci* (In Press)

613. Sandberg A A, Rosenthal H E. Estrogen receptors in the pancreas. *J*   4.5
      Steroid Biochem 1974; 5: 969–975

614. Sander E G, Warner R G, Harrison H N, Loosli J K. The stimulatory   2.7
      effect of sodium butyrate and sodium propionate on the development of
      rumen mucosa in the young calf. *J Dairy Sci* 1959; 42: 1600–1605

615. Sandler J A, Clyman R I, Manganiello V C, Vaughan M. The effects of   5.3
      serotonin (5-hydroxytryptamine) and derivatives of guanosine 3′.5′
      monophosphate in human monocytes. *J Clin Invest* 1975; 55: 431–435

616. Sassier P, Bergeron M. A method for the study of the inhibition of DNA   2.3
      synthesis by rabbit tissue extracts. *Can J Physiol Pharmacol* 1976; 54:
      367–372

617. Sassier P, Bergeron M. Specific inhibition of cell proliferation in the   2.3, 3.2
      mouse intestine in-vivo by an aqueous extract of rabbit small intestine.
      Cell Tissue Kinet 1977; 10: 223–231

618. Sassier P, Bergeron M. Specific inhibition of cell proliferation in the   2.3
      mouse intestine in-vivo by an aqueous extract of rabbit colon. *Cell Tissue*
      Kinet 1978; 11: 641–656

619. Sassier P, Bergeron M. Existence of an endogenous inhibitor of DNA   2.3
      synthesis in rabbit small intestine, specifically effective on cell prolifera-
      tion in adult mouse intestine. *Cell Tissue Kinet* 1980; 13: 251–261

620. Sato F, Muramatsu S, Tsuchihashi S et al. Radiation effects on cell   2.1, 2.5, 3.2
      populations in the intestinal epithelium of mice and its theory. *Cell*
      Tissue Kinet 1972; 5: 227–235

621. Sawicki W, Blaton O, Pindor M. Spatial distribution of DNA-   1.3
      synthesising cells in colonic crypts of the guinea pig. *Am J Anat* 1977;
      148: 417–425

622. Sawicki W, Rowinski J. Periodic acid-Schiff reaction combined with   1.3
      quantitative autoradiography of 3H-thymidine or 35S-sulfate-labelled
      epithelial cells of colon. *Histochemie* 1969; 19: 288–294

623. Sawicki W, Rowinski J. Proliferation kinetics in epithelium of guinea-   1.3
      pig colon. I. Variations depending on crypt length and its localisation.
      Cell Tissue Kinet 1970; 3: 375–383

624. Sawicki W, Rowinski J, Blaton O. Proliferation kinetics in epithelium   1.3
      of guinea-pig colon. II. Distribution of proliferating and specialised cells
      along various crypts. *Cel Tissue Kinet* 1971; 4: 225–232

625. Sbarbati R. Quantitative aspects of the embryonic growth of the intestine   1.2
      and stomach. *J Anat* 1979; 129: 795–803

626. Schauer A, Kunze E, Boxler K. Generationszeitzyklus von 1,2   5.1
      Dimethylhydrazin-induzierten Adenocarcinomen des Rattencolon.
      Naturwissenschaften 1971; 58: 221

627. Schauer A, Völlnagel T H, Wildanger F. Cancerisierung des Ratten-   5.2
      darmes durch 1,2-Dimethylhydrazin. *Z Ges Exp Med* 1969; 150: 87–93

628. Schenk E A, Samloff I M. Clinical and morphologic changes following   6.3
      gluten administration to patients with treated celiac disease. *Am J Path*
      1968; 52: 579–593

629. Scheving L E, Burns E R, Pauly J E, Tsai T-H. Circadian variation in   2.2

cell division of the mouse alimentary tract, bone marrow and corneal epithelium. *Anat Rec* 1978; 191: 479–486

630 Schneiderman M A. Digestive system cancer among persons subjected to occupational inhalation of asbestos particles. A literature review with emphasis on dose response. *Environ Health Perspect* 1974; 9: 307–311 5.5

631. Schnorr B, Vollmerhaus B. Das Oberflächenrelief der Pansenschleimhaut bei Rind und Ziege. *Zentrabl Veterinaermea* 1967: A14: 93–104 2.7

632. Schnorr B, Vollmerhaus B. Das Blutgefäs system des Pansens von Rind und Ziege. *Zentrabl Veterinaermed* 1968; 15: 799–828 2.7

633. Schoental R. Induction of intestinal tumours by N-ethyl-N-nitrosourethane. *Nature* 1965; 208: 300 5.1

634. Schoental R, Bousted J P M. Tumours of the intestines induced in rats by intraperitoneal injections of N-methyl- and N-ethyl-N-nitrosourethanes. *Br J Cancer* 1968; 22: 316–323 5.1

635. Schultz B, Haack V, Schmeer A C, Maurer W. Autoradiographic investigation of the cell kinetics of crypt epithelia in the jejunum of the mouse. *Cell Tissue Kinet* 1972–5: 131–145 1.1

636. Scott J F, Fraccastoro A P, Taft E B Jr. Studies in histochemistry: 1. Determination of nucleic acids in microgram amounts of tissue. *J Histochem Cytochem* 1956; 4: 1–10 4.4

637. Seelig L L, Winborn W B, Weser E. Changes in gastric glandular kinetics after small bowel resection in the rat. *Gastroenterology* 1978; 74: 1–6 2.2

638. Selikoff J, Hammond E C, Churg J. Asbestos exposure, smoking and neoplasia. *JAMA* 1968; 204: 106–112 5.5

639. Selikoff I J, Hammond E C, Churg J. Mortality experience of asbestos insulation workers 1943–68. In: Shapiro H A, ed. *Pneumoconiosis Proc Intl Conf Johannesburg 1969*. Capetown, Oxford University Press 1970: 180–186 5.5

640. Seller A F, Stevens C E, Dobson A, McLeod F D. Arterial blood flow to the ruminant stomach. *Am J Physiol* 1964; 207: 371–377 2.7

641. Shank R C, Magee P N. Similarities between the biochemical actions of cycasin and dimethylhydrazine. *Biochem J* 1967; 105: 521–527 5.1

642. Shellito P C, Peterson Dahl E, Terpstra O T, Malt R A. Postresectional hyperplasia of the small intestine without bile and pancreatic juice. *Proc Soc Exp Biol Med* 1978; 158: 101–104 4.4

643. Shimizu H, Toth B. Autoradiographic study of tissue-bound C14-1,2-dimethylhydrazine di-HCl in mice. *Fed Proc* 1973; 32: 825 abs 5.1

644. Shiner M. Jejunal biopsy tube. *Lancet* 1956; i: 85 6.3

645. Shiner M. Electron microscopy of jejunal mucosa. *Clinics in Gastroenterology* 1974; 3: 33–53 6.3

646. Shipley R E. Symposium on sitosterol concentration. *Trans NY Acad Sci* 1955; 18: 111–118 6.5

647. Shirakawa S, Luce J K, Tannock I, Frei E. Cell proliferation in human melanoma. *J Clin Invest* 1970; 49: 1188–1199 1.3

648. Shrader R E, Ferlatte M I, Zemen F J. Early postnatal development of the intestine in progeny of protein-deprived rats. *Biol Neonate* 1977; 31: 181–198 2.6

649. Shultz G, Shultz K, Hardman J G. Effects of norepinephrine on cyclic 5.3

nucleotide in the ductus deferens of the rat. *Metabolism* 1975; 24: 429–437

650. Shuster S, Watson A J, Marks J M. Small intestine in psoriasis. *Br Med J* 1967; 3: 458–460   6.3

651. Shuster S, Watson A J, Marks J M. Coeliac syndrome in dermatitis herpetiformis. *Lancet* 1968; i: 1101–1106   6.3

652. Sigdestad C P, Bauman J, Lesher S. Diurnal fluctuations in the numbers of cells in mitosis and DNA synthesis in the jejunum of the mouse. *Exp Cell Res* 1969; 58: 159–162   1.1, 1.4, 5.5

653. Sigdestad C P, Lesher S. Circadian rhythm in the cell cycle time of mouse intestinal epithelium. *J Interdiscipl Cycle Res* 1972; 3: 39–46   3.3

654. Simmons J L, Fishman P H, Freese E, Brady R O. Morphological alterations and ganglioside sialyltransferase activity induced by small fatty acids in Hela cells. *J Cell Biol* 1975; 66: 414–424   2.7

655. Simpson D P P. ³²P uptake in DNA nucleotide after partial hepatectomy and after unilateral nephrectomy. *Am J Physiol* 1961; 201: 523–525   2.3

656. Snodgrass D R, Angus K W, Gray E W, Menzies J D, Paul G. Pathogenesis of astrovirus infection in lambs. *Arch Virol* 1979; 60: 217–226.   6.2

657. Snodgrass D R, Ferguson A, Allan F, Angus K W, Mitchell B. Small intestinal morphology and epithelial cell kinetics in lamb rotavirus infections. *Gastroenterology* 1979; 76: 477–481   6.2

658. Soumarmon A, Cheret A M, Lewin M J. Localisation of gastrin receptors in intact isolated and separated rat fundic cells. *Gastroenterology* 1977; 73: 900–903   2.2

659. Spatz M. Carcinogenicity of methylazoxymethanol (MAM) in guinea pigs and hamsters (abstr). *Tenth Intl Cancer Cong Houston.* 1970: 24–25   5.4

660. Spector M H, Levine G M, Deren J J. Direct and indirect effects of dextrose and amino acids on gut mass. *Gastroenterology* 1977; 72: 706–710   4.4

661. Spencer R P, Coulombre M J. Quantitative approaches to intestinal growth. *Growth* 1965; 29: 323–330   2.2

662. Spjut H J, Noall M N. Colonic neoplasms induced by 3:2′dimethyl-4 aminodiphenyl. In: Burdette W J ed. *Cancer of the Colon and Antecedent Epithelium.* Springfield, Illinois: Charles C Thomas 1970: 280–288   5.1

663. Spjut H J, Spratt J S Jr. Endemic and morphologic similarities existing between spontaneous colonic neoplasms in man and 3:2′dimethyl 1-4-aminobiphenyl induced colonic neoplasms in rats. *Ann Surg* 1965; 161: 309–324   5.2

664. Sporn M B, Dunlop N M, Newton D L, Smith J M. Prevention of chemical carcinogenesis by vitamin A and its synthetic analogs (retinoids). *Fed Proc* 1976; 35: 1332–1338   6.1

665. Spratts J S, Acherman L V, Moyer C A. Relationship of polyps of the colon to colonic cancer. *Ann Surg* 1958; 148: 682–696   5.2, 6.4

666. Springer P, Springer J, Oehlert W. Early stages of DMA induced carcinoma of the small and large intestine of the rat. *Z Krebsforsch* 1970; 74: 236–240   5.1, 6.1

667. Springer P, Springer J, Oehlert W. Die Vorstufen des 1,2-Dimethyl-hydrazin-induzierten Dick-und Dunndarm-carcinoms der Rat. *Z Krebsforsch* 1970; 74: 236–240   5.2

668. Steel G G. *Growth Kinetics of Tumours*. Oxford, Clarendon Press 1977:   6.3
81–85

669. Steel G G, Adams K, Barrett J C. Analysis of the cell population kinetics   1.3
of transplanted tumours of widely-differing growth rate. *Br J Cancer*
1966; **20**: 784–800

670. Steel G G, Hanes S. The technique of labelled mitoses: analysis by   1.3, 5.3
automatic curve-fitting. *Cell Tissue Kinet 1971*; 4: 93–105

671. Stern J B, Sobel H J. Jejunal carcinoma with cells resembling Paneth   3.2
cells. *Arch Path* 1961; **72**: 47–50

672. Stevens R H, Loven D P, Osbourne J W, Prall J P, Lawson A J. Cyclic   5.3
nucleotide concentrations in 1,2-dimethylhydrazine induced rat colon
adenocarcinoma. *Cancer Lett* 1977; 4: 27–33

673. Stewart H L, Lorenz E. Histopathology of induced precancerous lesions   5.1
of the small intestine of mice. *J Natl Cancer Inst* 1947; 7: 239–268

674. Stillstrom J. Grain count corrections in autoradiography. *Int J Appl*   2.6
Radiat Iso 1963; 14: 113–118

675. Stoffels G L, Preumont A M, Reuck M de. Nuclear binding of tritiated   6.4
actinomycin in surface epithelial cells from normal stomach and atrophic
gastritis. *Gut* 1978; **19**: 870–874

676. Stoffels G L, Preumont A M, Reuck M de. Cell differentiation in human   6.4
gastric glands as revealed by nuclear binding of tritiated actinomycin.
Gut 1979; **20**: 693–697

677. Stormshak F, Leake R, Wertz N, Gorski J. Stimulatory and inhibitory   4.5
effects of estrogen on uterine DNA synthesis. *Endocrinology* 1976; **99**:
1501–1511

678. Storrie B, Puck T T, Wenger L. The role of butyrate in the reverse   2.7
transformation reaction in mammalian cells. *J Cell Physiol* 1978; **94**:
69–75

679. Straus E. Radioimmunoassay of gastrointestinal hormones. *Gastroenterol-*   2.2
ogy 1978; **74**: 141–152

680. Straus E, Gerson C D, Yalow R S. Hypersecretion of gastrin associated   4.4
with the short bowel syndrome. *Gastroenterology* 1974; **66**: 175–180

681. Straus E, Yalow R S. Cholecystokinin in the brains of obese and   2.2
non-obese mice. *Science* 1979; **203**: 68–69

682. Strober W. An immunological theory of gluten-sensitive enteropathy.   6.3
In: McNicholl B, McCarthy C F, Fottrell P F, eds. *Perspectives in coeliac*
disease. Lancaster, MTP Press Ltd 1978: 169–182

683. Stumpf W E, Sar M. The heart: A target organ for estradiol. *Science* 1977;   4.5
196: 319–321

684. Subbuswamy S G, Gibbs N M, Ross C F, Morson B C. Goblet cell   3.2
carcinoid of the appendix. *Cancer* 1974; **34**: 338–344

685. Sunter J P, Appleton D R, Rodriguez M S B de, Wright N A, Watson A J.   1.4
A comparison of cell proliferation at different sites within the large bowel of
the mouse. *J Anat* 1979; **129**: 833–842

686. Sunter J P, Appleton D R, Wright N A, Watson A J. Kinetics of   2.1, 5.1
changes in the crypts of the jejunal mucosa of dimethylhydrazine treated
rats. *Br J Cancer* 1978; **37**: 662–672

687. Sunter J P, Appleton D R, Wright N A, Watson A J. Pathological   5.1, 5.2
features of the colonic tumours induced in rats by the administration of
1,2 dimethylhydrazine. *Virchows Archiv (Cell Pathol)* 1978; **29**: 211–223

688. Sunter J P, Watson A J, Wright N A, Appleton D R. Cell proliferation   1.4, 5.1, 5.5
at different sites along the length of the rat colon. *Virchows Archiv (Cell Pathol)* 1979; 32: 75–87

689. Sunter J P, Wright N A, Appleton D R. Cell population kinetics in the   1.1, 1.4, 2.1
epithelium of the colon of the male rat. *Virchows Archiv (Cell Pathol)* 1978; 26: 275–287

690. Sylven B, Bois I. Protein content and enzymatic assays of interstitial   5.2
fluid from some normal tissues and transplanted mouse tumors. *Cancer Res* 1960; 20: 831–836

691. Symons L E A. Kinetics of epithelial cells and morphology of villi and   5.1
crypts in the jejunum of the rat infected by the nematode *Nippostrongylus brasiliensis*. *Gastroenterology* 1965; 49: 158–168

692. Szemeredy Gy, Raul R. Alteration of the ruminal mucosa and its relation   2.7
to the hepatic abscesses in bulls fed high energy and low fibre diets. *Acta Vet Acad Sci Hung* 1976; 26: 313–324

693. Takahashi M, Hogg J O, Mendelsohn M L. The automatic analysis of   5.3
FLM curves. *Cell Tissue Kinet* 1971; 4: 505–518

694. Tamate H. The anatomical studies of the stomach of the goat. II. The   2.7
post-natal changes in the capacities and the relative sizes of the four divisions of the stomach. *Tohoku J Agr Res* 1957; 8: 65–77

695. Tamate H, Fell B F. Cell deletion as a factor in the regulation of rumen   2.7
epithelial population. *Vet Sci Commun* 1978; 1: 359–364

696. Tamate H, Kikuchi T. Electron microscopic study on parakeratotic   2.7
ruminal epithelium in beef cattle. *Jap J Vet Sci* 1978; 40: 21–30

697. Tamate H, Kikuchi T, Sakata T. Ultrastructural changes in the ruminal   2.7
epithelium after fasting and subsequent refeeding in the sheep. *Tohoku J Agr Res* 1974; 27: 142–155

698. Tamate H, McGilliard A D, Jacobson N L, Getty R. Effect of various   2.7
diets on the anatomical development of the stomach in the calf. *J Dairy Sci* 1962; 45: 408–420

699. Tamate H, McGilliard A D, Jacobson N L, Getty R. The effect of   2.7
various diets on the histological development of the stomach of the calf. *Tohoku J Agr Res* 1964; 14: 171–193

700. Tamate H, Nagatani T, Yoneya S, Sakata T, Muira J. High incidence of   2.7
ruminal lesions and liver abscess in the beef associated with intensive fattening in Miyagi Prefecture. *Tohoku J Agr Res* 1973; 23: 184–195

701. Tannenbaum S R, Fett D, Young V R, Land P D, Bruce W R. Nitrite   6.1
and nitrate are formed by endogenous synthesis in human intestine. *Science* 1978; 200: 1487–1489

702. Tannock I F. A comparison of the relative efficiencies of various   1.4, 5.5, 6.3
metaphase arrest agents. *Exp Cell Res* 1967; 47: 345–356

703. Tannock I F. The relation between cell proliferation and the vascular   1.3, 5.1
system in a transplanted mouse mammary tumour. *Br J Cancer* 1968; 22: 258–273

704. Tchernitchin A, Tchernitchin X. Characterization of the estrogen   4.5
receptors in the uterine blood eosinophil leukocytes. *Experientia* 1976; 32: 1240–1242

705. Teichman R K, Hill F C, Rayford P L, Thompson J C. Effect of growth   2.2
hormone on serum, antral and duodenal gastrin in hypophysectomised rats. *Gastroenterology* 1977; 72: 1139

706. Terpstra O T, Peterson-Dahl E, Ross J S, Williamson R C N, Malt R A. 5.4
Distal colonic hyperplasia after colostomy closure: a promoter of chemical
carcinogenesis. *Surg Forum* 1979; 30: 130–131

707. Thrasher J D. Age and the cell cycle in mouse colonic epithelium. *Anat* 1.4
Rec 1967; 157: 621–626

708. Thrasher J D, Greulich R C. The duodenal progenitor population. I. 2.6
Age related increase in the duration of the cryptal progenitor cycle. *J Exp*
Zool 1965; 159: 39–46

709. Thrasher J D, Greulich R C. The duodenal progenitor population. III. 3.1
The progenitor cell cycle of principal, goblet and Paneth cells. *J Exp Zool*
1966; 161: 9–20

710. Thurnherr N, Deschner E E, Stonehill E H, Lipkin M. Induction of 3.3, 5.1, 5.2,
adenocarcinomas of the colon in mice by weekly injections of 1,2 6.1
dimethylhydrazine. *Cancer Res* 1973; 33: 940–945

711. Tilson M D. Compensatory hypertrophy of the gut in an infant with 4.4
intestinal atresia. *Am J Surg* 1972; 123: 733–734

712. Tilson M D, Livstone E M. Radioautography of heterotopic autografts of 4.4
ileal mucosa in rats after partial enterectomy. *Surg Forum* 1975; 26:
383–394

713. Tilson M D, Michaud J T, Livstone E M. Early proliferative activity in 5.4
the left colon of the rat after partial small-bowel resection. *Surg Forum*
1976; 27: 445–446

714. Tilson M D, Walton R, Livstone E M. Starvation overrides humoral 4.4
stimuli for adaptive growth of the ileum in parabiotic rats (abstr) *Clin*
Res 1975; 23: 579

715. Tilson M D, Wright H K. Villus hyperplasia in parabiotic rats (abstr.). 4.4
Clin Res 1971; 19: 405

716. Timbrell V. Characteristics of UICC standard reference samples of 5.5
asbestos. In: Shapiro H A, ed. *Pneumoconiosis Proc Intl Conf Johannesburg,*
1969. Capetown, Oxford University Press 1970: 28–36

717. Toback F G, Lowenstein L M. Uridine metabolism during normal and 2.3
compensatory renal growth. *Growth* 1974; 38: 17–34

718. Toback F G, Lowenstein L M. Thymidine metabolism during normal 2.3
and compensatory renal growth. *Growth* 1974; 38: 35–44

719. Toft D, Gorski J. A receptor molecule for estrogens: isolation from the 4.5
rat uterus and preliminary characterization. *Proc Natl Acad Sci USA*
1966; 55: 1574–1581

720. Toth B, Malick L. Production of intestinal and other tumors by 5.2
1,2-dimethylhydrazine dihydrochloride in mice. II. Scanning electron
microscopic and cytochemical study of colonic neoplasms. *Br J Exp*
Pathol 1976; 57: 696–705

721. Toth B, Malick L, Shimizu H. Production of intestinal and other tumors 5.1, 5.2
by 1,2 dimethylhydrazine dihydrochloride in mice. I. A light and
transmission electron microscopic study of colonic neoplasms. *Am J*
Pathol 1976; 84: 69–86

722. Touloukian R M, Wright H K. Intrauterine villous hypertrophy with 4.4
jejunoileal atresia. *J Pediatr Surg* 1973; 8: 779–784

723. Trautman A, Fiebiger J. *Fundamentals of the Histology of Domestic Animals.* 2.7
Translated by Habel R E and Bieberstein E L. Ithaca: Comstock
Publishing Associates 1952

724. Trier J S, Browning Th D. Epithelial-cell renewal in cultured duodenal   2.1, 6.3
biopsies in celiac sprue. *N Engl J Med* 1970; **283**: 1245–1250

725. Troughton W D, Trier J S. Paneth and goblet cell renewal in mouse   3.1, 3.2
duodenal crypts. *J Cell Biol* 1969; **41**: 251–268

726. Tubiana M, Frindel E, Croizat H, Vassort F. Study of some factors   4.2
influencing the proliferation and differentiation of the multipotential
hemopoietic stem cells. In: *Control of Proliferation in Animal Cells.
Cold Spring Harbor Conference on cell proliferation* 1974; **1**: 933–944

727. Turcot J, Despres J P, Pierre F. Malignant tumors of the central nervous   6.1
stystem associated with familial polyposis of the colon. *Dis Colon Rectum*
1959; **2**: 465–468

728. Tutton P J M. Control of epithelial cell proliferation in the small   2.3, 3.2
intestinal crypt. *Cell Tissue Kinet* 1973; **6**: 211–216

729. Tutton P J M. Variations in crypt cell cycle time and mitotic time in the   2.6
small intestine of the rat. *Virchows Archiv (Cell Pathol)* 1973; **13**: 68–78

730. Tutton P J M. Proliferation of epithelial cells in the jejunal crypts of   2.2, 2.6
adrenalectomized and adrenocortical hormone treated rats. *Virchows
Archiv (Cell Pathol)* 1973; **13**: 227–232

731. Tutton P J M. The influence of serotonin on crypt cell proliferation in   2.2, 5.3
the jejunum of rat. *Virchows Archiv (Cell Pathol)* 1974; **16**: 79–87

732. Tutton P J M. The influence of histamine on epithelial cell proliferation   2.2, 5.3
in the jejunum of rat. *Clin Exp Pharmacol Physiol* 1976; **3**: 369–373

733. Tutton P J M. The influence of thyroidectomy and of tri-iodothyronine   2.2
administration on epithelial cell proliferation in the jejunum of rat.
Virchows Archiv (Cell Pathol) 1976; **20**: 139–142

734. Tutton P J M. Neural and endocrine control systems acting on the   2.1, 5.3
population kinetics of the intestinal epithelium. *Med Biol* 1977; **55**:
201–208

735. Tutton P J M. Control of epithelial cell proliferation in the small   5.3
intestine—the villous longistat. *J Anat* 1978; **128**: 638

736. Tutton P J M, Barkla D H. Cell proliferation in the descending colon of   2.1, 5.1,
dimethylhydrazine treated rats and in dimethylhydrazine induced   5.2, 5.3, 5.4
adenocarcinomata. *Virchows Archiv (Cell Pathol)* 1976; **21**: 147–160

737. Tutton P J M, Barkla D H. A comparison of cell proliferation in normal   5.1, 5.3
and neoplastic intestinal epithelium following either biogenic amine
depletion or monoamine oxidase inhibition. *Virchows Archiv (Cell Pathol)*
1976; **21**: 161–168

738. Tutton P J M, Barkla D H. The influence of adrenoreceptor activity on   2.2, 5.1, 5.3
cell proliferation in colonic crypt epithelium and in colonic adenocarcinomata. *Virchows Archiv (Cell Pathol)* 1977; **24**: 139–146

739. Tutton P J M, Barkla D H. Cytotoxicity of 5,6-dihydroxytryptamine in   5.3
dimethylhydrazine-induced carcinomas of rat colon. *Cancer Res* 1977; **37**:
1241–1244

740. Tutton P J M, Barkla D H. Cell proliferation in dimethylhydrazine   5.1
induced colonic adenocarcinoma following cytotoxic drug treatment.
Virchows Archiv (Cell Pathol) 1978; **28**: 151–156

741. Tutton P J M, Barkla D H. The influence of serotonin on the mitotic rate   5.3
in the colonic crypt epithelium and in colonic adenocarcinoma in rat.
Clin Exp Pharmacol Physiol 1978; **5**: 91–94

742. Tutton P J M, Barkla D H. Stimulation of cell proliferation by histamine   5.3

H_2 receptors in dimethylhydrazine-induced adenocarcinomata. *Cell Biol Int Rep* 1978; 2: 199–202

743. Tutton P J M, Barkla D H. The influence of prostaglandin analogues on epithelial cell proliferation and xenograft growth. *Br J Cancer* 1980; 41: 47–51   5.3

744. Tutton P J M, Helme R D. Stress induced inhibition of jejunal crypt cell proliferation. *Virchows Archiv (Cell Pathol)* 1973; 15: 23–34   2.6

745. Tutton P J M, Helme R D. The influence of adrenoreceptor activity on crypt cell proliferation in the rat jejunum. *Cell Tissue Kinet* 1974; 7: 125–136   2.2, 2.3, 2.6, 5.3

746. Tutton P J M, Steel G G. The influence of biogenic amines on the growth of xenografted human colorectal carcinoma. *Br J Cancer* 1979; 40: 743–749   5.3

747. Utsunomiya J, Iwana T, Ichikawa T, Miyanga T, Hirayama T. Present status of familial polyposis of the colon in Japan. In: Farber E, et al, eds. *Pathophysiology of Carcinogenesis in Digestive Organs.* University of Tokyo Press 1977: 305–311   6.1

748. Varghese A J, Land P, Furrer R, Bruce W R. Evidence for the formation of mutagenic N-nitroso compounds in the human body. *Proc Am Assn Canc Res* 1977; 18: 80   6.1

749. Vassort F, Frindel E, Tubinana M. Effects of hydroxyurea on the kinetics of colony forming units of bone marrow in the mouse. *Cell Tissue Kinet* 1971; 4: 423–431   4.2

750. Vassort F, Winterholer M, Frindel E, Tubiana M. Kinetic parameters of bone marrow stem cells using in vivo suicide by tritiated thymidine or by hydroxyurea. *Blood* 1973; 41: 789–796   4.2

751. Veale A M O. Intestinal polyposis. *Eugenics Laboratory Memoir Series* 40, London: Cambridge University Press 1965   6.1

752. Verly W G, Deschamps Y, Desrosiers M, Pushpatadam J. The hepatic chalone. I. Assay method for the hormone and purification of the rabbit liver chalone. *Can J Biochem* 1971; 49: 1376–1383   2.3

753. Vollmer E P, Gordon A S. Effect of sex and gonadotropic hormones upon the blood picture of the rat. *Endocrinology* 1941; 29: 828–837   4.5

754. Wagner J C. Epidemiology of diffuse mesothelial tumors: evidence of an association from studies in South Africa and the United Kingdom. *Ann NY Acad Sci* 1965; 132: 128–138   5.5

755. Walker R. The contribution of intestinal endotoxin to mortality in hosts with compromised resistance: a review. *Exp Hematol* 1978; 6: 169–184   4.3

756. Walker-Smith J A. *Diseases of the small intestine in childhood.* Tunbridge Wells: Pitman Medical Publishing Co. 1979   6.2

757. Walpole A J, Williams M H C, Roberts D C. The carcinogenic action of 4 aminodiphenyl and 3:2'-dimethyl 4-amino-diphenyl. *Br J Ind Med* 1952; 9: 255–263   5.1

758. Walpole A L, Williams M H C, Roberts D C. Bladder tumours induced in rats of two strains with 3:2' dimethyl-4-aminodiphenyl. *Br J Cancer* 1955; 9: 170–176   5.1

759. Walsh J H, Gorssman M I. Gastrin. *N Engl J Med* 1978; 292: 1324–1332, 1337–1384   2.2

760. Ward J M. Morphogenesis of chemically induced neoplasms of the colon and small intestine in rats. *Lab Invest* 1974; 30: 505–513   5.1, 5.2, 5.4

761. Ward J M, Rice J M, Roller P P, Wenk M L. Natural history of   5.4
      intestinal neoplasms induced in rats by a single injection of methyl
      (acetoxymethyl) nitrosamine. *Cancer Res* 1977; 37: 3046–3052
762. Ward J M, Weisburger E K. Intestinal tumors in mice treated with a   5.4
      single injection of N-nitroso-N-butylurea. *Cancer Res* 1975; 35:
      1938–1943
763. Ward J M, Yamamoto R S, Brown C A. Pathology of intestinal   5.1, 5.2
      neoplasms and other lesions in rats exposed to azoxymethane. *J Natl
      Cancer Inst* 1973; 51: 1029–1035
764. Warner R G, Flatt W P. In: Dougherty R W, ed. *Physiology of Digestion*   2.7
      in the Ruminant. Washington DC: Butterworth 1965: 24–38
765. Warren P M, Pepperman M A, Montgomery R D. Age change in small   2.2
      intestinal mucosa. *Lancet* 1978; ii: 849
766. Watanabe K, Reddy B S, Wong C Q, Weisburger J H. Effect of dietary   5.1
      undegraded carrageenan on colon carcinogenesis in F344 rats treated
      with azoxymethane or methylnitrosourea. *Cancer Res* 1978; 38:
      4427–4430
767. Watne A L, Lai H L, Mance T, Core S K. Fecal steroids and bacterial   6.1
      flora in polyposis coli patients. *Am J Surg* 1976; 131: 42–46
768. Watson A J, Wright N A. Morphology and cell kinetics of the jejunal   1.1, 6.3
      mucosa in untreated patients. *Clinics in gastroenterology* 1974; 3: 11–31
769. Watson A J, Wright N A. Crypt cell kinetics in convoluted jejunal   6.3
      mucosa. In: Hekkens W Th J M, Peña A S, eds. *Coeliac disease*. Leiden:
      Stenfert Kroese 1974: 151–154
770. Wattenberg L W. Inhibition of carcinogenic and toxic effects of   6.1
      polycyclic hydrocarbons by phenolic antioxidants and ethoxygens. *J Natl
      Cancer Inst* 1972; 48: 1425–1430
771. Wattenberg L W. Inhibition of dimethylhydrazine-induced neoplasia of   6.1
      the large intestine by disulfiram. *J Natl Cancer Inst* 1975; 54: 1005–1006
772. Wattenberg L W. Inhibition of chemical carcinogenesis. *J Natl Cancer*   6.1
      Inst 1978; 60: 11–18
773. Wattenberg L W, Fiala E S. Inhibition of 1,2 dimethylhydrazine-   6.1
      induced neoplasm of the large intestine in female CGI mice by carbon
      disulfide: brief communication. *J Natl Cancer Inst* 1978; 60: 1515–1517
774. Weekes T E C. Effects of pregnancy and lactation in sheep on the   2.7
      metabolism of propionate by the ruminal mucosa and on some enzymic
      activities in the ruminal mucosa. *J Agr Sci Camb* 1972; 79: 409–421
775. Weibel E R. Principles and methods for the morphometric study of the   2.1
      lung and other organs. *Lab Invest* 1963; 12: 131–155
776. Weinstein W M. Epithelial cell renewal of the small intestinal mucosa.   2.3
      Med Clin North Am 1974; 58: 1375–1386
777. Weisburger J H. Colon carcinogens: their metabolism and mode of   5.1, 5.4
      action. *Cancer* 1971; 28: 60–70
778. Weisburger J H, Reddy B S, Wynder E L. Colon cancer: its epidemiol-   5.4
      ogy and experimental production. *Cancer* 1977; 40: 2414–2420
779. Weiss P, Kavanau J L. A model of growth and growth control in   1.1, 2.5
      mathematical terms. *J Gen Physiol* 1957; 41: 1–47
780. Wells G A H. Mucinous adenocarcinoma of the ileum in a rat. *J Pathol*   5.1
      1971; 103: 271–275
781. Werner B, Heer K de, Mitschke H. Cholecystectomy and carcinoma of   6.5

the colon. *Z Krebsforsch* 1977; **88**: 223–230

782. Weser E, Heller R, Tawil T. Stimulation of mucosal growth in the rat   4.4
     ileum by bile and pancreatic secretions after jejunal resection. *Gastroen-
     terology* 1977; 73: 524–529

783. Weser E, Hernandez M H. Studies of small bowel adaptation after   2.1, 4.4
     intestinal resection in the rat. *Gastroenterology* 1971; 60: 69–75

784. Whitmore G F, Gulyas S, Botund J. In: *Cellular Radiation Biology*   4.3
     (Symposium). 18th Annual Symposium on Fundamental Cancer
     Research. Baltimore: Williams and Watkins 1965; 423–441

785. Wiebecke B, Heybowitz S, Löhrs U, Eder M. Der Einfluss des Hungers   1.1
     auf die Proliferations-Kinetic der Dünn und Deckdarmschleimhaut der
     Maus. *Virchows Archiv (Cell Pathol)* 1969; 4: 164–175

786. Wiebecke B, Krey U, Löhrs U, Eder M. Morphological and autoradiog-   5.1, 5.2
     raphical investigations on experimental carcinogenesis and polyp
     development in the intestinal tract of rats and mice. *Virchows Archiv
     (Pathol Anat)* 1973; 360: 179–193

787. Wiebecke B, Löhrs U, Gimmy J, Eder M. Erzeugung von Darmtumoren   5.2, 5.2
     bei Mausen durch 1,2 Dimethylhydrazin. *Z Ges Exp Med* 1969; 149:
     277–278

788. Wiernik G, Plant M. The origin and kinetics of goblet cells in the   3.1
     human jejunum during irradiation. *Br J Radiol* 1971; 44: 348–356

789. Wilbanks G D, Richart R M, Terner J Y. DNA contents of cervical   6.1
     intraepithelial neoplasm studies by two wavelength Feulgen
     cytophotometry. *Am J Obstet Gynaecol* 1967; 98: 792–799

790. Wild D. Cytogenetic effects in the mouse of 17 chemical mutagens and   5.1
     carcinogens evaluated by the micronucleus test. *Mutat Res* 1978; 56:
     319–327

791. Wilkins T D, Hackman A S. Two patterns of neutral steroid conversion   6.1
     in the feces of normal North Americans. *Cancer Res* 1974; 34:
     2250–2254

792. Williamson R C N. Intestinal adaptation. I. Structural, functional and   4.4, 5.4
     cytokinetic aspects. *N Engl J Med* 1978; 298: 1393–1402

793. Williamson R C N. Intestinal adaptation. 2. Mechanisms of control. *N*   4.4, 5.4
     Engl J Med 1978; 298: 1444–1450

794. Williamson R C N, Bauer F L R. Evidence for an enterotropic hormone: 4.4
     compensatory hyperplasia in defunctioned bowel. *Br J Surg* 1978; 65:
     736–739

795. Williamson R C N, Bauer F L R, Ross J S, Malt R A. Proximal   4.4, 5.4
     enterectomy stimulates distal hyperplasia more than bypass or pancreac-
     ticobiliary diversion. *Gastroenterology* 1978; 74: 16–23

796. Williamson R C N, Bauer F L R, Ross J S, Malt R A. Contributions of   2.2, 4.4, 5.4
     bile and of pancreatic juice to cell proliferation in ileal mucosa. *Surgery*
     1978; 83: 570–576

797. Williamson R C N, Bauer F L R, Ross J S, Oscarson J E A, Malt R A.   5.1, 5.4
     Promotion of azoxymethane-induced colonic neoplasia by resection of the
     proximal small bowel. *Cancer Res* 1978; 38: 3212–3217

798. Williamson R C N, Bauer F L R, Ross J S, Watkins J B, Malt R A.   5.4
     Enhanced colonic carcinogenesis with azoxymethane in rats after pan-
     creaticobiliary diversion to mid small bowel. *Gastroenterology* 1979; 76:
     1386–1392

799.   Williamson R C N, Bauer F L R, Terpstra O T, Ross J S, Malt R A.   5.4
        Contrasting effects of subtotal enteric bypass, enterectomy and colectomy
        on azoxymethane-induced intestinal carcinogenesis. *Cancer Res* 1980; 40:
        538–543

800.   Williamson R C N, Buchholtz T W, Malt R A. Humoral stimulation of   2.2, 4.4
        cell proliferation in small bowel after transection and resection. *Gastroen-
        terology* 1978; 75: 249–254

801.   Wimber D R, Lamerton L F. Cell population studies on the intestine of   3.2, 6.3
        continuously irradiated rats. *Radiat Res* 1963; 18: 137–146

802.   Wimber D E, Quastler H, Stein O L, Wimber D R. Analysis of tritium   4.2
        incorporation into individual cells by autoradiography of squash prepara-
        tions. *J Biophys Biochem Cytol* 1960; 8: 327–331

803.   Winawer S, Lipkin M. Cell proliferation kinetics in the gastrointestinal   6.1
        tract of man. IV. Cell renewal in intestinalized gastric mucosa. *J Natl
        Cancer Inst* 1969; 42: 9–17

804.   Winneker R C, Tompkins M, Westenberger P, Harris J. Morphological   5.1
        studies of chemically induced colon tumor in hamsters. *Exp Mol Pathol*
        1977; 27: 19–34

805.   Withers H R. Regeneration of intestinal mucosa after irradiation. *Cancer*   3.2
        1971; 28: 75–81

806.   Withers H R. Colony forming units in the intestine. In: Cairnie A B,   3.2
        Lala P K, Osmond D G, eds. *Stem Cells of Renewing Cell Populations*. New
        York: Academic Press 1976: 33–40

807.   Withers H R, Elkind M M. Dose-survival characteristics of epithelial cells   4.2
        of mouse intestinal mucosa. *Radiology* 1968; 91: 998–1000

808.   Withers H R, Elkind M M. Radiosensitivity and fractionation response   4.3
        of crypt cells of mouse jejunum. *Radiat Res* 1969; 38: 598–613

809.   Withers H E, Elkind M M. Microcolony survival assay for cells of mouse   3.1, 3.2, 4.2,
        intestinal mucosa exposed to radiation. *Int J Radiat Biol* 1970; 17:   4.3
        261–267

810.   Withers H R, Mason K, Reid B O et al. Response of mouse intestine to   4.3
        neutrons and gamma rays in relation to dose fractionation and division
        cycle. *Cancer* 1974; 34: 39–47

811.   Woo Z H, Nygaard K. Small-bowel adaptation after colectomy in rats.   4.4
        Scand J Gastroenterol 1978; 13: 903–910

812.   Wright E G, Lord B I. Production of stem cell proliferation stimulators   2.2
        and inhibitors by haematopoietic cell suspensions. *Biomedicine* 1978; 28:
        156–160

813.   Wright N A. The cell population kinetics of repopulating cells in the   1.1, 3.2
        intestine. In: Lord B I, Potten C S, Cole R J, eds. *Stem Cells and Tissue
        Homeostasis*. Cambridge: University Press 1978: 335–358

814.   Wright N A, Al-Dewachi H S, Appleton D R, Watson A J. Cell   1.1, 3.2, 5.5
        population kinetics in the rat jejunal crypt. *Cell Tissue Kinet* 1975; 8:
        361–368

815.   Wright N A, Al-Dewachi H S, Appleton D R, Watson A J. The effect of   2.2
        single and of multiple doses of prednisolone tertiary butyl acetate on cell
        population kinetics in the small bowel of the rat. *Virchows Archiv (Cell
        Pathol)* 1978; 28: 339–350

816.   Wright N A, Appleton D R. The metaphase arrest technique: a critical   1.4
        review. *Cell Tissue Kinet* (In Press)

817. Wright N A, Appleton D R, Marks J, Watson A J. Cytokinetic studies   1.1, 6.3
of crypts in convoluted human small-intestinal mucosa. *J Clin Pathol*
1979; 32: 462–470

818. Wright N A, Morley A R, Appleton D R. Variation in the duration of   1.1, 1.4, 2.1,
mitosis in the crypts of Lieberkühn of the rat; a cytokinetic study using   4.2, 5.5
vincristine. *Cell Tissue Kinet* 1972; 5: 351–364

819. Wright N A, Morley A R, Appleton D R. The effect of testosterone on   1.1, 1.3, 2.2
cell proliferation and differentiation in the small bowel. *J Endocrinol*
1972; 52: 161–175

820. Wright N A, Watson A J. The morphogenesis of the flat avillous mucosa   6.3
of coeliac disease. In: Hekkens W Th J M, Pena A S, eds. *Coeliac Disease*.
Leiden: Stenfert Kroese 1974: 141–150

821. Wright N, Watson A, Morley A, Appleton D, Marks J, Douglas A. The   1.1, 2.3, 6.3
cell cycle time in the flat (avillous) mucosa of the human small intestine.
Gut 1973; 14: 603–606

822. Wright N, Watson A, Morley A, Appleton D, Marks J. Cell kinetics in   1.1, 2.3, 6.3
flat (avillous) mucosa of the human small intestine. *Gut* 1973; 14:
701–710

823. Wright N, Watson A, Morley A, Appleton D, Marks J, Douglas A. The   2.1, 6.3
measurement of cell production rates in the crypts of Lieberkuhn. An
experimental and clinical study. *Virchows Archiv (Pathol Anat)* 1974;
364: 311–323

824. Wynder E L, Reddy B S. Colon cancer prevention: today's challenge to   6.1
biomedical scientists and clinical investigators. *Cancer* 1977; 40:
2565–2571

825. Wynder E L, Shigematsu T. Environmental factors in cancer of the colon   5.4
and rectum. *Cancer* 1967; 20: 1520–1561

826. Yalow R S. Radioimmunoassay: a probe for the fine structure of biologic   2.2
systems. *Science* 1978; 200: 1236–1245

827. Yau H C, Cairnie A B. Cell survival characteristics of intestinal stem   3.1
cells and crypts of γ-irradiated mice. *Radiat Res* 1979; 80: 92–107

828. Yeh K-Y. Cell kinetics in the small intestine of suckling rats. I.   2.2, 2.6
Influence of hypophysectomy. *Anat Rec* 1977; 188: 69–76

829. Yeh K-Y, Moog F. Development of the small intestine in the   2.6
hypophysectomized rat. I. Growth, histology and activity of alkaline
phosphatase, maltase and sucrase. *Dev Biol* 1975; 47: 156–172

830. Yeh K-Y, Moog F. Development of the small intestine in the   2.2
hypophysectomized rat. II. Influence of cortisone, thyroxine, growth
hormone and prolactin. *Dev Biol* 1975; 47: 173–184

831. Yeh K-Y, Moog F. Influence of the thyroid and adrenal glands on the   2.2, 2.6
growth of the intestine of the suckling rat, and on the development of
intestinal alkaline phosphatase and disaccharidase activities. *J Exp Zool*
1977; 200: 337–348

832. Zajicek G. The intestinal proliferon. *J Theor Biol* 1977; 67: 515–   1.1
521

833. Zedeck M S, Grab D J, Sternberg S S. Differences in the acute response   5.1, 5.4
of the various segments of rat intestine to treatment with the intestinal
carcinogen methylazoxymethanol acetate. *Cancer Res* 1977; 37: 32–36

834. Zedeck M S, Sternberg S S. A model system for studies of colon   5.2
carcinogenesis: tumor induction by a single injection of methylazoxy-

methanol acetate. *J Natl Cancer Inst* 1974; **53**: 1419–1421

835. Zedeck M S, Sternberg S S, Poynter R W, McGowan J. Biochemical and   5.1
pathological effects of methylazoxymethanol acetate, a potent carcinogen. *Cancer Res* 1970; **30**: 801–812

836. Zimmerman E G. Peptides of the brain and gut: introductory remarks.   2.2
Fed Proc 1979; **38**: 2286–2287

837. Zucoloto S, Wright N, Bramble M, Record C. Assessment of villus and   1.1
crypt population sizes in human small intestinal biopsies. *Gut* 1979; **20**:
A921

838. Zufarov K A, Baibekov I M. Electron microscopic and radioautographic   5.4
investigation of colonic epithelium in rats after jejunectomy. *Arkh Anat
Histol Embryol* 1972; **60**: 36–45